Register Now for Online Access to Your Book!

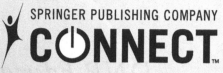

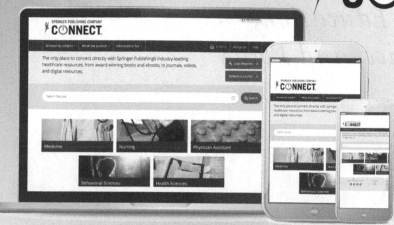

Your print purchase of *DNP Education, Practice, and Policy, Second Edition* **includes online access to the contents of your book**—increasing accessibility, portability, and searchability!

Access today at:

http://connect.springerpub.com/content/book/978-0-8261-4019-7 or scan the QR code at the right with your smartphone and enter the access code below.

YCRUS4X2

Scan here for quick access.

If you are experiencing problems accessing the digital component of this product, please contact our customer service department at cs@springerpub.com

The online access with your print purchase is available at the publisher's discretion and may be removed at any time without notice.

Publisher's Note: New and used products purchased from third-party sellers are not guaranteed for quality, authenticity, or access to any included digital components.

SPRINGER / PUBLISHING COMPANY

View all our products at springerpub.com

DNP Education, Practice, and Policy

Stephanie W. Ahmed, DNP, FNP-BC, DPNAP, holds the role of executive director for Clinical Effectiveness at Brigham & Women's Hospital, in Boston, Massachusetts. In this capacity, Dr. Ahmed has a key role as clinical leader of the discipline of nursing and is actively engaged in the organization's quality and care redesign initiatives. She is a nurse practitioner and coordinated the complex care of the nation's first partial face transplant patient at the Brigham. Recognizing the value of the DNP to expand the leadership skills of the advanced practice nurse, she completed a DNP in administration. She has served as an assistant professor of Nursing at the University of Massachusetts Graduate School of Nursing, in Worcester, Massachusetts, where she taught Trends in Nursing and instruction and oversight for the DNP residency program. She has served in both faculty and lecture roles in various Boston-based nursing programs including the MGH Institute of Health Professions where she taught Adult Primary Care Seminar and Professional Issues in Nursing, and at Simmons College where she served as faculty for Leadership and Management in the Clinical Setting. Dr. Ahmed has been involved in leadership roles with several professional societies, including the Massachusetts Coalition of Nurse Practitioners, where she has served as president and legislative chair, leading the organization's legislative filings for nurse practitioner full-practice authority. Acknowledged nationally for her work to advance nursing practice and a commitment to interdisciplinary team work, Dr. Ahmed is a fellow of the National Academies of Practice and holds the title of Distinguished Practitioner. She has published in peer-reviewed journals and has been an invited speaker both nationally and internationally. Engaged in post-doctoral studies at the Watson Caring Science Institute in Colorado, Dr. Ahmed is a Watson Scholar with a deep belief that human caring will humanize the healthcare system and offer clinicians a framework upon which joy in practice can be encountered.

Linda C. Andrist, PhD, RN, WHNP, is a professor emerita at the MGH Institute of Health Professions School of Nursing, Boston. She directed the DNP program from 2007 to 2011, when she became assistant dean and then retired as associate dean for academic affairs and program innovation. She was instrumental in curriculum development. She taught courses relevant to the DNP project, such as Knowledge and Inquiry, Doctoral Practicum, Project Development, and Residency. She continues to supervise DNP projects. Dr. Andrist previously coordinated the women's health nurse practitioner program at the institute and was one of the authors of the National Organization of Nurse Practitioner Faculties Nurse Practitioner Primary Care Competencies in Specialty Areas: Adult, Family, Gerontological, Pediatrics, and Women's Health (2002). Dr. Andrist has many years of practice as a women's health nurse practitioner in reproductive healthcare and has been teaching at the graduate level for more than 30 years. She was a Commission on Collegiate Nursing Education accreditation site visitor and a consultant to the Ohio Board of Regents for accreditation of new DNP programs. She was a 2010–2011 fellow in the American Association of Colleges of Nursing Leadership for Academic Nursing programs. Dr. Andrist has over 30 publications in peer-reviewed and invited book chapters. She is one of the coauthors of *A History of Nursing Ideas.*

Sheila M. Davis, DNP, ANP-BC, FAAN, is the chief of clinical operations and chief nursing officer at Partners In Health, an international nongovernmental organization working in 10 countries providing comprehensive healthcare and services for the poor globally. Dr. Davis led the organization's Ebola response in West Africa during the 2014 to 2015 epidemic. Dr. Davis is on the faculty at the University of California at San Francisco School of Nursing and is a frequent lecturer at a number of schools of nursing, including MGH Institute of Health Professions, Duke, Emory, and Northeastern. Dr. Davis had a clinical practice as an APN (DNP) in the Infectious Diseases clinic MGH, Boston from 1997 to 2014 and continues to oversee clinical practice at global sites. She was selected as a Robert Wood Johnson Executive Nurse Fellow as part of the 2012 to 2015 cohort and is the recipient of numerous awards and honors. She cofounded a nurse-run nongovernmental organization working in South Africa on a rural nurse-run clinic and orphan feeding program in an urban township. Her publications include 26 papers, 10 abstracts, and two book chapters. Dr. Davis is deeply involved with Association of Nurses in AIDS/ HIV Care (ANAC), was the founding/elected president of the Washington, DC chapter, and has been a locally, nationally, and internationally invited speaker on AIDS/HIV for ANAC since the mid-1980s. She has presented on a number of topics in global health, emergency response, and infectious diseases nationally and internationally.

Valerie J. Fuller, PhD, DNP, AGACNP-BC, FNP-BC, FAANP, holds dual roles as an assistant professor of nursing at the University of Southern Maine and assistant professor of surgery at Tufts University School of Medicine, Medford, Massachusetts. She works clinically in vascular surgery at Maine Medical Center in Portland, Maine where she also serves as a certified advanced practice wound ostomy nurse, certified foot care RN, and RN first assistant. In addition to her clinical work, Dr. Fuller is actively engaged in nursing regulation and healthcare policy at both the state and national levels. She is the president of the Maine State Board of Nursing, where she also serves as the APRN representative, and is a member of the board of directors at the National Council of State Boards of Nursing (NCSBN). She is the 2017 recipient of the Elaine Ellibee award, which recognizes board presidents who have made significant contributions to NCSBN. She is the Maine state representative to the American Association of Nurse Practitioners and the past president of the Maine Nurse Practitioner Association. In 2015, she was selected as a Maine Hanley Health Leadership Fellow, which recognizes Maine healthcare leaders, and is a fellow in both the American Association of Nurse Practitioners and the National Academies of Practice. The focus of her DNP and PhD research was on postoperative delirium and delirium education.

DNP Education, Practice, and Policy

Mastering the DNP Essentials for Advanced Nursing Practice

SECOND EDITION

Stephanie W. Ahmed, DNP, FNP-BC, DPNAP

Linda C. Andrist, PhD, RN, WHNP

Sheila M. Davis, DNP, ANP-BC, FAAN

Valerie J. Fuller, PhD, DNP, AGACNP-BC, FNP-BC, FAANP

SPRINGER PUBLISHING COMPANY

Springer Publishing Company, LLC
11 West 42nd Street
New York, NY 10036
www.springerpub.com

Acquisitions Editor: Margaret Zuccarini
Compositor: diacriTech, Chennai

ISBN: 978-0-8261-4018-0
ebook ISBN: 978-0-8261-4019-7
Instructor's PowerPoint ISBN: 978-0-8261-3668-8

Instructor's Materials: Qualified instructors may request supplements by emailing textbook@springerpub.com

18 19 20 21 22 / 5 4 3 2 1

The author and the publisher of this Work have made every effort to use sources believed to be reliable to provide information that is accurate and compatible with the standards generally accepted at the time of publication. The author and publisher shall not be liable for any special, consequential, or exemplary damages resulting, in whole or in part, from the readers' use of, or reliance on, the information contained in this book. The publisher has no responsibility for the persistence or accuracy of URLs for external or third-party Internet websites referred to in this publication and does not guarantee that any content on such websites is, or will remain, accurate or appropriate.

Library of Congress Cataloging-in-Publication Data
Names: Ahmed, Stephanie W., editor. | Andrist, Linda C., editor. | Davis,
   Sheila M., editor. | Fuller, Valerie J., editor.
Title: DNP education, practice, and policy : Mastering the DNP Essentials
   for Advanced Nursing Practice / [edited by] Stephanie W. Ahmed, Linda C. Andrist,
   Sheila M. Davis, Valerie J. Fuller.
Description: Second edition. | New York, NY : Springer Publishing Company,
   [2018] | Includes bibliographical references and index.
Identifiers: LCCN 2017056809| ISBN 9780826140180 | ISBN 9780826140197 (e-book)
Subjects: | MESH: Advanced Practice Nursing | Education, Nursing, Graduate |
   Nurse Practitioners | Evidence-Based Nursing | Nurse's Role | Leadership
Classification: LCC RT82.8 | NLM WY 128 | DDC 610.7306/92—dc23
LC record available at https://lccn.loc.gov/2017056809

Contact us to receive discount rates on bulk purchases.
We can also customize our books to meet your needs.
For more information please contact: sales@springerpub.com

Printed in the United States of America.

For my mother, Dorothy, the nurse who provided my earliest instruction in carative theory and for the millions of patients across the United States, who deserve a truly patient-centered transformation of their healthcare system.
—Stephanie W. Ahmed

To all of my students—past and present—with whom I proudly share our excitement about shaping the future of nursing.
—Linda C. Andrist

To all of the nurses working at Partners In Health sites in Haiti, Sierra Leone, Liberia, Rwanda, Lesotho, Malawi, Mexico, Peru, Russia, Navajo, Rosebud, and Boston who work with our patients, families, and communities around the world. I am honored and humbled to work with you every day.
—Sheila M. Davis

In memory of my father, Alfred R. Fuller, who proved that the difference between the possible and the impossible lies in a person's determination.
—Valerie J. Fuller

Contents

SECTION V: INTRODUCTION: POLICY, POLITICS, AND THE DNP
Stephanie W. Ahmed

Contributors

Jeffrey M. Adams, PhD, RN, NEA-BC, FAAN Senior Nurse Scientist, Center for Nursing Excellence, Brigham and Women's Hospital, Boston, Massachusetts; Executive Director, Workforce Outcomes Research and Leadership Development Institute (WORLD-Institute), Arizona State University, Tempe; Arizona Principal, Jeff Adams, LLC, Belmont, Massachusetts

Stephanie W. Ahmed, DNP, FNP-BC Nursing Director, Ambulatory, Brigham and Women's Hospital, Boston, Massachusetts; Assistant Professor of Nursing, University of Massachusetts, Graduate School of Nursing, Worcester, Massachusetts

Linda C. Andrist, PhD, RN, WHNP Professor Emerita, Former Associate Dean for Academic Affairs and Program Innovation, MGH Institute of Health Professions, School of Nursing, Boston, Massachusetts

Pamela A. Bessmer, DNP, AGACNP-BC, CNL, CRNP Nurse Practitioner, Division of Cardiac Surgery, University of Maryland Medical Center, Baltimore, Maryland

Elaine Bridge, DNP, MBA, RN Vice President of Clinical Operations, Partners eCare, Partners HealthCare, Boston, Massachusetts

Christine Buckley, DNP, MBA, RN Associate Chief Nursing Officer for Women and Children's Services, University of Massachusetts Memorial Medical Center, Worcester, Massachusetts

Edna Cadmus, PhD, RN, NEA-BC, FAAN Executive Director, New Jersey Collaborating Center for Nursing; Clinical Professor, Specialty Director-Leadership Tracks, School of Nursing, Rutgers, The State University of New Jersey, Newark, New Jersey

Ann H. Cary, PhD, MPH, RN, FNAP, FAAN Dean and Professor, School of Nursing and Health Studies, University of Missouri–Kansas City, Kansas City, Missouri

Lisa Colombo, DNP, MHA, RN   Senior Vice President for Patient Care Services and Chief Nursing Officer, UMass Memorial Medical Center, Worcester, Massachusetts; Associate Dean of Clinical Practice, UMass Graduate School of Nursing, Worcester, Massachusetts

John T. Connors, Major, USAF, DNP, FNP-BC   Family Nurse Practitioner, Joint Base Anacostia Bolling Clinic, 579th Medical Group, Washington, DC

Inge Corless, RN, PhD, FAAN   Professor, MGH Institute of Health Professions, School of Nursing, Boston, Massachusetts

Katherine Crabtree, PhD, FAAN, APRN-BC   Retired Professor, Former Associate Dean, University of Portland School of Nursing, Portland, Oregon

Sheila M. Davis, DNP, ANP-BC, FAAN   Chief of Clinical Operations, Chief Nursing Officer, Partners In Health, Boston, Massachusetts

Christina Dempsey, MSN, MBA, RN, CNOR, CENP, FAAN   Senior Vice President, Chief Nursing Officer, Press Ganey Associates, Inc., Springfield, Missouri

Marianne Ditomassi, DNP, MBA, RN, NEA-BC, FAAN   Executive Director, Nursing & Patient Care Services, Operations and Magnet Recognition, Massachusetts General Hospital, Boston, Massachusetts

Susan Doyle-Lindrud, DNP, ANP, DCC   Assistant Professor, School of Nursing, Columbia University, New York, New York

Jeanette Ives Erickson, DNP, RN, FAAN   Chief Nurse Emerita, Distinguished Paul M. Erickson Chair in Nursing, Massachusetts General Hospital, Boston, Massachusetts

Valerie J. Fuller, PhD, DNP, AGACNP-BC, FNP-BC, FAANP   Assistant Professor of Nursing, University of Southern Maine, Portland, Maine; Assistant Professor of Surgery Tufts University School of Medicine Boston, Massachusetts

Debra J. Gillespie, PhD, RN   Evaluation Faculty, Western Governors University, Salt Lake City, Utah; Adjunct Faculty, University of Southern Maine, Portland, Maine; Co-owner, Nursing Knowledge Solutions, LLC, Brownfield, Maine

Joanne Hogan, DNP, RN   Vice President, Population Health, Complex Care Management, Boston Medical Center Health System, Boston, Massachusetts

Kristina Hyrkäs, PhD, LicNSc, MNSc, RN   Director, Center for Nursing Research and Quality Outcomes, Maine Medical Center, Portland, Maine; Adjunct Professor, University of Southern Maine, Portland, Maine

Debra Kramlich, PhD, RN, CNE, CCRN-K   Assistant Professor of Nursing, University of New England, Portland, Maine; Co-owner, Nursing Knowledge Solutions, LLC, Brownfield, Maine

Jeffrey Kwong, DNP, MPH, ANP-BC, FAANP   Associate Professor, School of Nursing, Columbia University, New York, New York

Paulette D. Long, DNP, CRNP, PNP-BC   Adjunct Associate Professor, Bachelor of Science in Nursing for Registered Nurses, University of Maryland University College, Adelphi, Maryland

Leah McKinnon-Howe, DNP, ANP-BC   Administrative Director and Nurse Practitioner, New England Conservatory of Music, Boston, Massachusetts; Affiliate Associate Professor, School of Nursing, Northeastern University, Boston, Massachusetts

Maura McQueeney, RN, MPH, DNP   President, Baystate Home Health/Post Acute Executive, Springfield, Massachusetts

Patrice Nicholas, DNSc, DHL (Hon.), MPH, RN, ANP, FAAN   Professor, School of Nursing, MGH Institute of Health Professions, Boston, Massachusetts; Director of Global Health and Academic Partnerships, Division of Global Health Equity, Center for Nursing Excellence, Brigham and Women's Hospital, Boston, Massachusetts

Stacey Ober, RN, JD   Nurse Attorney and Executive/Legislative Agent, Craven & Ober, Policy Strategists, LLC, Boston, Massachusetts

Rollie Perea, DNP, RN, ANP-BC   Nurse Practitioner, Care Well Urgent Care, Northborough, Massachusetts

Patricia A. Polansky, MS, RN   Director, Program Development and Implementation, Center to Champion Nursing in America (CCNA) an initiative of the AARP Foundation, AARP, and the Robert Wood Johnson Foundation (RWJF), Washington, DC

Cenean Walls Raphemot, Captain, USAF, DNP, PMHNP-BC   Psychiatric Nurse Practitioner/Competent Medical Authority, 31st Medical Group, Aviano Air Base, Italy

John Roberts, DNP, ANP-BC   Clinical Information Specialist, Harbor Health Systems, Boston, Massachusetts

Michael Sanchez, DNP, CRNP, FNP-BC   Assistant Professor, Johns Hopkins University, School of Nursing, Baltimore, Maryland

Anna E. Schoenbaum, DNP, RN   Director, Enterprise Clinical Applications, Information Services and Technology, University of Maryland Medical System, Baltimore, Maryland; Faculty Associate, School of Nursing, University of Maryland, Baltimore, Maryland

Lisa Sgarlata, DNP, RN, MS, FACHE   Chief Patient Care Officer, Chief Nurse Executive, Lee Health, Fort Myers, Florida

Claire Simeone, DNP, FNP   Family Nurse Practitioner, San Francisco Department of Public Health; Zuckerberg San Francisco General Hospital and Trauma Center, Department of Psychiatry, Division of Substance Abuse and Addiction Medicine, San Francisco, California

Margie H. Sipe, DNP, RN, NEA-BC   Director, DNP Program; Assistant Professor, School of Nursing, MGH Institute of Health Professions; Nursing Program Director, Center for Nursing Excellence, Brigham and Women's Hospital, Boston, Massachusetts

Maureen Sroczynski, DNP, RN   President/CEO Farley Associates, Inc., Norton, Massachusetts; Nurse Expert/Consultant, Center to Champion Nursing in America (CCNA) an initiative of the AARP Foundation, AARP, and the Robert Wood Johnson Foundation (RWJF), Washington, DC

Theresa Trivette, DNP, RN   Assistant Vice President, Quality and Risk Management, Florida Hospital Tampa, Adventist Health System, Tampa, Florida

Judith Webb, DNP, ANP-BC, Palliative Care NP-BC   Retired Associate Professor, University of North Carolina, Chapel Hill, School of Nursing, Chapel Hill, North Carolina

Marjorie S. Wiggins, DNP, MBA, RN, FAAN, NEA-BC   Senior Vice President for Patient Care Services and Chief Nursing Officer, Maine Medical Center, Portland, Maine

Sarah Wilkie, MS   Project Specialist, Quality, Safety, and Value, Partners HealthCare, Boston, Massachusetts

Karen Anne Wolf, PhD, ANP-BC, DFNAP   Adjunct Professor, Samuel Merritt University, Oakland, California; Consultant, Wolf Health Professions Education, Lewisburg, Pennsylvania

Laura J. Wood, DNP, RN, NEA-BC   Senior Vice President, Patient Care Operations, Chief Nursing Officer, Boston Children's Hospital, Boston, Massachusetts

Karen Lynn Yarbrough, DNP, CRNP   Director, Comprehensive Stroke Center Neurology, University of Maryland Medical Center, Baltimore, Maryland

Preface

In 2011, in response to those national discussions around health reforms that mandated universal access to healthcare coverage and further, a demand that this be achieved with also recognizing cost containments and improved outcomes, the Institute of Medicine (IOM) issued a call to action with the release of its report *The Future of Nursing: Leading Change, Advancing Health.* As nurses are the most prevalent of healthcare providers in the setting of a national physician shortage, the discipline was best positioned to respond to what had become a national crisis. The American healthcare system was then, and continues to be, in an agonal state. Nurses were called to partner and lead in transforming the healthcare system, and were further encouraged to practice to the full extent of their education and training—it was clear the IOM was looking to the discipline to make a strong impact on the U.S. healthcare system. Doctors of nursing practice (DNP) will be the change agents, and as Cary queries in Chapter 2, "Could the DNP be the future in *The Future of Nursing* report?" We think so.

We offer this text as food for thought and to serve as a guide for students as well as DNPs engaged in advanced practice in the following specialty areas: leadership, policy, and information technology. Presented in a framework that addresses *DNP education, practice, and policy*, the text seeks to challenge the reader, and is at times provocative. We hope the content will stimulate discussion at many levels.

Ahmed and Wolf retrace the rich history of advanced nursing practice in Section I, offering the reader a sense of how societal forces, much as those today, have long contributed to the shaping of advanced nursing practice. Transporting the reader to the present, this section further addresses the evolution of the DNP in the context of contemporary healthcare challenges and culminates in a discussion of how the DNP can influence the essential changes identified in *The Future of Nursing* reports (2011, 2015). With recognition of the national drivers to improve access, quality, and satisfaction, Dempsey takes us beyond the outcomes, highlighting that a truly person-centered transformation of the U.S. healthcare system will require us to look broadly at the patient's experience of care.

Section II takes the reader through the process of clinical scholarship, beginning with Andrist and Crabtree's definition of clinical scholarship and the evolution of students into scholars. They discuss how the role of the DNP is to generate nursing knowledge from practice. Sipe and Andrist continue with the process of carrying out the culminating piece of scholarship in DNP education programs—the DNP Scholarly Project. Nurse executives and administrators contributed examples of the DNP projects they were involved with while advanced practice DNPs share their experience of the challenges and opportunities presented during the DNP Project experience. It is hearing the student voice that makes this section particularly strong.

Section III explores the application of the DNP essential, the role and continual evolution of the nursing profession. Seven DNP graduates who work in different practice settings discuss their real-life experiences in integrating their learnings from their education, and further outline opportunities and challenges they have experienced since graduation. The DNP will be a leader in healthcare, and Doyle-Lindrud and Kwong give concrete guidance on how to gain valuable leadership experience in the clinical setting. Ives-Erickson, Ditomassi, and Adams take leadership to the next level in their chapter discussing the unique skill set needed for the Executive Nurse Leader. Webb and McKinnon discuss finding our voices and defining ourselves as DNPs and O'Dell shares highlights from multiple years of the DNP community survey.

Section IV highlights three important essentials of the DNP curriculum: evidence-based practice (EBP), information technology, and outcomes measurement. In Chapter 12, Fuller, Gillespie, and Kramlich provide an overview of EBP and share a new nursing framework to assist practitioners in moving evidence into practice. In Chapter 13, Wiggins and Hyrkäs discuss the organizational barriers and facilitators of implementing EBP and the theories and methods that can be used to promote change. In Chapter 14, Schoenbaum reviews the essential role that information technology plays in transforming healthcare. In the final chapter in this section, Colombo discusses outcomes measurement and its importance in driving processes of care that will result in better outcomes for patients and healthcare organizations. An understanding of these essentials prepares the DNP graduate to lead at the highest level in both the clinical and organizational environment.

The final section of this text addresses policy, politics, and the DNP. The *Code of Ethics for Nurses* (ANA, 2015) requires nursing to evolve practice beyond the bedside, engaging in the advancement of policy as a form of nursing praxis that serves to protect the health of the public and reduce health disparities. Offered in the context of today's pressing health reform agendas, Ober and Wilkie establish a foundational understanding of advocacy and the necessary skills required for the DNP-prepared nurse to advance health policy. From the modernization of state licensing laws to federal workforce initiatives, the agendas of the major U.S. professional nursing organizations are outlined and offered to provide the reader with role-specific-related opportunities to act as a collective for the purpose of advancing nursing practice and health. With recognition that healthy communities are created by intention, Sroczynski, Cadmus, and Polansky demonstrate that health policy can be leveraged in tandem with cross-sector collaboration to impact those sociopolitical structures that contribute to health inequities. Cosmopolitan in their approach and shifting away from acute care models, the authors encourage nursing to extend its influence beyond the traditional, to consider those social inputs including housing, employment, and education, which have been identified to have influence on health and health behaviors. In this way, not only will the healthcare delivery system be transformed, but so too will the communities in which patients and families reside.

In addition to the book, as a resource for faculty, we have provided chapter-based PowerPoint presentations. To obtain an electronic copy of these materials, faculty should contact Springer Publishing Company at textbook@ springerpub.com.

Stephanie W. Ahmed
Linda C. Andrist
Sheila M. Davis
Valerie J. Fuller

■ REFERENCE

American Nurses Association. (2015). *Code of Ethics for Nurses with Interpretive Statements.* Silver Spring, MD: Author.

Acknowledgments

The editors wish to acknowledge the many committed people who have served to both inspire us and support us as we have embarked on this literary journey. We are indebted to the following:

- In memorial—Joyce Clifford, RN, PhD, FAAN, whose influence helped to develop the framework upon which this text was developed for exploring the DNP in the context of education, practice, and policy
- The Massachusetts General Hospital (MGH) Institute of Health Professions School of Nursing faculty and leadership who conceived and implemented an innovative DNP program and had faith in the first three students. Thank you especially to former Associate Dean Dr. Linda C. Andrist, professor emerita, who directed the DNP program from 2007 to 2011 and championed the program and former Dean Marjorie Chisholm, EdD, RN, CS, ABPP.
- All DNP students, past, present, and future, who share in our excitement of shaping the future of nursing
- The Department of Nursing and the patients at Brigham and Women's Hospital, for your support and inspiration
- The nurses, surgeons, and support staff in the Department of Surgery and Richards 3, Maine Medical Center, Portland, Maine
- Sally Rankin and Kathy Crabtree who never fail to inspire and support
- The staff, patients, and communities from the Partners In Health sites worldwide
- The Massachusetts Coalition of Nurse Practitioners

Finally, much gratitude is due to our families, spouses, and friends who offered endless love and support, thereby making this process possible.

SECTION ONE

Through the Looking Glass: The Growth and Development of Doctor of Nursing Practice Roles

STEPHANIE W. AHMED

Whoever wishes to foresee the future must consult the past; for human events ever resemble those of preceding times.
—Niccolo Machiavelli

Contemporary healthcare challenges include escalating costs, poor access to care coupled with a rise in number of older Americans, and the birth of a quality movement that has created a demand for improved outcomes and transparency. From Nightingale in the Crimea to the new doctorate of nursing practice (DNP) graduate of today, nursing history provides testimony to the strong impact such societal forces have historically exerted upon the shaping of nursing education, practice, and policy.

Seeking to mitigate the impact of current U.S. healthcare challenges, Congress proposed and implemented the much-debated Affordable Care Act. Seeking a solution, the Institute of Medicine (IOM, 2011) released a landmark report titled *The Future of Nursing: Leading Change, Advancing Health*. With an acknowledgement that nurses are the most prevalent of healthcare providers and therefore best positioned to make a strong impact on the ailing U.S. healthcare system, the IOM issued a national call to remove those barriers that prohibit nurses to optimally respond to the evolving healthcare needs of the nation. Issuing an imperative, the IOM (2011) acknowledged that to advance the national healthcare agenda, nurses must be permitted to practice to the full extent of their education and training, and further, positioned to lead and advance health.

In 2015, the IOM convened a committee to assess progress toward achieving its overarching goals for nursing. It acknowledged that while progress has been made in some areas, significant opportunities remain to position the nursing workforce to transform America's healthcare system.

The march forward has been slow. With leadership reflected in the curriculum, the DNP nurse is prepared to lead such a change. However, in order to best understand how we arrived at this present juncture, it is helpful to reflect back upon our history and take notice of how through the years nurses have challenged the constraints of their scope of practice, expanding skill sets in an effort to best meet the needs of society.

In this section, the reader is offered a thoughtful explanation of the history of advanced practice, while jointly being engaged around the IOM reports (2011, 2015) as compass, propelling the DNP closer to the intended future of nursing.

■ REFERENCES

Institute of Medicine. (2011). *The future of nursing: Leading change, advancing health.* Washington, DC: U.S. Government Printing Office.

Institute of Medicine. (2015). *Assessing progress on the institute of medicine report future of nursing.* Retrieved from http://www.nationalacademies.org/hmd/~/media/Files/Report%20Files/2015/AssessingFON_releaseslides/Nursing-Report-in-brief.pdf

Evolution to Revolution: Positioning Advanced Practice to Influence Contemporary Healthcare Arenas

STEPHANIE W. AHMED AND KAREN ANNE WOLF

The evolution of the doctorate of nursing practice (DNP) degree occurred rapidly in the United States. Forged by a coalition of nursing organizations, the DNP degree emerged in the midst to calls for greater accountability in the healthcare system. The DNP curricula are reflective of this concern and the belief that leadership by advanced practice nurses can make a substantial contribution to improve healthcare system costs, quality, and access. While educational parity of advanced nursing practice (ANP) with other health professions is justified, the most compelling rationale and sustaining drive for the DNP is the need for transparency and change in the healthcare system. APRNs, historically subordinated to medicine as "mid-level providers," now lay claim to greater practice liberty. Emboldened by support from groups such as the Institute of Medicine (IOM) and the Robert Wood Johnson Foundation, advanced practice nurses have been seeking to take a central role in evolving the healthcare delivery system. The United States is one of the few developed nations that historically has not offered healthcare coverage to its citizens, and Americans are now being challenged to evaluate the concept of health both as a value and a human right. While the nation grapples with coverage and Washington considers how to shift the cost of care, it has become obvious that the unintended consequence of health reform is access to healthcare coverage without access to care. A 2017 physician access survey demonstrates that nationally, wait times for new patients seeking appointments in cardiology, dermatology, obstetrics-gynecology, orthopedic surgery, and family medicine have increased 30% since 2014 (Merritt Hawkins, 2017).

In the context of a national physician shortage, resources to advance the larger national healthcare agenda simply have not been available. As policy changes in health reform remain central, it is evident that APRNs cannot afford to be passive.

Advanced practice nurses are challenged to break from the patterns of the past and assert their claims to practice leadership.

The history of advanced practice nursing demonstrates the discipline's commitment to meeting societal and healthcare system's needs. However, over the past 20 years, growing concern about "how" needs are met has reframed our professional accountability. As healthcare costs escalated and the perceived quality of care declined, healthcare quality, long measured by process and structural characteristics, shifted toward practice outcomes. By 1990, health research began to focus on the outcome measures (Epstein, 1990). Many of our physician colleagues went "back to school" to study health financing and economics, outcome research, and epidemiology. The measurement of clinical practice outcomes is now a central component of healthcare. Among the stresses of system changes and demand for greater accountability, innovations in advanced practice education have flourished.

■ REFLECTIONS FROM OUR PAST

The evolution of ANP is both chaotic and continuous. Looking back over the past century, the development of roles in ANP is marked by different chronologies and practice patterns. A diversity of ANP roles emerged out of the complexity of the nursing educational and practice environments. Despite the apparent differences, there are common themes that have shaped their trajectory, including (a) the adaptation of nursing practice to meet the needs of society, (b) the transfer of knowledge and skills and role negotiation between nursing and medicine, and (c) the influence of a dialectical culture of managerialism and professionalism in shaping nursing roles. Both sides are evident in the unique history of advanced practice roles.

The development of advanced practice roles has reshaped nursing, forging new opportunities for autonomy in practice. At the same time, changes in nursing roles have brought to light the political and economic constraints faced when pursuing such practice. Nursing has been defined and redefined in modern history in relation to hospitals and medicine. This initial set of conditions provides the basis for the constraints and barriers that advanced practice roles have faced. For most of modern history, APRNs have repeatedly stretched the acceptable boundaries of nursing to meet societal needs and institutional demands, only to be asked to recoil when economic and political pressures mounted. Advanced practice roles such as midwifery, nurse anesthesia, clinical nurse specialist (CNS), and nurse practitioner (NP) found the path to legitimacy twisted and strewn with obstacles often placed by forces external to the discipline and at times from within. Some nurse leaders resisted the development of advanced practice roles, arguing that this eroded the professional identity, whereas others embraced the opportunity and new identities. Repeat efforts by groups such as the American Medical Association (AMA) have attempted to block the APRNs legislation; yet, many APN roles were shaped by close educational and practice partnerships with physicians.

Advanced nursing practice, reflective of nursing, shares a history that is also marked by distinctly gendered roles, as well as class and racial differentiation of roles (Hines, 1994). The feminization of nursing in America was both a source of strength and a constraint. While nurses forged their way to engage in caring work, they were also restrained from engaging in self-advocacy for much of their first century. A culture of paternalism and institutional policies constrained nursing power (Ashley, 1976).

■ NURSING, SOCIAL JUSTICE, AND THE DRIVE TO MEET SOCIETAL NEEDS

Nursing has been characterized as having a strong ethic of service. The profession grew in tandem with social reformism. Nurses attribute this to the foundation laid by Florence Nightingale. Best known for her work in addressing the care of hospitalized soldiers during the Crimean War, her efforts extended beyond hospital reformism to address the health of the poor in the British Empire (Rafferty & Wall, 2010). Nightingale's concern for vulnerable populations and their environment (Beck, 2006; Dossey, Selanders, Beck, & Atwell, 2005) is the foundation for advance nursing practice. The ethic of service was also a legacy of the religious and military culture of early hospitals. The advancement of professional nursing in the United States perpetuated this legacy through the system of hospital schools of nursing, which created a contradiction, as nurses were "ordered to care" (Reverby, 1987).

While much of nursing was rooted in hospitals, most nurses educated in the early part of the 20th century worked in the community doing private duty nursing or in public health nursing. The surge of immigration and industrialization was well underway. Public health and nursing practice in settings such as the Henry Street Settlement House and the Frontier Nursing Service provided outreach to populations at risk, and embraced efforts toward social justice and advocacy (Drevdahl, 2002; Jenkins, 2006). The work of nurses in outreach to underserved urban and rural settings created a foundation for the evolution of advanced practice roles.

■ KNOWLEDGE AND SKILL TRANSFER

The growth in knowledge and technology has reshaped nurses' roles over the past 150 years. From thermography to genetic testing, there has been a consistent transfer of knowledge between nursing and medicine. For much of nursing history, the transfer of technology has expanded the scope of nursing responsibility and the work of patient care. While physicians may have initially controlled diagnostics and therapeutic interventions, as Sandelowski (2000) notes, more often than not, it was nurses who operationalized them. Nurses were expected to contribute their skill in assessing patients' status without making judgment. However, it became clear to many nurses and physicians that the boundaries of practice were much more fluid, and once knowledge and skills have crossed the boundary, they do not recede (Allen, 1997). The continuous flow of technology in healthcare has reshaped nursing work with greater demand for information management. But along with information comes the question of how it is to be used. As nurses gained competence in knowledge and skills, they were challenged to reject a passive stance and actively use their expertise in patient care. For the nurse anesthetist, it was through the administration and regulation of anesthesia; for midwives in the care of mothers, through the prenatal to the postnatal period; and for NPs and CNSs through engagement in the management of patients with acute and chronic health challenges.

■ DIALECTICAL CULTURES OF MANAGERIALISM AND PROFESSIONAL NURSING

From the well-known work of Nightingale to the more recent emergence of professional models of nursing practice, nursing identity was fused to hospitals. By the mid-20th century, hospitals became the centerpiece of the U.S. healthcare system and nursing education was viewed as a means to supply hospitals with a ready supply of nursing workers. Despite efforts to advance nursing education through raising standards and accreditation, the education of nurses in diploma schools of nursing subordinated education to hospital interests until the 1960s. Hospital and medical paternalism subordinated nursing, and a good nurse followed orders within the hospital hierarchy (Ashley, 1976). Efforts to move nursing education into colleges and universities were directed at preparing nursing superintendents to manage hospitals and teach in schools of nursing. The oversight of the day-to-day management of hospitals gave nurses the power to protect and further structure their expertise, and to set the basis for nursing definition and professionalism efforts (Abbott, 1988). By claiming hospital nursing as the primary basis for professionalization, nursing further intertwined with medicine, which further thwarted efforts to achieve autonomy in practice. Over time, as hospital bureaucracy grew and became highly corporatized, nursing knowledge and skills were subjugated to organizational rationality (Wolf, 2006). For the first half of the 20th century, the slow march to professional practice took nurses into management and away from direct patient care.

By mid-century, nurses began to work more consistently as staff nurses (Reverby, 1987). Collegiate nursing education grew along with efforts to advance nursing knowledge and skills. The dialectic of managerialism and professionalism converged in the role of the institutionally based CNS. By the late 1960s, nurses, empowered by the unified interests of nursing and feminism, began to organize and reclaim professionalism. Educational programs were developed to support clinician expertise, with formalized movement to universities supported through federal legislation and monies. By the end of the 1970s, the expanded scope of nurses' practice was slowly codified by state laws, professional certification developed, and APRNs organized to advance their professional interests.

■ NURSE-MIDWIFERY

Before professional nursing and allopathic medicine, midwifery was a major source of healthcare in the United States. Midwives, historically trained through apprenticeships, lost ground to physician "male midwives." With medicalization, childbearing was viewed as a problem to be controlled (Wertz & Wertz, 1977). As medicine and professional nursing grew in status and power, efforts mounted to abolish midwives. The ideological battle to professionalize and control childbearing practices served both the interests of nursing and medicine. While medicine viewed the "granny midwife" as competition, the nursing community viewed midwifery as a threat to professionalization. Nursing joined forces with physicians in a campaign to eliminate the midwife in the name of social reformism (Dawley, 2001). Midwives were made scapegoats for the rise in maternal mortality. The mortality was in fact due to the increased physician use of unclean equipment such as forceps (Varney, Kriebs, & Gegor, 2004). Nursing leaders began a movement to claim midwifery services within the scope of nursing practice. Nurses began to train as midwives under the umbrella of public health nursing. The scope of nurse-midwifery expanded to become maternity care, financially supported by the Children's Bureau and the Sheppard-Towner Act. Nurse-midwifery took off slowly, providing care to immigrant and poor women in urban areas such as New York City and Philadelphia and rural areas such as Appalachia. Lay-midwifery practice was largely eliminated and/or forced underground. Physicians, freed from the threat of lay-midwifery, achieved legitimacy with wealthier patients. Nurse-midwives, in such settings, became subordinated to physicians by law and practice, serving as the physicians' eyes (Varney et al., 2004).

Nurse-midwives attempted to follow the path to professionalism. Training schools were opened in major cities; standards were set first in the 1930s and again in the 1960s. The first unifying organization, the American College of Nurse-Midwives (ACNM), was formed in the 1940s. As the nurse-midwives began to pursue legitimacy in education and practice in the 1950s, the number of programs in midwifery remained small, and it was overshadowed by the "scientific" approach of medicine. By the 1960s, legal recognition of nurse-midwives was limited to only Kentucky, New Mexico, and New York. By the 1970s, nurse-midwives were rediscovered as the women's movement reframed pregnancy and childbearing as natural life experiences rather than pathological states. The public demand for nurse-midwives increased, further fueled by the growth of federally qualified health centers and a shortage of obstetrician–gynecologists. A 1971 joint statement between the ACNM and the American College of Obstetricians and Gynecologists voiced support for nurse-midwives as members of the obstetrical team but also reinforced physician supervision over the team. The 1980s ushered in a new era of regulation with legal recognition for nurse-midwives in all states by the end of the decade (Rooks, 1997).

The quest to obtain prescriptive authority and third-party reimbursement moved nurse-midwives to align more closely with other advanced practice nurses. The nurse-midwives achieved the latter, first through the federal CHAMPUS (Civilian Health and Medical Program of the Uniformed Services) program for military dependents and then Medicaid payments in many states. The 1990s led to a gain in prescriptive authority, which was authorized state by state for the certified nurse-midwives (CNMs) alongside other APRNs (Hamric, Hanson, Tracey & O'Grady, 2014).

Over the past few decades, nurse-midwives not only gained legitimacy but also challenged the constraints of their historic scope for practice. Nurse-midwives took on technology in hospital centers, managing increasingly high-risk patients in collaborative relations with physicians. The infusion of technology into midwifery shifted the "natural-birthing" stance of midwifery. Because of changing practice patterns, there was an increase in cost of the malpractice insurance. The high costs of malpractice insurance further constrained the availability of sites for practice, as well as the education of nurse-midwives. The move to managed care in the 1990s has brought midwifery practices under new scrutiny. Constraints on choices continue to marginalize midwifery services (Brodsky, 2008). The demands on healthcare systems to reduce cost and improve quality and safety through evidence-based practice have further challenged nurse-midwifery practice (Sinclair, 2010). Nurse-midwifery is now more often than not, practiced in institutional settings with the scope of practice constrained by requirements of collaboration with an OB/GYN or in some instances regulatory restrictions requiring clinical practice within a "healthcare system" (Ahmed et al., 2014). These regulations have moved CNMs out of community settings, altered working partnerships in family practice settings and further served to prohibit independent practice. The Joint Commission defines CNMs and other APRNs as "any individual permitted by law and by the organization to provide care, treatment and services without directions" (The Joint Commission, 2017). While state regulations may grant authority for independent practice, too often the language of institutional practice agreements is more restrictive, calling for supervision rather than collaboration. This further impedes access to CNMs by restricting their ability to admit and discharge patients. A consequence of institutional controls and hospital-based birthing is the disturbing trend toward increased medicalization of childbirth, with cesarean births once again on the rise. The development of alternative settings of nurse-midwifery practice, such as birthing centers demonstrate lower rates of medical intervention such as cesarean births, with shortened recovery times and less cost to the healthcare system (Thornton, McFarlin, & Park, 2017).

While the American Congress of Obstetricians and Gynecologists (ACOG) acknowledges that access to quality maternal care is essential to maternal child health, they also recognize physician demand has not been able to keep pace and underserved areas exist nationally (ACOG, 2015). One solution has been to advance legislation that would permit the designation of maternity care shortage areas and further allow members of the Public Health Service to respond to the need. The nurse-midwife, similar to other advanced practice roles, offers society an effective option to address the demands for improved access, quality, and contained costs. Trained not only for the provision of gynecologic and obstetric care, CNMs are educated to provide the full complement of primary care services for women of childbearing years and across the life span. However, with variation in practice and autonomy across the states, optimization of the CNM workforce will require uniform removal of barriers to practice including institutional, governmental, and those imposed by insurers who may restrict CNMs from primary care provider (PCP) status.

■ NURSE ANESTHESIA

The role of the nurse anesthetist is acknowledged as the first advanced practice role to emerge with formal recognition in the United States. The nursing role in the administration of anesthetics arose from 1861 to 1865, during the Civil War, when Catherine S. Lawrence and other nurses provided anesthesia for surgeons operating on the wounded (American Association of Nurse Anesthetists [AANA], n.d.-b).

Wartime experience would be repeated throughout history, as nurses provided anesthesia to meet the needs of injured soldier-patients and expanded both the knowledge base and skills of the nurse. Nurse anesthetists have been a consistent presence working in the United States and abroad to train and care for military troops. In the late 1870s, Sister Mary Bernard, a catholic nursing sister at St. Vincent's Hospital in the industrial and shipping center of Erie, Pennsylvania, became the first nurse known to specialize in anesthesia. The practice of anesthesia continued as nurses were schooled on the job in hospitals from Philadelphia to Chicago. The need for professional anesthetists was discussed across the country, as surgery outcomes were compromised at the "hands of skilled anesthetizers" (Galloway [1899] cited in Harris & Hunzikar-Dean, 2001). Nurses and the wives of physician–surgeons frequently provided the anesthesia, as few physicians were willing to accept the limited fee provided from the surgeon for services (Harris & Hunzikar-Dean, 2001). Formal nurse anesthesia education developed as discovery of new agents and techniques made surgery and the demand for anesthesia "administrators" more common in hospitals. Industrialization and the tandem growth of hospitals would expand the role across the United States. In 1893, Alice Magaw began her practice in nurse anesthesia at Mayo Clinic, and was later proclaimed the "Mother of Anesthesia" by Dr. Charles H. Mayo. Magaw, a leader nurse anesthetist, published the first major paper in a medical journal (Magaw, 1900) by a nurse on anesthesia practices. The Lakeside Hospital in Cleveland, Ohio, became the site of the school of anesthesia in 1915, under the direction of Agatha Hodgins. The Lakeside alumni association evolved to become the Organization of Nurse Anesthesia. Typical of professionalization efforts, the subsequent organization, the Association of Nurse Anesthetists, began an official publication. In 1952, the association was granted the authority to serve as the accrediting agency for schools of anesthesia. Post–World War II (WWII) and the Korean conflict, the growing complexity and economics of surgery made anesthesia more viable and attractive (AANA, n.d.-b; Hamric et al., 2014).

During the 1950s, medical practitioners began to enter into anesthesia in greater numbers, setting the stage for future challenges to the nurse authority and creating the image of anesthesia as a main field of practice. The development of all-male nurse anesthesia programs followed in the late 1950s, leading to nurse anesthesia becoming the area of nursing most inclusive for men (Hamric et al., 2014). Nurse anesthesia, like other advanced practice roles, established practice ahead of regulation. The passage of regulation was difficult, as the field of anesthesia, once ignored by medicine as a specialty, became one of interest. As the government, through programs such as Medicare and Medicaid, joined the realm of payers for surgical services, regulation and challenges to nurse anesthesia practice grew. The nurse anesthetists responded by raising the educational association standards to a master's degree. This elevation in requirements occurred during a period of program closure and growing physician opposition.

For over 40 years, the AANA met in conjunction with the American Hospital Association meetings, evidence of the central role that surgery and nurse anesthesia played in hospital growth and prosperity (Hamric et al., 2014). The practice of holding meetings in tandem ended in 1976, and with the divergence, physicians mounted efforts to take control over anesthesia practice. One such effort is physician support for the development of nonnursing-based anesthesia associate programs as well as efforts to require regulations that require tight supervision of nurse anesthetists under state regulation. A second effort is at the level of federal and state regulation with ongoing policy debates about the autonomy and supervision by physicians. The context for state regulation was set at the federal level in 2001 by the Centers for Medicare and Medicaid Services (CMS), which offered flexibility to the governors of states to "opt out" of the reimbursement requirement that the administration of anesthesia be overseen by either a surgeon or anesthesiologist (Dulisse & Cromwell, 2010). Opting out "required that states: (1) consult the state boards of medicine and nursing about issues related to access to and the quality of anesthesia services in the state, (2) determine that opting out is consistent with state law, and (3) determine that opting out is in the best interests of the state's citizens" (CMS & U.S. Department of Health and Human Services, 2001). By 2005, there were 14 states that had chosen to opt out. An analysis of Medicare data gathered between 1999 and 2005 explored the likelihood of death and complications from anesthesia. It was examined in the context of state opt-out status and by provider groups including MD solo, certified registered nurse anesthetist (CRNA) solo, and team-based anesthesia delivery (MD with a CRNA). The evidence demonstrated that opting out of oversight did not correlate with increased deaths or complications. By 2017, only 18 states have "opted out" of the federal physician supervision requirement (AANA, n.d.-a). The safety of the CRNA solo model of care was strongly supported and should inform policy implications that enhance access to CRNA driven care (Dulisse & Cromwell, 2010).

■ CLINICAL SPECIALISTS

The emergence of CNS marked an expansion of specialty practice in nursing. Nurses have typically evolved their practice along specialty lines, seeking out individual opportunities to develop competence in specialty practice. In the early decades of the 20th century, specialty practice included areas such as public health, maternity care, and pediatrics. In the post–WWII period, primed by the development of new knowledge and technologies, interest in the formal process and recognition of specialization was generated (Christman, 1968). Peplau (1965), viewed as the mother of the psychiatric CNS role, states that the role originated in 1938. The concept of an expert clinician was proposed by Frances Reiter in 1943 as a generic title for a nurse with clinical competence demonstrated in function, depth of understanding, and breadth of service. The nurse clinician and nurse clinical specialist have been used synonymously through the years and reflect a common focus on specialized knowledge and function (Reihl & McVay, 1973; Reiter, 1966).

As the role of CNS evolved, more and more of the CNS practice was institutionally bound to hospitals. By mid-century, the CNS role began to parallel medical specialization in areas such as medical–surgical, pediatric, or psychiatric nursing. Clinical specialists were hired into roles based on their education, knowledge, and skills. Certification was not yet developed or required (Hudspeth, 2011). During the 1970s, despite the lack of consensus among the discipline over the CNS role, the number increased dramatically along with graduate education funding. By the mid-1970s, the American Nurses Association (ANA) advocated for the master's degree as a requirement for the CNS (ANA Congress for Nursing Practice, 1974). Despite the growing number of nurses educated in CNS roles, confusion over the role persisted. Some CNSs were working in direct care roles or as members of physician-led teams in specialty practice and their clinical practice was influenced and reshaped by the transfer of specialized knowledge skills. The direct care of clinical specialist appealed to many CNSs as a means to expand access and address the needs of patients in crisis. The psychiatric CNSs exemplified this trend with practices that, more often than not, provided care to underserved populations. A larger number of CNSs were expert consultants to nursing staff, bridging clinical expertise with managerialism at the unit or nursing service level. The CNS working in areas such as gerontology, psychiatry, and cardiovascular nursing has supported the development of implementation of guidelines and rational systems of care. The inability to show direct cost saving through the integration of the CNS in nursing services remained a persisting problem.

CNSs organized and sought legitimacy through certification. Certification slowly evolved beginning in the late 1970s but was not the panacea; except for the psychiatric CNS, certification was rarely required by employers. By the 1980s, psychiatric CNS aligned with nurse-midwives and NPs in the pursuit of legislative goals for reimbursement and prescriptive authority (Lyon, 2000). This move supported the successful campaign for legislative and regulatory changes in many states. In the past two decades, there has been increasing debate about the future of psychiatric CNS role as NP programs have added psychiatric specialties (Jones & Minarik 2012; Lego & Caverly, 1995). Psychiatric clinicians, historically more autonomous than other CNS colleagues, are finding their practice model eroded. The changing practice patterns in psychiatric and mental health including the growing role of prescribing pharmacotherapeutics has reshaped practice expectations for the psychiatric APRN. The psychiatric APRN, unlike CNS colleagues in institutional settings, are increasingly involved in direct and reimbursable care, but in collaboration and supervision with physician colleagues.

As changes in hospital reimbursement constrained budgets, the hospital-based CNS became an easy target, as their role did not generate income for the hospital systems. In many institutions, the CNS positions were eliminated or combined into administrative or teaching positions such as unit-based clinical teaching, nurse managers, and/or case managers. By 1990, CNSs found themselves at an economic disadvantage to NPs, whose clinical skill set, including prescriptive authority, contributed to their success in securing positions in specialty practices. Given advances in pharmacotherapeutics and eligibility for billing, prescriptive authority became increasingly important. Thousands of clinical specialists returned to school to seek NP certification. Within the advanced practice community, there was an increasing talk about the blended role of CNS–NP (Hamric et al., 2014).

The medical outcomes era was well underway by the time the first major wave of CNS completed their NP education. The release of the 2001 IOM report, *Crossing the Quality Chasm* (IOM, 2001), generated close attention on system improvements for quality and safety. A decade after, there was fear that the CNS might become extinct; renewed focus on the CNS as nursing change agent ensued.

The 2004 National Association of Clinical Nurse Specialists (NACNS) statement on CNS practice and education reaffirmed the importance of preparing the CNS with skills in leadership, collaboration, and consultation; professionalism; ethical practice; and professional citizenship. The NACNS further elaborated these in 2010 as it outlined new core competencies such as (a) direct care; (b) consultation; (c) systems leadership; (d) collaboration; (e) coaching; (f) research including interpretation, use, translation, evaluation, and conduct; and (g) ethical decision making, moral agency, and advocacy. These were presumed to occur with leadership, collaboration, and consultation; professionalism; ethical practice; and professional citizenship (NACNS, 2010b). The CNS role continued to be broadly focused on specialty knowledge for populations, nursing staff education, consultation, and organizational change (Sparacino, 2005).

The 2010 passage of the Patient Protection and Affordable Care Act raised questions once again on the economic viability of the CNS role. As many CNSs were working in direct care roles in areas such as gerontology, oncology, palliative care, and maternal child health, NACNS (2010a) reaffirmed the position that CNSs are valuable members of primary care teams. Brenda Lyon, former chairperson of the American Association of CNS legislative/regulatory committee, noted the following: "although several barriers to CNS practice were identified in the analysis, the two most prevalent were (1) not recognizing CNS practice at all or requiring a CNS to meet requirements to practice as an NP and (2) requiring a CNS to be certified in specialty areas even in the absence of availability of CNS certification in the specialty." The development of the 2008 consensus report on ANP did not resolve the regulatory issues for the CNS (NACNS, 2008). Many CNSs practice in states that do not recognize or require certification. At the federal level, the CNS role continues to lack recognition as APN and instead, CNSs are included with RNs (NACNS, 2004).

Despite gains in professional legitimacy, the role of the CNS continues to be at risk. The future of CNS practice, constrained by fiscal trends, requires a political savvy to maneuver the straits of healthcare reforms, such as the Patient Protection and the Affordable Care Act. The CNS has the potential to help reshape health systems to guide chronic care and patients' transitions inside and out of hospitals.

■ NURSE PRACTITIONERS

The NP was the last of the direct practice advance nursing roles to develop in the 20th century. The history of NPs is commonly dated back to 1965 with the opening of the pediatric NP program by Loretta Ford and Henry Silver, MD, in Colorado. In reality, the NP role evolved after decades of expanding nursing practice in community settings such as public health and outpatient centers (Norris, 1977). The formal creation of the role was observed by Loretta Ford to legitimize the reality of nurses practice (Fairman, 2008). In the 1960s, the great society movement led to a dual concern for easing social tensions with major policy reforms. These included the development of new forms of healthcare payment under Medicare and Medicaid, as well as the development of new settings of care such as community health centers. As Medicare and Medicaid policies created an unprecedented demand for healthcare services, interest in a new expanded role grew. Primary care physicians were few and far between, as the culture of medicine placed greater value on specialization and resultantly, diverted physicians into more lucrative areas of surgery and medical specialties. The growing shortage of general practitioners and the limited availability of pediatricians created an opportunity for the first programs for pediatric NPs (Andrews, Yankauer, & Connelly, 1970).

Many nurses had already demonstrated the ability and a willingness to take on the assessment and management of patients with common acute and chronic healthcare needs. NP education began with support from medicine, causing many leaders in nursing to cast a jaundiced eye on NPs. The NP movement took off, just as the nursing profession and feminist ideology converged, offering a critical view and fear of further subjugation. As the numbers of NPs grew and gained positive reviews from patients and collaborating physicians, efforts to sustain the movement took shape through policy making. With the support of federal funding, the nursing profession began to acknowledge NPs, opening the doors in the 1970s to offer training, first as certificate programs and a few years later, as graduate programs. Nursing organizations such as the ANA and their state constituent organizations, despite ambivalence, facilitated NP practice groups' efforts. Legal recognition of NP practice was slowly achieved on a state-by-state basis. This also helped to advance efforts to establish standards and certification. At the national level, NPs organized as the American Academy of Nurse Practitioners (AANPs) in 1985 as a "unified way to network and advocate for NP issues." This was the first national organization created to advocate politically for NPs of all specialties. This step in organizing NPs helped to advance legislation and set standards of practice. Regulatory efforts at the state level were initially sought to recognize and control the scope of practice and later of prescriptive practices and reimbursement (Keeling, 2007). The varieties of state policy outcomes vary widely, as evidence of the strength of physician attempts to assert control and nursing power to resist this. NP autonomy of practice became a goal but elusive to NPs in most states. Barbara Safriet (1992), in the *Yale Law Journal*, argued for greater consistency in criteria for NP education and practice. As NPs demonstrated the ability to provide cost-effective quality care, the public and private insurance markets began to open to NP practice.

■ APRN REGULATION

APRNs have been recognized by the IOM (2011), the National Governor's Association (2012) and other key stakeholders as essential to enhancing access to care for patients. To engage in APN requires the legal authority to evaluate patients, diagnose, order and interpret diagnostic tests, and initiate and manage treatments including prescriptive practice (AANP, 2017). When there are no legal or regulatory restrictions imposed and the oversight for this practice occurs exclusively under the licensure authority of the respective state's board of nursing, this is referred to as Full Practice Authority (FPA; AANP, 2017). Nursing practice, however, is regulated at the state level and resultantly, the authority of APRNs varies from state to state with arbitrarily imposed restrictions creating unnecessary barriers to accessing the care delivered by this important segment of the healthcare workforce. In 2008, seeking to create a uniform and transparent approach to APRN licensure, 48 nursing organizations including the National Council of State Boards of Nursing (NCSBN) and advance practice professional organizations, educational and regulatory bodies came together to endorse a report titled the "Consensus Model for APRN Regulation: Licensure, Accreditation, Certification, & Education (LACE)" (APRN Consensus Work Group & the National Council of State Boards of Nursing APRN Advisory Committee, 2008). The Consensus Model, together with NCSBN's (2017) FPA aligned "APRN Model Legislation," provide a foundation for a uniform practice environment that promotes the mobility of nurses across state lines and further, access to the unrestricted care of APRNs. Despite a reported goal to align all state and federal regulations with the LACE recommendations by 2015 (Stanley, 2012), efforts to revise and pass state regulations are progressing slowly across the United States.

A beleaguered United States Veterans Administration (VA) issued a ruling that would authorize FPA for those NPs, CNSs, and CNMs who are employed within a VA system and acting within scope (Department of Veterans Affairs [DVA], 2016) irrespective of state limitations. A little discussed exception however, the ruling also includes language that is a nod to the concept of "state supremacy" and defers to state law regarding the authority to prescribe and administer controlled substances (DVA, 2016). Challenged to meet the timely access demands of U.S. veterans, this ruling will expand access to cost-effective, high-quality, APRN-driven care with limitations. The ability to alleviate human suffering, including the management of pain, is foundational to APRN practice. While the VA's progress toward FPA represents a significant movement toward the NCSBN model and a victory for advancing APRN practice, the omission of CRNAs and inclusion of prescriptive limitations in the ruling demonstrate that at both the state and national levels, there is still work to be done to modernize licensing laws. Such advancements are often hampered under the guise of consumer protection and restrict the ability of APRNs to respond to the public demand for care (McMichael, 2017). Higher political spending on behalf of physician interest groups has been demonstrated to correlate with restrictive licensing laws for NPs. Further, the ability of nursing groups to effect licensing law changes has been documented as small (McMichael, 2017). Achieving uniformity with respect to FPA will require a high degree of political will, consumer engagement, and importantly, interprofessional partnerships.

■ BEYOND DIRECT CARE: ENGAGING IN ANP

APN, as defined by the NCSBN (2011) in the Campaign for APRN Consensus, includes the previously introduced direct care roles of the CRNA, CNM, CNS, and the certified nurse practitioner (CNP). However, there is an acknowledgment that new and emerging nursing roles will continue to evolve and perhaps, in some instances, even migrate away from direct patient care, which has long been the hallmark of advanced practice. Nurses engaged in administration, policy work, or the emerging role of the informatics nurse specialist provide us with such example. The inclusion of these diverse roles under the umbrella of *engaging in ANP* is an acknowledgment of the broad sphere of influence and specialized nature of the work undertaken by nurses practicing in these areas.

NURSING ADMINISTRATION

The ANA developed *Nursing Administration: Scope and Standards of Practice* (2009), which outlines competencies and provides a framework for the administrative practice of nurses today. Nurse administrators are RNs responsible for communicating the shared vision of an organization, and they further orchestrate and influence the work of others toward the achievement of important organizational outcomes (ANA, 2009).

Because of her appointment to the position of superintendent of the Upper Harley Street Hospital, Florence Nightingale is often credited with developing the management role in nursing. Like much of nursing, history suggests that it is unlikely that this role would have developed outside of the influence of the social and political forces of the time (Wildman & Hewiston, 2009). Historically, female superintendents held responsibility for the oversight of nursing practice, as was chronicled by Nightingale. However, the literature suggests that similar structures of nursing workforce oversight existed among 19th-century religious sisterhoods, alluding to the idea that some early form of nursing management may have predated

Nightingale. Despite this ambiguity, what remains significant today is that this structure of clinical oversight establishes a foundation for the nurse management role and precedence that nurses are responsible for the management of other nurses (Wildman & Hewiston, 2009).

From Nightingale to Clifford, who served as the senior vice president and nurse-in-chief of the Beth Israel Deaconess Hospital in Boston, Massachusetts, and who is credited with the development of a professional nursing model that is considered the benchmark for professionalism in nursing, history is rich with examples of nurses engaged in administration and leadership. Early nursing leaders often lacked formalized management training; however, the 1899 development of a "Hospital Economy" certificate program at Teachers College at Columbia University in New York represented an important step toward formalizing the education of the nurse administrator (Alexander, 1997). Designed to train nurses for administrative positions in hospitals, the Columbia program is credited with establishing the foundation for early baccalaureate and master's degree programs (Alexander, 1997).

Over the years, the migration of nurses from the bedside to the boardroom has been both tenuous and tentative. In the early 1900s, the AMA reported that more than 1,500 charitable or church-affiliated institutions were being managed by nurses (Alexander, 1997). However, secondary to an evolving perception that nurses lacked the acumen necessary to lead, the presence of women in hospital leadership began a trajectory of decline, often substituted by men who possessed proficiency in business and medicine (Alexander, 1997).

The march for nurse administrators to evolve their roles and maintain organizational footing was slow and required significant help from private funders, including the Kellogg Foundation and, later, the Commonwealth Fund (Alexander, 1997). During the 1950s, graduate programs for nursing administration became more prevalent. However, as greater value was placed on increasing the body of nursing knowledge and developing the clinical practice, academic opportunities for nursing administration again began to decline. It was not until the 1970s and 1980s that interdisciplinary master's programs in nursing administration were developed within university schools of business, public health, and healthcare administration. Eventually, with recognition that management within the nursing services required improvement, dual-degree programs such as the MSN/MBA were initiated. These degree programs provided a long-overdue opportunity for the nurse administrator role to flourish as this degree soon became the preparation of choice for the nurse executive, producing a master's prepared nurse with an MBA (Alexander, 1997).

The contemporary role of the nurse administrator has evolved from the "head nurse" with a defined unit-based responsibility to include executive-level roles with broad organizational influence and responsibility such as the vice president of Patient Care Services, chief nursing officer (CNO), chief executive officer (CEO), chief operating officer (COO), or dean (ANA, 2009). Certification for nursing administration has been offered through the American Nurse Credentialing Center (ANCC) since 1979. However, in 2008, the organization announced that the certification title would be changed to the nurse executive certification with basic and advanced competencies. With broad applicability across diverse administrative roles, this move was designed to both align and contemporize the nurse administrator title with current healthcare culture and remains standard today (ANCC, 2008). Despite such changes in titles and a high public trust rating, a recent Gallup poll suggests that the nurses remain largely absent at the highest decision-making levels and lack a meaningful presence in the boardroom when compared to physician colleagues (Khoury, Blizzard, Wright Moore, & Hassmiller, 2011). A national coalition of professional nursing organizations established the goal of placing 10,000 nurses on governing boards by 2010 (Sachs & Hurwitz, 2014). Clearly, there is much work to be done to move nurses out of the margins of healthcare leadership.

■ EMERGING ROLES FOR ADVANCED PRACTICE

Over the past two decades, the restructuring of healthcare systems toward consolidation and integration of services has led to new roles such as case managers and informatics nurse specialists. The support for such roles has risen amid expanding governmental regulations to address quality and safety. Both roles represent a significant solution toward addressing the healthcare system dysfunctions that contribute to injuries and high costs of rehospitalization.

Case management or care management, acknowledged as an advanced practice role function, is in transition to become a distinct role for nurses engaged in advanced practice. In 2012, the ANA released "The Value of Nursing Care Coordination," a white paper. Creating clarity on which elements of practice constitute "care coordination," the focus included ensuring that the patient's needs and/or preferences are met and supported across people, functions, and sites. The document served to highlight both the qualitative and quantitative benefits of RN coordination of care in a highly fragmented healthcare system including decreased emergency department admissions, lower Medicare costs, enhanced ability to self-manage disease, and importantly, improved patient satisfaction. Speaking not only to the coordination of care, the paper further addresses the importance of a primary care delivery model offered in the context of an integrated multidisciplinary team (Camicia, Chamberlain, Finnie, Nalle, Lindeke, Lorenz, & McMenamin (2013). Health reform has strengthened the impetus of case management with a shift toward value-based payment models and reimbursement for the coordination of care. With recognition of the need to ensure a seamless transition of care across the continuum, and the increased acuity in the ambulatory setting, the aforementioned creates a case for the inclusion of nurse care managers in Patient-Centered Medical Home (PCMH) models. As healthcare institutions tackle new mandates in chronic disease management and care transitions, nurse care management has an opportunity to demonstrate greater expertise and control over healthcare decision making. Graduate-level education programs for case management are emerging throughout the United States and master's-level case management certification is now offered by the ANCC.

Nursing informatics has slowly become integrated into nursing education and practice. The first documented computer technology course was offered in New York for undergraduate nursing students in 1976 (Guenther, 2006). Over time, nurses have assumed increasingly larger roles in the management of health-related data, but the phrase "nursing informatics" reportedly did not appear in the literature until 1985. A decade later, the ANA defined nursing informatics as a specialty and published the *Scope of Practice in Nursing Informatics* and *Nursing Informatics Standards of Practice* (Guenther, 2006). The ANA (1994) defined nursing informatics as "the specialty that integrates nursing science, computer science and information science in identifying, collecting, processing and managing data and information to support nursing practice, administration, education, research and the expansion of nursing knowledge."

The evolution toward a nursing informatics specialty necessitated that the nursing informatics roles evolve from the already well-established medical and healthcare informatics specialties (Guenther, 2006). As core content and competencies for nursing informatics have become better developed, there has been an emergence of coursework to support the growing specialty. Offering the first certifying exam in November of 1995, the ANCC remains the official certifying organization for informatics nurse specialists (Tietze, 2008). Although certification was offered, it is important to note that it was not until 2001 that the ANA's *Scope of Practice in Nursing Informatics* and *Nursing Informatics Standards of Practice* were integrated and the *Scope and Standards of Nursing Informatics* was published (Guenther, 2006). Accordingly, it is with this process that the ANA set the stage to truly legitimize the specialty and define nursing informatics; the integration of nursing, computer, and information sciences to manage and communicate data, knowledge, and nursing practice (Guenther, 2006). An additional necessity is the integration of such data to support decision making across all healthcare roles and settings (Tietze, 2008).

Reinforced by the tendency for chief information officers (CIOs) to value technology, the early roles for the information nurse specialists were largely related to the insertion of technology into practice settings (Staggers, 2002). Today, there are numerous programs across the country preparing nurses to engage in the advanced practice of nursing informatics, and their graduates have prominent roles in staff education, quality, and safety, as well as the protection of the privacy and confidentiality of patients (Tietze, 2008). Informatics nurse specialists are integral to ensuring the delivery of safe patient care and may serve as systems analysts, consultants, programmers, researchers, or decision support/outcomes managers (Tietze, 2008). Indeed, the roles are likely to continue to evolve as the infusion of technology and the need to effectively manage data continue to exert an impact upon the dynamic healthcare environments in which nurses are engaged in practice. The leveraging of technology to show value for nursing and health services includes predictive modeling and clinical decision making as well as tracking population health outcomes. Nursing expertise is essential in the construction of informatics systems to assure that nursing and essential patient-related indicators are explicitly included and measured across settings of care. Recent trends include the acceleration of intervention research by nurse informatics researchers and other APRNs (Carrington, 2016). This trend has been fueled in part by the development of the DNP focus on informatics as well as changing health policies.

■ DNP: PREPARING ANP FOR THE FUTURE—OR IS THE FUTURE NOW?

The move to a practice doctorate for ANP is again a response by nursing to societal demands and anticipated challenges. There is no question that the master's-prepared nurses have demonstrated well-documented outcomes that include safe, cost-effective care and high patient satisfaction rates (Guadagnino, 2008; Newhouse et al., 2011). The American Association of Colleges of Nursing (AACN, 2004) makes the case for reshaping the education for APN, citing demographic imperatives, and population health trends. In 2006, as the AACN was considering the transformative shift of specialty education to the doctoral level, the U.S. Census Bureau reported that the number of Americans with employer-based access to health insurance had markedly declined, and an estimated 47 million Americans were then living without health insurance (Johnson, 2007). In 2010, the U.S. Census Bureau (2012) reported the number of uninsured had increased to 49.9 million and in the current state, despite the passage of universal healthcare coverage, the healthcare system is no better positioned to meet the access needs of the people.

Further complicating matters, the United States is potentially facing a geriatric crisis, as unprecedented growth in the number of older adults is anticipated (Centers for Disease Control and Prevention [CDC] and the Merck Company Foundation, 2007). As societal and healthcare advances in prevention have reduced the threat of infectious diseases, a demographic shift toward longevity and chronic disease has emerged. The number of Americans aged 65 or older is predicted to double, and by 2030, this population could reach a staggering 71 million older adults with documented healthcare costs significantly exceeding that of a younger demographic (CDC and Prevention & the Merck Company Foundation, 2007). An examination of healthcare outcomes for Medicare beneficiaries suggests that there is a strong case for cost-containment and coordinated care if we are to meet the healthcare needs of an aging population (Jencks, Williams, & Coleman, 2009). An analysis of Medicare claims data revealed that one fifth of discharged Medicare beneficiaries were readmitted within 30 days. Those readmitted had a longer than average length of stay and many had not had postdischarge follow-up—a clear case for improved access and coordination of care. The estimated cost of unplanned hospital readmissions in 2004 alone was a staggering $17.4 billion (Jencks et al., 2009). In the backdrop is an IOM report (Kohn, Corrigan, & Donaldson, 2000) that estimates as many as 98,000 Americans die annually because of errors in care. While the Affordable Care Act extended healthcare coverage to 22 million Americans (Association of American Medical Colleges, 2017), access to primary care is limited by a shortage of primary care physicians and unnecessary regulatory constraints placed on the practice of advance practice nurses. A report by the Association of American Medical Colleges (2017) projects that the country will experience a shortage of between 40,800 and 104,900 physicians by 2030, including both primary care and specialty-trained MDs.

While the decline in both primary and specialty physicians can lead to rationing, delays in access, and fragmentation of care, there is the potential that expanded use of advanced practice nurses may be able to stave off such deleterious trends. Without better utilization, the fragmented healthcare system will likely be ill-positioned to meet the complex medical needs of an aging U.S. population (Schwartz, Basco, Grey, Elmore, & Rubenstein, 2005). The increased complexities of the healthcare environment, coupled with a rising population of older Americans and decreased access to care, can be cited as major drivers in the nation's healthcare crisis, the direction of health reforms, and the need to move specialty education in nursing to the doctoral level.

Citing concern related to the quality and safety of patient care delivery, as well as the increasing complexity of the current healthcare system, the AACN published the *Essentials of Doctoral Education for Advanced Nursing Practice* (2006) and issued a call for transformational change in the educational preparedness for nurses practicing at the most advanced level in nursing. With a recommended implementation date of 2015, the AACN boldly asserted that nurses effectively engaged in practice at advanced levels would require doctoral-level preparedness. At that time, identified benefits of repositioning specialty education to the doctoral level further included closing the gap on evolving advance nursing competencies for practice, leadership, and faculty shortages (AACN, 2006).

Having borne witness to the rise and fall of the DNP and doctor of nursing science (DNSc) degrees, a practice-oriented doctorate was not novel for nursing. However, of significance, the AACN-proposed DNP would impact broadly the scope of ANP, and the AACN Position Statement on the Practice Doctorate in Nursing (AACN, 2004) was foundational in defining it as

> nursing intervention that influences health care outcomes for individuals or populations, including the direct care of individual patients, management of care for individuals and populations, administration of nursing and health care organizations, and the development and implementation of health policy. Preparation at the practice doctorate level includes advanced preparation in nursing, based on nursing science, and is at the highest level of nursing practice. (p. 3)

Given the divergence from direct clinical care in scope, framing the DNP as a "clinical doctorate" may be a misnomer. Reflecting upon this broad definition, the DNP-prepared nurse is either an APRN with specialization in direct patient care, or a nurse with a specialized focus in administration, healthcare policy, informatics, or population-based care who is engaged in practice at an aggregate, systems, or organizational level (AACN, 2006). This move by the AACN to ensure the inclusion and doctoral preparation of nurses engaged in "indirect care" roles under the rubric of ANP thoughtfully ensures the migration of these roles toward a formalized plan of education. The aforementioned strategizes to develop the transformational leaders needed to respond to an evolving healthcare crisis, assuming greater responsibility for patient and organizational outcomes. Such a move is not merely good for patients but further positions the larger body of nursing professionals toward better representation with respect to ongoing national healthcare-related discussions and, further, to be responsive to evolving healthcare needs. With consideration of the diverse roles that nurses engaged in advanced practice assume, DNP curricula are designed to meet both foundational competencies considered core to engaging in ANP, as well as specialty content (AACN, 2006).

While nursing continues to ruminate around the very basics, including standardizing education requirements for entry-level practice, the IOM (2011), recognizing the complexity of the current healthcare environment, issued a report entitled *The Future of Nursing: Leading Change, Advancing Health.* This landmark piece of work, funded by the Robert Wood Johnson Foundation, offers strong recommendations with implications for nursing practice at all levels. Significant attention has been paid to the need to reconceptualize existing nursing roles, innovate, attract, and retain new nurses, and increase the numbers of nursing faculty. Attuned to the need to strategize to develop and retain nursing faculty, the IOM (2011) issued a call to double the number of nurses with a doctoral degree by 2020. Alarmingly, this call to action was issued at a time when the AACN (2011) has acknowledged that in 2010, more than 1,200 qualified doctoral applicants were denied entry into programs. These denials were largely attributed to the faculty shortage. If nursing is to succeed in preparing greater numbers of nurses at the doctoral level, there is no question that preparing DNPs will be essential to the successful attainment of such a goal.

■ SUMMARY

While initially the DNP-prepared nurse was conceived as a nurse of the future, positioned to deliver evidence-based direct care, manage systems and lead quality initiatives, integrate technology into care delivery systems and models, and further impact organizations and policy at the highest levels—all critical to transforming our broken healthcare system and ensuring the health of the nation, it becomes increasingly apparent that the future is now. ANP is juxtaposed between the sociopolitical issues driving the healthcare environment, increased demand for access with an imperative to enhance quality and contain cost. In this context, the demand for advanced education is likely to increase and further contribute to the evolution of nursing roles. The DNP challenges both the master's degree as the cornerstone of nursing specialty education and the traditional outcomes of doctoral education, where clinical research has historically been the hallmark.

The second decade of the 21st century shepherded in a new era of healthcare policy and debate. The passage of the Patient Protection and Affordable Care Act catapults nurses, particularly advanced practice nurses, into a new prominence in healthcare. As advanced practice nurses seek to expand practice into a variety of settings and secure reimbursement for their services, they must be prepared to demonstrate effective outcomes of care (Newhouse et al., 2011). The DNP, with the emphasis on practice-based research, supports the attainment of a higher level of accountability in healthcare (Florczak, 2010). The future of ANP rests on a rich and complex history of nursing practice. The DNP presents an opportunity to renegotiate and legitimize the APRN role in the evolving healthcare system. With this opportunity comes the challenge to hold onto our values and to transcend the age of intra- and interprofessional politics to participate fully in the healthcare system change.

■ REFERENCES

Abbott, A. (1988). *A system of professions, an essay on the division of expert labor.* Chicago, IL: University of Chicago Press.

Ahmed, S. W., Alves, S., Beal, M., Carr, K. K., Carter, D., & Consalvi, C. (2014, November). *The advanced practice nurse in Massachusetts. Massachusetts Action Coalition for Nursing* Report. Retrieved from http://www.mass.edu/nahi/documents/REPORT-APRN%20 in%20MA-111814-FINAL.pdf

Alexander, C. C. (1997). The nurse executive in the 21st century: How do we prepare? *Nursing Administration Quarterly, 22,* 76–82.

Allen, D. (1997). The nursing–medical boundary: A negotiated order. *Sociology of Health and Illness, 19,* 498–520.

American Association of Colleges of Nursing. (2004, October). *AACN position statement on the practice doctorate in nursing.* Retrieved from http://www.aacnnursing.org/Portals/42/ News/Position-Statements/DNP.pdf

American Association of Colleges of Nursing. (2006, October). *The essentials of doctoral education for advanced nursing practice.* Retrieved from http://www.aacnnursing.org/ Portals/42/Publications/DNPEssentials.pdf

American Association of Colleges of Nursing. (2011). 2011 *annual report: Shaping the future of nursing education.* Retrieved from http://www.aacn.nche.edu/aacn-publications/ annual-reports/AR2011.pdf

American Association of Nurse Anesthetists. (n.d.-a). *Fact sheet concerning state opt-outs and November 13, 2001 CMS Rule.* Retrieved from https://www.aana.com/ advocacy/state-government-affairs/federal-supervision-rule-opt-out-information/ fact-sheet-concerning-state-opt-outs

American Association of Nurse Anesthetists. (n.d.-b). Timeline of AANA history, pre AANA. Retrieved from http://sharepoint.aana.com/resources2/archives-library/Pages/Timeline -of-AANA-History-Pre-AANA.aspx

American Association of Nurse Practitioners. (2017). State practice environment. Retrieved from https://www.aanp.org/legislation-regulation/state-legislation/state-practice-environment

American Congress of Obstetricians and Gynecologists. (2015). ACOG applauds intro-duction of the improving access to Maternity Care Act. Retrieved from https:// www.acog.org/About-ACOG/News-Room/Statements/2015/ACOG-Applauds -Introduction-of-the-Improving-Access-to-Maternity-Care-Act

American Nurses Association. (1994). *The scope of practice for nursing informatics.* Washington, DC: American Nurses Publishing

American Nurses Association. (2009). *Nursing administration: Scope and standards of practice.* Silver Spring, MD: Nursesbooks.org.

American Nurses Association Congress for Nursing Practice. (1974). *Definition: Nurse prac-titioner, nurse clinician and clinical nurse specialist.* Kansas City, MO: American Nurses Association Practice.

American Nurse Credentialing Center. (2008, April 24). ANCC updates nursing administration certifications and credentials. Retrieved from http://nursecredentialing. org/Documents/Certification/Articles/NurseExecAnnouncement.aspx

Andrews, P., Yankauer, A., & Connelly, Y. (1970). Changing the patterns of ambulatory pediatric caretaking: An action-oriented training program for nurses. *American Journal of Public Health*, *60*, 870–879.

APRN Consensus Work Group & the National Council of State Boards of Nursing APRN Advisory Committee. (2008). *Consensus model for APRN regulation: Licensure, accreditation, certification & education*. Retrieved from https://www.ncsbn.org/Consensus_ Model_for_APRN_Regulation_July_2008.pdf

Ashley, J. A. (1976). *Hospital, paternalism and the role of the nurse*. New York, NY: Teachers College Press.

Association of American Medical Colleges. (2017, July 20). Improving the health care system. Retrieved https://news.aamc.org/for-the-media/article/aca-health-coverage

Beck, D. M. (2006). Nightingale's passion for advocacy: Local to global. In L. Andrist, P. Nicholas, & K. Wolf (Eds.), *A history of nursing ideas* (pp. 473–487). Sudbury, MA: Jones & Bartlett.

Brodsky, P. (2008). Where have all the midwives gone? *Journal of Perinatal Education*, *17*, 48–51.

Camicia, M., Chamberlain, B., Finnie, R. R., Nalle, M., Lindeke, L. L., Lorenz, L., & McMenamin, P. (2013). The value of nursing care coordination: A white paper of the American Nurses Association. *Nursing Outlook*, *61*(6), 490e–501e.

Carrington, J. M. (2016). Trends in nursing informatics research and the importance of the nurse administrator. *Nursing Administration Quarterly*, *40*(2), 184.

Centers for Disease Control and Prevention & the Merck Company Foundation. (2007). *The state of aging and health in America*. Retrieved from http://www.cdc.gov/Aging/pdf/ saha_2007.pdf

Centers for Medicare and Medicaid Services & U.S. Department of Health and Human Services. (2001, November 13). Medicare and Medicaid programs; Hospital conditions of participation: Anesthesia services. Final rule (to be codified at 42 C.F.R. pts. 416, 482, 485). 66 Fed. Reg. 56,762–56,763.

Christman, L. (1968). The nurse clinical specialist. *Hospital Progress*, *49*, 14–16.

Dawley, K. (2001). Ideology and self-interest, nursing, medicine and the elimination of the nurse-midwife. *Nursing History Review*, *9*, 99–126.

Department of Veterans Affairs. (2016). VA grants full practice authority to advanced practice registered nurses. Retrieved from https://www.va.gov/opa/pressrel/pressrelease.cfm?id=2847

Dossey, B. M., Selanders, L., Beck, D. M., & Atwell, A. (2005). *Florence Nightingale today: Healing leadership and global action*. Silver Spring, MD: Nursebooks.org.

Drevdahl, D. (2002). Social justice or market justice? The paradoxes of public health partnerships with managed care. *Public Health Nursing*, *19*, 161–169.

Dulisse, B., & Cromwell, J. (2010, August 1). No harm found when nurse anesthetists work without supervision by physicians. *Health Affairs*, *29*(8), 1469–1475.

Epstein, L. (1990). The outcomes movement—Will it get us where we want to go? *New England Journal of Medicine*, *323*(4), 266–270.

Fairman, J. (2008). *Making room in the clinic, nurse practitioners and the evolution of modern health care*. Piscataway, NJ: Rutgers University Press.

Florczak, K. (2010). Research and the doctor of nursing practice: A cause for consternation. *Nursing Science Quarterly*, *23*, 13–17.

Galloway, D. H. (1899, May 29). The anesthetizer as a specialist. *The Philadelphia Medical Journal*, 1173.

Guadagnino, C. (2008).Growing role of nurse practitioners. Medicalnews.com retrieved from https://physiciansnews.com/2008/05/22/growing-role-of-nurse-practitioners

Guenther, J. T. (2006). Mapping the literature of nursing informatics. *Journal of the Medical Library Association*, *94*, E92–E98.

Harris, N., & Hunzikar-Dean, J. (2001). The art of open-drop ether. *Nursing History Review*, *9*, 159–184.

Hamric, A. B., Hanson, C. M., Tracy, M. F., & O'Grady, E. T. (2014). *Advanced practice nursing: An integrative approach* (5th ed.). Philadelphia, PA: Elsevier/Saunders.

Hines, D. C. (1994). The intersection of race, class and gender in the nursing profession. In E. D. Baer (Ed.), *Enduring issues in American nursing* (pp. 25–36). New York, NY: Springer Publishing

Hudspeth, R. (2011). Changes for the valuable clinical nurse specialist: A regulatory conundrum. *Nursing Administration Quarterly*, *35*, 282–284.

Institute of Medicine. (2001). *Crossing the quality chasm*. Washington, DC: National Academies Press.

Institute of Medicine. (2011). *The future of nursing: Leading change, advancing health*. Washington, DC: National Academies Press.

Jenkins, M. (2006). Nursing centers and the autonomy of nursing work. In L. Andrist, P. Nicholas, & K. Wolf (Eds.), *A history of nursing ideas* (pp. 319–332). Sudbury, MA: Jones & Bartlett.

Jencks, S. F., Williams, M. V., & Coleman, E. A. (2009). Rehospitalizations among patients in the Medicare fee-for-service program. *New England Journal of Medicine*, *360*, 1418–1428.

Johnson, T. D. (2007). Census bureau: Number of U.S. uninsured rises to 47 million Americans are uninsured: Almost 5 percent increase since 2005. Retrieved from http://getinsuredintime.blogspot.com/2011/10/census-bureau-number-of-us-uninsured.html

Jones J. S., & Minarik P. A. (2012). The plight of the psychiatric clinical nurse specialist: The dismantling of the advanced practice nursing archetype. *Clinical Nurse Specialist*, *26*, 121–124.

Keeling, A. (2007). *Nursing and the privilege of prescription 1893–2000*. Columbus, OH: The Ohio State University Press.

Khoury, C., Blizzard, R., Wright Moore, L., & Hassmiller, S. (2011). Nursing leadership from bedside to boardroom: A Gallup national survey of opinion leaders. *Journal of Nursing Administration*, *41*(7/8), 299–305.

Kohn, L. T., Corrigan, J. J., & Donaldson, M. S. (Eds.). (2000). *To err is human: Building a safer health system*. Washington, DC: National Academy of Sciences.

Lego, S., & Caverly, S. (1995). Coming to terms: Psychiatric nurse practitioner versus clinical nurse specialist. *Journal of the American Psychiatric Nurses Association*, *1*(2), 61–65.

Lyon, B. (2000). Enhancing the public's access to CNS services: Model statutory and regulatory language for CNS practice. *Clinical Nurse Specialist*, *14*, 156–157.

Magaw, A. (1900). Observations on 1092 cases of anesthesia from January 1, 1989 to January 1, 1900. *St. Paul Medical Journal*, *2*, 306–311.

McMichael, B. J. (2017, May 01). The demand for healthcare regulation: The effect of political spending on occupational licensing laws. *Southern Economic Journal*, *84*(1), 297–316. doi:10.1002/soej.12211

Merritt Hawkins. (2017). Physician appointment wait times and Medicare and Medicaid acceptance rates. Retrieved from https://www.merritthawkins.com/news-and-insights/thought-leadership/survey/survey-of-physician-appointment-wait-times

National Association of Clinical Nurse Specialists. (2004). *Statement on clinical nurse specialist practice and education* (2nd ed.). Harrisburg, PA: Author.

National Association of Clinical Nurse Specialists. (2010a). Clinical nurse specialists—Practitioner contributing to primary care: A briefing paper. *Clinical Nurse Specialist, 24,* 271–272.

National Association of Clinical Nurse Specialists. (2010b). Organizing framework and core competencies. Retrieved from http://nacns.org/LinkClick.aspx?fileticket=22R8AaNmrUI%3d&tabid=139

National Association of Clinical Nurse Specialists. (2016, July 26). Failure to classify clinical nurse specialists as APRNs is 'out of step with the nursing and health care communities,' nurse leader warns [Press release]. Retrieved from http://nacns.org/2016/07/failure-to-classify-clinical-nurse-specialists-as-aprns-is-out-of-step-with-the-nursing-and-health-care-communities-nurse-leader-warns/

National Council of the State Boards of Nursing. (2017). NCL model legislation and rules. Retrieved from https://www.ncsbn.org/95.htm

National Governor's Association. (2012). *The role of nurse practitioners in meeting increasing demand for primary care.* Retrieved from https://www.nga.org/cms/home/nga-center-for-best-practices/center-publications/page-health-publications/col2-content/main-content-list/the-role-of-nurse-practitioners.html

Newhouse, R., Stanik-Jutt, J., White, K., Johantgen, M., Bass, E., Zangaro, G., . . . Weiner J. P. (2011). Advanced practice nurse outcomes 1990–2008: A systematic review. *Nursing Economics, 29,* 1–21.

Norris, D. M. (1977). One perspective on the nurse practitioner movement. In A. Jacox & D. Norris (Eds.), *Organizing for independent nursing practice* (pp. 21–33). New York, NY: Appleton-Century-Crofts.

Peplau, H. E. (1965). Specialization in professional nursing. *Nursing Science, 3,* 268–287.

Rafferty, A. M., & Wall, R. (2010). An icon for today and iconoclast for today. In S. Nelson & A. M. Rafferty, *Notes on Nightingale, the influence and legacy of a nursing icon* (pp. 130–143). Ithaca, NY: Cornell University Press.

Reihl, J., & McVay, J. (1973). *The clinical nurse specialist: Interpretations.* Appleton, WI: Century Crofts.

Reiter, F. (1966). The nurse-clinician. *American Journal of Nursing, 66*(2), 274–280.

Reverby, S. (1987). *Ordered to care: The dilemma of American nursing, 1850–1985.* New York, NY: Cambridge University Press.

Rooks, J. (1997). *Midwifery and childbirth in America.* Philadelphia, PA: Temple University Press.

Sachs, A., & Hurwitz, J. (2014, November 17). National coalition launches effort to place 10,000 nurses on governing boards by 2020. Retrieved from http://www.nursingworld.org/FunctionalMenuCategories/MediaResources/PressReleases/2014-PR/Effort-to-Place-Nurses-on-Governing-Boards.html

Safriet, B. J. (1992). Health care dollars and regulatory sense: The role of advance practice nursing. *Yale Journal of Regulation, 9,* 417–477.

Sandelowski, M. (2000). The physician's eyes: American nursing and the diagnostic revolution in medicine. *Nursing History Review, 8,* 2–38.

Schwartz, M. D., Basco, W. T., Grey, M. R., Elmore, J. G., & Rubenstein, A. (2005). Rekindling student interest in generalist careers. *Annals of Internal Medicine, 142,* 715–724.

Sinclair, M. (2010). Moving midwifery research forward in the revolutionary information and high-tech era. *Evidence Based Midwifery, 8,* 111.

Sparacino, P. (2005). The clinical nurse specialist. In A. Hamric, J. Spross, & C. Hanson (Eds.), *Advanced practice nursing: An integrative approach* (3rd ed., pp. 414–446). Philadelphia, PA: Saunders.

Staggers, N. (2002). The evolution of definitions for nursing informatics: A critical analysis and revised definition. *Journal of the American Medical Informatics Association, 9,* 255–261.

Stanley, J. M. (2012). Impact of new regulatory standards on advanced practice registered nursing: The APRN consensus model and LACE. *Nursing Clinics of North America, 47,* 241–250. Retrieved from http://www.nursing.theclinics.com/article/S0029-6465(12)00025-4/abstract

The Joint Commission. (2017). Ambulatory care program: The who, what, when, and where's of credentialing and privileging. Retrieved from https://www.jointcommission .org/assets/1/6/AHC_who_what_when_and_where_credentialing_booklet.pdf

Thornton, P., McFarlin, B. L., Park, C., Rankin, K., Schorn, M., Finnegan, L., & Stapleton, S. (2017). Cesarean outcomes in U.S. birth centers and collaborating hospitals: A cohort comparison. *Journal of Midwifery and Women's Health, 62*(1), 40–48. doi: 10.1111/jmwh.12553

Tietze, M. (2008, August). Nursing informatics: What's it all about? Retrieved from http://www.uta.edu/ced/static/onlinecne/CEAugust08.pdf

U.S. Census Bureau. (2012). Highlights: 2010. Retrieved from https://www.census.gov/prod/2012pubs/p60–243.pdf

Varney, H., Kriebs, J. M., & Gegor, J. M. (2004). *Varney's midwifery* (4th ed.). Sudbury, MA: Jones & Bartlett.

Wertz, R., & Wertz, D. (1977). *Lying in: A history of childbirth in America.* New York, NY: Free Press.

Wolf, K. (2006). The slow march to professional practice. In L. Andrist, P. Nicolas, & K. Wolf (Eds.), *A history of nursing ideas* (pp. 305–318). Boston, MA: Jones & Bartlett.

Wildman, S., & Hewiston, A. (2009). Rediscovering a history of nursing management: From Nightingale to the modern matron. *International Journal of Nursing Studies, 46*(12), 1650–1661.

How Will the DNP Contribute to the "Future" in The Future of Nursing (2011, 2015) Reports?

ANN H. CARY

Aim high, aim for something that will make a difference.
> —(Drucker & Maciariello, 2006, p. 111)

■ MANDATE FOR CHANGE: PRELUDE TO REDESIGNING HEALTHCARE IMPACT

Four key messages framed the eight recommendations in *The Future of Nursing* (2011) to the public as well as the (2016) subsequent assessment report:

- Nurses should practice to the full extent of their education and training.
- Nurses should achieve higher levels of education and training through improved educational systems that promote seamless academic progression.
- Nurses should be full partners with other health professionals in redesigning healthcare in the United States.
- Effective workforce planning and policy require better data collection and an improved information infrastructure. (Institute for Medicine [IOM], 2010, 2011, p. 4)

An intriguing dimension of these original key messages was that while addressing nursing specifically there remains today explicit recognition of the interdependent, interprofessional, and systemic changes among all providers and policymakers to assure any successful healthcare transformation (Altman, Butler, & Shern, 2016). The doctor of nursing practice (DNP) provider and the national guidelines (American Association of Colleges of Nursing [AACN], 2006, 2015) for DNP programs are critical to assure that DNPs and their impact on systems reflect knowledge of the science and practice of systems thinking and application in real-world venues. Strategy, leadership, teamwork, policy competencies, and informatics knowledge and translation, implementation, and evaluation science are minimal requisites to successfully innovate all of the components of a redesigned healthcare system. Education, practice, workforce data modeling and surveillance, policy, and effective, intentional interprofessional teamwork preparation and practice are domains of action embedded in these messages. Following are some of the issues that undergird the key messages by the IOM (2011, 2016), Robert Wood Johnson Foundation (RWJF), and AACN.

FULL PRACTICE TO THE LIMITS OF CREDENTIALS, TRAINING, AND EDUCATION

State and federal regulatory models and institutional restrictions for advanced practice registered nurse (APRN) practice have created a barrier to the ability of DNPs to practice to the full extent of preparation (Fauteux, Brand, Fink, Frelick, & Werrlein, 2017). Disciplinary "guilds" indirectly work to assure that any economic redistribution of income potential among interprofessional providers is prevented in order to maintain adequate levels of an expected disciplinary standard of living. Organizations, payers, and insurers maintain policies that may prevent the DNP provider from being credentialed or privileged as well as set reimbursement rules for direct or "incident to" reimbursement in fee for service models. Should value-based and bundled reimbursement be fully executed, the reimbursement gap may become less of an issue. In the majority of cases, the entity that pays the provider for service decides how they will value the DNP provider, even though the DNP may have outcomes that are equal to or better than another provider. Newhouse and coauthors published a systematic review of the literature on whether nurse practitioners and certified midwives who worked collaboratively with physicians had patient outcomes similar to physicians working without APRNs. Their review encompassed 18 years of literature and found that outcomes were similar and sometimes better, depending on the patient population and setting (Newhouse et al., 2011). In fact, in 2017, the RWJF publication *Charting Nursing's Future* featured a composite of research related to removing barriers to APRN practice that serves as an important brief with respective evidence of both outstanding outcomes of APRN providers and the gaps in access to care, cost, and quality that are created when full scope of practice is absent in healthcare systems and policies. In this publication, 22 states had full practice authority, up from 13 when the 2011 IOM report was published, and other states are working toward it. Additionally, changes by the Veterans Health Administration in 2016, which allows three of the four APRN providers to be granted full practice authority, portends progress toward a tipping point in federal, state, and institutional regulations.

Institutional policies limit nurses at both the bedside and in the boardroom. However, barriers to full practice are not limited to nurse providers (DNPs or PhDs) with the highest credentials. All members of the healthcare team who are credentialed also work in organizations that place boundaries around their unique and overlapping practice abilities. This is achieved through institutional policies that guide actual "institutional" scopes of practice and memberships on key policy boards such as medical privileging committees and boards of directors. In fact, AACN (2016) illustrated that one of the six pillars, *Embracing a new vision for academic nursing*, recognized the key to influence and policy change was in nurse participation in health systems governance and on governing boards. This participation can be a key role for a DNP provider. Few organizations have evaluated frameworks in which the work of providers at the lowest-paid level are matched to their competency to perform work based on training and education, from community worker and health coach to bedside nurse, DNP, and physician.

The IOM (2016) *Assessing Progress . . .* report noted that while some progress had been made in the states, federal rules, and some businesses to meet the IOM recommendations, action should be taken to broaden any working coalition on *The Future of Nursing* recommendations to include more diverse stakeholders—other health professions, policymakers, and the community—thus reinforcing the common ground among all to achieve healthcare outcomes for patients by removing barriers to practice, increasing collaboration, and working other issues to improve the systematic provision of care (p. 24).

SEAMLESS ACADEMIC PROGRESSION TO ENSURE HIGHER EDUCATIONAL PREPARATION WITHIN THE DISCIPLINE

The fault line within nursing between levels of preparation for entry into practice at one end and the debate about the PhD versus DNP as an appropriate academic and practice scholar at the other end fractures the ability of nurses to speak with one voice in their role as a full partner in the future of healthcare. In an RWJF 2010 Gallup poll, opinion leaders ranked doctors and nurses first and second in providing trusted information, but noted that nurses who had relatively weak influence on increasing access to care were not perceived as important decision players or revenue assets and did not speak with one voice on national issues. However, these same opinion leaders suggested that nurses should demonstrate more leadership and higher expectations (RWJF, 2010). Only one RN licensure is provided for multiple routes of entry whereby eligibility relies on at least three degree/diploma pathways or only a graduate degree. In addition, nurses earn multiple "professional initials" as testimony to advanced practice or specialty designations and academic credentials. These are clearly not understood or differentiated by the public and, in many cases, within the profession.

While the Consensus Model for APRNs (2008) has been supported by all 50 states, implementation is slow as it winds through the state regulatory review processes. The majority of nurses (80%) who are educated for licensure at the associate degree level do not seek graduate preparation even if they eventually earn a BSN (Aiken, Cheung, & Olds, 2009) and, thus, are not optimally prepared to provide higher levels of care to patients or amass the knowledge to generate or translate research/science on nursing or healthcare. Similarly, these nurses are not eligible to assume faculty positions, APRN, and/or DNP positions to provide advanced care and educate the next generation of nurses, nor are they easily able to sit equitably with highly educated peers to influence next-generation practices, governance, and policies. Various levels of nursing degree programs maintain themselves as silos in which the ability of the nurse to transition between levels is fraught with redundant requirements and lengthy curriculums to satisfy perceived higher education requirements. It is likely that a nurse who earns an associate degree (AD) and then seeks a bachelor of science in nursing (BSN) degree will spend much longer total time to achieve the BSN post–high school than to earn the BSN degree initially. The 2016 IOM *Assessing Progress* report noted that efforts toward the baccalaureate degree had moved the dial from approximately 50% to 53% of nurses—shy of the 80% goal for 2020. While the numbers of BSN and BSN completion programs grew, the majority of employers do not require the BSN. Attention to the quality of expanded programs should be monitored to ensure patients experience improved outcomes noted by this workforce. The IOM (2016) report suggests strengthening academic pathways through community colleges and 4-year programs; that employers play a critical role in providing fiscal and logistical support for progression to the BSN; and that transition-to-practice residencies for entering and advance practice providers be created and funded to reduce turnover and improve onboarding results for quality practice.

The current nursing licensure/certification renewal process is often predicated on continuing education courses that do not demonstrate sufficient evidence of additional learning or behavioral competency. Some states have no requirements for continuing education. Thus, much of the skill development of nurses who decline to seek higher educational preparation is "just-in-time" or on-the-job training, which can vary tremendously by region and institution in terms of quality practice expectations. Lifelong learning, while providing lip service, has not been a consistent expectation for high-value practice.

Access to progress in degree attainment is enhanced with the availability of distance and online educational programs. These provide convenient access from distance sites and flexibility in schedules to accommodate multiple commitments of the nurse and assure a more user-friendly path for educational advancement. The need to redesign educational pathways, articulation requirements, dual enrollment options, and entry to terminal degree pathways efficiently can align easily with healthcare systems redesign.

The rate of knowledge explosion in healthcare and nursing demands that curriculum content reflect immediate advancements. Nursing education is constantly challenged to anticipate and teach the latest in science, practice, and technology to assure that students and graduates access knowledge rapidly for translation to patients and systems (Benner, Sutphen, Leonard, & Day, 2009). The DNP graduate has acquired such capabilities as a hallmark of his or her educational competencies and thus is an optimal clinical and theoretical teacher for all levels of students and as preceptors for new students, graduates, nurse residency programs, and team consultants as providers learn the process for rapid acquisition of specific knowledge, skills, and behaviors for improved competence.

A more recent tension developing among both PhD and DNP degree programs has been illustrated by Dreifuerst et al. (2016) in their research conducted with 548 current students or recent graduates of doctoral programs. While the overall numbers of doctorally prepared nurses remain low in the profession, DNP graduates are showing a steep rise compared to the PhD graduates whose numbers have leveled off. Even though nearly all PhD graduates and as many as 60% of DNP graduates are in faculty roles, the faculty shortage does not seem to be abating. Most PhD programs emphasize that the graduate is prepared as a nurse scientist, whereas most DNP programs emphasize the graduate is prepared as an advanced clinician who uses research utilization for practice and administration activities. Both PhD and DNP program *Essentials* do not emphasize pedagogy theory nor education research (AACN, 2006, 2010). In fact, the AACN (Task Force on the Implementation of the DNP, 2015) white paper *Current Issues and Clarifying Recommendations* for the DNP indicates:

> Practice as a nurse educator should not be included in the DNP practice hours. The focus of a DNP program, including practicum and DNP Project, should not be on the educational process, the academic curriculum, or on educating nursing students. (p. 10)

However, the IOM recommendation to double the number of doctoral-prepared nurses who are also available to teach students as well as to practice in their roles as nurse scientists and/or advanced clinician and systems agents seems to suggest reconciliation between PhD and DNP graduates employment and the curricular infusion of pedagogy theory, research, and practice to prepare them for academic roles in which they are likely to be employed. Any doctoral preparation as a PhD or DNP that adds specific content to prepare the graduate to excel in their role as an educator and/or academic faculty will strengthen the faculty supply and help to reduce the faculty shortage in nursing.

FULL PARTNERSHIP IN SYSTEMS REDESIGN

Full partnerships necessarily imply equitable accountability for assuring the process and outcomes for systems design. All partners must come to the table with an exquisite capacity to negotiate and leverage their professional assets, communicate a vision, contribute resources, create and maintain energy, and provide influence, power, and stamina to achieve the desired redesign impact. The ability to work in collaborative, hierarchial, and interprofessional groups will be critical to a successful effort.

A 2011 survey of 1,000 hospitals found nurses were woefully lacking in representation on hospital boards, accounting for only 6% compared to 20% for physicians. This number of nurses on boards actually declined to 5% in 2014 (American Hospital Association [AHA], 2014). Improvement in collection of data about nurses on boards of healthcare-related organizations, in addition to other seminal organizations and businesses engaged in creating a *Culture of Health* movement in communities, will be critical to measuring success of nurses. A national effort to compile and populate this data is funded by RWJF and has at least 20 organizational members. The goal of the coalition is to have 10,000 nurses on governing boards by 2020 (nursesonboardscoalition.org).

Earlier reference was made to the opinion leaders survey results (RWJF, 2010), questioning the effectiveness of nurses to successfully influence change in healthcare systems. However, interprofessional preparation and practice is fraught with uneven science outcomes across systems, as well as a disciplinary climate of "silo mentality," and in some cases, "imagined" boundaries of unique competencies and delayed care delivery due to inadequate team processes. Interprofessional teams as a fulcrum in the educational and provider culture appear to suffer from a lack of implementation leadership within systems of care for populations. Catalysts for selecting the power brokers in systems redesign have typically been achieved through the alignment of organizational consultants, healthcare administrators, chief financial officers, and medical committees. Evidence of the effectiveness of nursing leadership in redesign has been revealed in TCAB (transforming care at the bedside) projects. TCAB is a national program that incentivizes nurses to lead process improvement for health and fiscal outcomes through small tests of change, rapid adoption, and improvement (Bolton & Aronow, 2009). Evaluations of systems that efficiently create, manage, and assure outcomes of interprofessional team structures, processes, and outcomes are emerging (e.g., the Department of Veterans Affairs [VA] system of organizing primary care providers into health teams and linking integrated information technology to teams and services; www.va.gov/health; Barr, 2002; Barr, Koppel, Reeves, Hammick, & Freeth, 2005; Reeves et al., 2008).

Systems redesign by nature requires the assessment of information flow, efficiency, and the ability of digitalization and health information technology (HIT) to improve quality of work, care, and system effectiveness. Healthcare is in the midst of a commitment to digital interoperability and digital workflow schemata to test and improve the impact. Nurse leaders must be engaged in the design and knowledgeable in the technologies and opportunities of application to support these HIT efforts if early success is to be achieved. Technology–digital workflow impacts how nurses and team members document, deliver, and review clinical care. Redesigned systems will incorporate computerized knowledge management and decision support that releases providers to address complex care and high-touch needs of patients not addressed by the technology. It also promotes the ability to provide many types of care without regard to location of the provider or the patient. Today, patient and population care is radically influenced by information technology and digitalization. Research shows how it influences the increase or decrease in documentation requirements (Thompson, Johnston, & Spurr, 2009) and quality indicators (DesRoches, Donelan, Buerhaus, & Zhonghe, 2008; Waneka & Spetz, 2009), and it is improved by the participation of nurses in the design. The Patient Protection and Affordable Care Act (ACA) and Health Care and Education Affordability Reconciliation Act (2010) contained incentives to assure the "meaningful use" of HIT by providers to improve patient care and to add to the aggregate picture of quality clinical care nationally. However, the future of these legislative mandates is being transformed into new healthcare proposals and mandates that will change the landscape of what was planned and what we know. In addition, precision medicine and healthcare is a critical intervening practice that has the opportunity to radically change what care is provided to whom in a very personalized manner. The DNP, having been educated in systems, informatics, and leadership, is well positioned to advance the concept of digital redesign within the redesign team and to gather the best evidence and science in care to translate these rapidly emergent findings to patients and systems.

In 2011, the Interprofessional Education Collaborative (IPEC) Expert Panel published a vision and explicated competencies of interprofessional collaborative practice as essential to safe, high-quality, accessible, patient-centered care. The initial IPEC paper was revised in 2016 by acknowledging the inclusion of public health population competencies (IPEC, 2016). Building on the concept of interprofessionality as a process to develop practice, the panel adopted the definition of D'Amour and Oandasan to describe it:

> the process by which professionals reflect on and develop ways of practicing that provide an integrated and cohesive answer to the needs of clients/family/ population . . . involves continuous interaction and knowledge sharing between professionals, organized to solve or explore a variety of education and care issues, all while seeking to optimize the patient's participation. . . . Interprofessional practice has unique characteristics in terms of values, codes of conduct, and ways of working. (D'Amour & Oandasan, 2005, p. 9)

Key challenges exist, however, to successfully operationalize full partnerships through interprofessional practices (IPs) in a redesigned system (IPEC, 2011, 2016). These include the following:

- The support of top leadership to dismantle barriers to design, education, and practice within an interprofessional concept.
- Limited professional schools within an institution and the need for outreach agreements to embrace interinstitutional collaboratives to achieve interprofessional training.
- Scheduling issues for conflicting classes/clinicals among the professional schools.
- Faculty development training and practice to articulate and integrate new behaviors and attitudes about processes of engagement in interprofessional culture.
- Early stage development of assessment instruments and metrics to capture processes and outcomes of IP.
- Regulatory expectations of "learning together to work together" need to be developed to affirm the concept and commit to transformational changes in accreditation and certification of institutions and providers.

Confounding issues can be solved through intentional solutions by all parties that value effective execution of healthcare delivery. The fact that IPEC membership has now been expanded to 20 disciplines is extraordinary and surely broadens the common ground among healthcare team members.

Exemplars of redesign efforts are described here from the IOM report (2011). Nurses are reminded that the ACA has also provided additional opportunities to advance "disruptive innovation" strategies in an effort to change healthcare delivery and practice through the creation and funding of the Center for Medicare and Medicaid Innovation (CMMI) within the Department of Health and Human

Services (DHHS). Four current initiatives that are receiving expanded funding support include accountable care organizations (ACOs), medical/health homes (MHHs), community health centers (CHCs), and nurse-managed health clinics (NMHCs). Each of these strategies needs to incorporate highly functioning interprofessional teams in which nurses are used as full partners in the design and operate to the full extent of their education and training. Interprofessional research teams are critical to assure that the production will incorporate nurse-sensitive indicators as well as collaborative indicators. The future of these options will rest with new legislative programs created in Congress. It is unclear what shape new opportunities will take until signed into law.

ACOs are structured around the coordination of primary care providers (including APRNs), hospitals, and some specialists. Payment models may include shared savings or capitated payments, and move well beyond the traditional fee for service, which encourages more service, redundancy, and costs. The goals of the ACO are to improve quality, contain growth and costs, and improve coordination of care (IOM, 2011; Exhibit 2.1).

MHHs are not a new concept; they were originally created by pediatricians in the 1960s. The ACA indicates that the interprofessional teams that include physicians, nurses, and other health professionals should support these structures. This particular type of primary care coordinates and provides comprehensive services, strengthens the relationship between provider and patient/family, and measures and monitors quality. As the IOM notes, the language in the ACA uses the terms medical/health sometimes interchangeably, allowing the interpretation by funders to exclude APRNs at will. The VA system uses this concept (primary care medical home) and has expanded it to include staff nurses who function as care managers and coordinators to provide health risk appraisals, as well as health promotion and disease prevention. Other terms for this model include patient-centered medical or health home (IOM, 2011; Exhibit 2.2).

CHCs have a proven record of providing high-value primary and preventive care for the underserved and have been allocated additional funds (in the billions) through ACA (IOM, 2011). CHCs offer comprehensive services for dental, mental, and behavioral health as well as access to pharmacies. Nurses have traditionally played a central role on the team as APRN primary care providers and in outreach and home care services. Outcome indicators show that CHC patients have fewer unmet needs, underutilize emergency department services, avoid hospitalizations, and have lower medical costs (NACHC, the Robert Graham Center and Capital Link, 2007; Exhibit 2.3).

EXHIBIT 2.1   DNP Leadership in ACOs

With a sufficient number of DNP providers in each ACO, can you envision the articulation of practices, data and systems requirements, technology, regulatory reform, and teamwork required to be successful in this environment?

ACO, accountable care organizations; DNP, doctor of nursing practice.

EXHIBIT 2.2   DNP Leadership in MHHs

- With a sufficient number of DNP providers in each MHH, can you envision your role, function, and effectiveness in planning the model, measuring the processes and outcomes, adjusting the system components for improvement, and disseminating the results for replication?
- Can you imagine the information technology needs, the training for interprofessional high-level functioning, and the cost and quality metrics that can inform replication and dissemination?
- How will your participation provide the value-added component to this model in terms of substitution and expansion of provider roles and scopes of practice?
- What will it take for DNPs to demonstrate leadership and a successful outcome for sustainable regulatory reform?

DNP, doctor of nursing practice; MHH, medical/health home.

EXHIBIT 2.3   DNP Leadership in CHCs

- With a sufficient number of DNP providers in each CHC, can you envision an expanded role for DNPs?
- What new skills do DNPs add to CHCs due to the education and training received in the DNP program?
- What disruptive innovations do you imagine could be provided to make the impact of CHCs on the community's health even more dramatic?
- What are the expanded metrics required to capture the impact of CHC care on the populations they serve?

CHC, community health center; DNP, doctor of nursing practice.

NMHCs have existed since the 1960s to serve Medicare and Medicaid recipients, the uninsured, and children in communities across the nation. Although run by nurses with APRNs providing primary care, NMHCs employ an array of healthcare providers including physicians, health educators, social workers, and outreach workers using a collaborative team model. Services may include primary care, family planning, mental/behavioral health, prenatal care, health promotion, and disease prevention (IOM, 2011). A major challenge for NMHCs is financial sustainability from patient revenues so that fiscal models employed in any redesign of a transformational healthcare system will dramatically impact the sustainability of a center. The ACA authorized $50 million to NMHCs funding in 2010 and additional sums as possible (NNCC, 2011).

EXHIBIT 2.4   DNP Leadership in Nurse-Managed Health Centers

- With a sufficient number of DNP providers in each NMHC, can you envision an expanded role for DNPs?
- What new skills do DNPs add to NMHCs due to the education and training received in the DNP program?
- What disruptive innovations do you imagine could be provided to make the impact of NMHCs on the community's health even more dramatic?
- What are the expanded metrics needed to capture the impact of NMHC care on the populations they serve?

DNP, doctor of nursing practice; NMHC, nurse-managed health clinic.

The National Nurse-Led Care Consortium (NNCC; n.d.) explicates the reasons nurse-managed centers are successful in patient care as follows:

- As a neighborhood initiative, they understand patient and community needs and earn their trust.
- NMHCs strive to identify and coordinate the social services that are essential to maintain all avenues of health support.
- By bringing care to the "people," NMHCs build community capacity in areas such as safety and violence abatement, after-school programs, and community advocacy.

Outcomes for improved patient care at lower costs in NMHCs give this model another dimension of credibility to funders. Regulatory and other disciplinary support will be necessary to advance this model. Clearly, national incentives through grants, demonstration projects, and other mechanisms will be the key to assure innovative projects by nurses, in interprofessional teams, and through strategic and thoughtful leadership (Exhibit 2.4).

BETTER WORKFORCE POLICY INFLUENCE THROUGH IMPROVED INFORMATION INFRASTRUCTURE

Health professions workforce data are critical to forecasting, planning, and resourcing the right mix, distribution, and competencies needed by a transformed healthcare system. Systematic and timely collection of data and new models of provider mix to supply efficacious and cost-effective care to more patients in the new era of healthcare are essential to its success. Workforce data provide the early warning mechanism for any "tsunami" of patients likely to overwhelm current achievements in quality, not to mention improvements that are at risk for failing in an overwhelmed system. While past efforts in workforce surveillance have yielded various modeling approaches, the science is far from precise. Often adjustments in assumptions are later discovered to mediate the implications of the data for programming and workforce policy decisions. The need for primary care providers is forecasted (Duchovny, Trachtman, & Werble, 2017) but the political will of self-interests among disciplines, new educational programs (DNP), and regulatory mandates will mediate the ability of workforce models to redesign sufficient incentives to meet the needs of populations needing primary care.

For example, a 2017 working paper from the Congressional Budget Office (CBO) estimates that the demand for primary care will increase by 18% from 2013 to 2023 due to growth in the population, degree of insurance coverage, and more rapid aging of the population (Duchovny et al., 2017). The use of telehealth delivery, changing reimbursements, more primary care residencies, and loan repayment are all variables that could increase the physician supply; whereas, the total supply of primary care providers could be increased through providers other than physicians when scopes of practice are fully allowable for APRNs and when retail clinics that are typically staffed by APRN—NPs and PAs—expand. Distribution demand is forecast to be in metropolitan counties due to faster population growth. Clearly, workforce data supply and demand of providers with similar scopes of practice need to be aligned for adequate systems design of care delivery.

The evidence that primary care can be provided by nonphysician APRN providers with equal or better outcomes for patients appear to get lost in the modeling assumptions. The impact of the DNP workforce on care and systems redesign is not yet evident since these providers are a relatively new entry to the healthcare system, although anecdotal examples exist. This disconnect between what is, what should be, and what will be is often traced to political "spin" on data as well as too many data variations and analysis options.

A balance of providers to impact the vision of the redesigned healthcare system must be achieved with careful attention to improved modeling for supply. The critical elements in such a system are included in Exhibit 2.5.

Demand can be created to match the supply, which can either harm or help the redesign impact.

EXHIBIT 2.5 Critical Elements in a Redesigned Healthcare System

- The necessary shift to ambulatory care
- Telehealth
- Information technology
- Prioritization of healthcare resource consumption among an increasingly diverse patient population
- Global market competition
- Newly prepared evidence-based providers and teams
- "Medicalization" of events in the life of a patient

The three key areas explicated for workforce data across the health professions in the IOM (2011, p. 261) report include the following:

1. Core data sets on healthcare workforce supply and demand
2. Surveillance of workforce market conditions
3. Healthcare workforce effectiveness research

Some of these areas are addressed in the ACA. Specifically, the law created but did not fund a National Health Workforce Commission (NHWC) to "develop and evaluate training activities to determine whether demand is being met, identify barriers to improved coordination at federal, state and local levels and recommend solutions" (p. 256). However, the National Center for Workforce Analysis (NWC) receives federal support as well as support from state and regional centers for improved data collection and analysis. Still, improvements are needed for accuracy in the state minimum data sets, collaborative data collection by nursing organizations, federal data in the American Community Survey and National Ambulatory Medical Care Survey, and the National Sample of Registered Nurses and Nurse Practitioners (IOM, 2016).

It is pertinent to recognize that a severe shortage of faculty is forecasted as the demand for educating health professions and nursing providers is realized (Kovner, Fairchild, & Jacobson, 2006). Fang and Kersten (2017) projected that faculty retirements for the next 10 years, beginning in 2015, will equal roughly one third of total faculty working in 2015. Educational systems must ready their resources today to be able to meet the production cycle of preparing new faculty for tomorrow. Creative models of faculty sharing, rapid preparation, and partnerships with the business community in strategic planning and execution will all be "on the table" as partial solutions.

Finally, the IOM *Assessing . . . Report* (2016) noted that specific emphases on ensuring a more diverse workforce and providing more culturally competent care is needed. While the supply of nurses who represent diverse racial, ethnic, gender, and socioeconomic backgrounds grew, the growth failed to match the characteristics of the U.S. population. When diverse providers are in the healthcare system, these providers are more likely to practice in similar communities which improves access and quality of care in those communities. New educational pathway supports, job placement, and retention efforts will need to be measured to understand critical factors of success to increase a diverse nursing workforce from all levels of education to all levels of practice.

Regulatory issues emerge when attempting to innovate in any of the key areas or to implement any of the recommendations noted in the following section. Disruptive innovation is just that; it questions and repositions all assumptions that maintain the current system. Transformational healthcare will require regulatory experimentation and timely responses. For each of the four key areas, successful solutions are at the mercy of regulatory and policy reforms. DNP graduates must always be thoughtful and action-oriented toward the policy and regulatory dimensions necessary to assure any redesign change is executed. By committing to be thoughtful strategists, their likelihood of success is greatly improved.

■ EIGHT RECOMMENDATIONS FOR TRANSFORMATION OF THE FUTURE OF NURSING

The eight original recommendations published by the IOM are repeated, practically verbatim, to preserve the consensus of the IOM committee for the reader (IOM, 2011, pp. 9–15).

1. **Remove scope of practice barriers**
   APRNs should be able to practice to the full extent of education and training. This will be possible with federal recognition by the Centers for Medicare and Medicaid Services, Office of Policy and Management; federal reimbursement models for APRN parity; institutional participation, which assures APRNs are eligible for credentialing and privileging; and state scopes of practice, which conform to National Council of State Boards Model Act. The Federal Trade Commission and the Antitrust Division of the Department of Justice should review existing and proposed state regulations for needless anticompetitive effects.

2. **Expand opportunities for nurses to lead and diffuse collaborative improvement efforts**
   Private and public funders, healthcare organizations (HCOs), nursing education programs, and nursing associations should expand opportunities for nurses to lead and manage collaborative efforts with interprofessional healthcare team members to conduct research and redesign and improve practice environments and health systems. Nurses must diffuse successful practices and identify administrative waste and redundancies to improve efficiencies. Nurses should be part of medical device and HIT design and evaluation teams. Nurses are capable of using their experiences to design entrepreneurial care systems.

3. **Implement nurse residency programs**
   State boards of nursing, accrediting bodies, the federal government, and HCOs should take actions that support nurses' completion of a transition-to-practice nurse residency program after they have completed a prelicensure or APRN degree program or when they transition to a new clinical practice area. Policymakers should redirect the Graduate Medical Education funding from diploma programs to support BSN and nurse residency programs.

4. **Increase the proportion of nurses with baccalaureate degrees to 80% by 2020**
   Academic nurse leaders should work together to increase the proportion of nurses with baccalaureate degrees from 50% to 80%. Higher education should partner with accrediting bodies, private and public funders, and employers to ensure funding, monitor progress, and increase diversity of students. The workforce must be prepared to meet the demands of diverse populations across the life span. Education and training with interprofessional

students and teams should be done early in the educational process to affirm the culture of team practice.

5. **Double the number of nurses with doctorates by 2020**
   Schools of nursing, with support from private and public funders, academic administrators, university trustees, and accrediting bodies should double the number of nurses with a doctorate to add to the cadre of nurse faculty, practitioners, and researchers. Attention should be directed to increasing diversity. Policymakers should monitor the progression of entry nurses through masters and doctoral programs and incentivize rapid and efficient matriculation. Higher education must create compensation packages to reward recruitment and retention of highly educated nurse faculty who are responsible to create and deliver the next generation of educational innovations in nursing.

6. **Ensure that nurses engage in lifelong learning**
   Accrediting bodies, schools of nursing, HCOs, and continuing competency educators from multiple health professions should collaborate to ensure that nurses, nursing students, and faculty continue their education to engage in lifelong learning. Competencies need to be refined to provide care for diverse populations across the life span. Special attention to the inclusion of interprofessional competency development in integrated disciplinary learning teams within delivery systems is the key to ensuring sustainable performance and improved quality improvements.

7. **Prepare and enable nurses to lead change to advance health**
   Nurses, nursing education programs, and nursing associations should prepare nurses for leadership at all levels in healthcare. Private and governmental healthcare decision makers should ensure that leadership positions are available and filled by nurses. Nurses should receive priority for inclusion on boards, executive teams, and other key leadership areas commensurate with their competencies. Leadership development must recognize the power of interprofessional development with others in the business and healthcare enterprise.

8. **Build an infrastructure for the collection and analysis of interprofessional healthcare workforce data**
   The National Health Care Workforce Commission, with oversight from the Government Accountability Office and the Health Resources and Services Administration (HRSA), should lead a collaborative effort to improve research and collection and analysis of data on healthcare workforce requirements. The Workforce Commission and HRSA should collaborate with state licensing boards, state nursing workforce centers, and the Department of Labor in this effort to ensure that the data are timely and publicly accessible.

It is worthwhile to read the details in the IOM *Future of Nursing* (2011, 2016) reports in entirety as each contains rich and solid research from which timely recommendations and degrees of progress emerge. The report challenges the responsibility and the accountability of the nursing profession to unify its position on policy, education, practice, leadership, and research to build logical propositions and articulate solid leverage for transformational change in healthcare today. It seeks allies, collaborators, and broader coalitions outside of nursing who commit to create the larger pie of healthcare access, quality, and value rather than continue a downward spiral by positioning each discipline for the size of the healthcare delivery piece. Patients and population health lose ground in the current politics of fragmented financing, education, and delivery systems.

■ COULD THE DNP BE THE FUTURE OF NURSING AND HEALTHCARE?

For many reasons, the answer is YES!

- The AACN (2006) *DNP Essentials* document, referenced to prepare nurses with the DNP, clearly articulates the areas of competence expected by DNP graduates. In doing so, it unifies and standardizes expectations for systems and advanced practice knowledge so that DNPs will translate science rapidly to improve healthcare delivery, policy, and leadership impact. Curriculum should be producing "big picture" change agents who are capable of testing disruptive innovations in systems and with populations, understanding replication implications, and rapidly disseminating these to other researchers, policymakers, and interested parties.
- The DNP has a vital "stake in the game" for regulatory reform within advanced practice, among other disciplinary regulations that impinge on full scope of practice, and within institutions and systems in which they practice. Leading the way in all of these areas in a coordinated manner will be critical to opening the window of policy reform necessary to execute transformational systems for healthcare.
- DNPs should be facile with information and knowledge to advance translation and implementation science as they redesign practice and systems. Traditional practices cannot be used as leverage against evidence-based practices if the DNP is to adhere to the ethical mandate of beneficence. All patients deserve a right to high-value healthcare and to expect high-performing providers. The DNP provider is mandated to bring expertise equitably to the patient, the institution, the system, policymakers, and team members.
- DNPs can make substantive contributions to study and execute the following key evidence gaps identified by the IOM (2011, pp. 274–277; 2016) to transform practice, education, and leadership:
  1. Studying personal and professional characteristics, knowledge, and skills most important to leaders of redesigned organizations and quality initiatives, including ACOs, MHHs, CHCs, NMHCs, and other innovative delivery systems which will evolve from new legislation.

2. Identifying spheres of influence used by nurses in healthcare decision making and on boards and healthcare committees at a variety of levels.

3. Identifying mentoring and coaching characteristics most successful in recruiting, retaining, and promoting optimal performance in interprofessional teams, by individual providers, and within an array of institutions.

4. Examining how alternative faculty/student ratios affect the acquisition of competence and student retention as well as the impact of distance technologies and simulation to expand capacity for educating a more highly competent nurse at every level and setting.

5. Identifying faculty, staff, environmental, and organizational characteristics that best support a diverse nurse population to successfully pursue and complete BSN, graduate, and doctoral degrees.

6. Testing new models of nursing education and residency options incorporating Benner et al.'s (2009) characteristics, interprofessional paradigms, continuing competence for lifelong learning, technology efficiencies, and benefit structures for attracting highly qualified nurses to faculty roles.

7. Comparing programs, providers, provider teams, and health exchange models on costs, quality, access, and impact of current and innovative delivery models.

8. Identifying and evaluating decision support technologies on care delivery, high-value performance, quality, provider satisfaction, and rapid dissemination of science to the bedside and articulating measures of "meaningful use" of HIT to nurses and the team.

9. Examining trends and the impact of innovations and incubators of redesign in which "concept to execution processes" are tested for efficacy, policy impact, human capital requirements, and community sustainability.

10. Testing the characteristics of translation research that improve uptake and sustainability for diverse communities, organizations, providers, financiers, and policymakers.
    • DNP and PhD providers can demonstrate the power of collaboration from the scientist and the executer "team" approach as they iteratively discover, test, refine, and evaluate bench and applied evidence in current and emergent care systems. Program planning and evaluation capabilities are strengthened with systematic approaches that yield both qualitative and quantitative outcomes.

The "future" of nursing is a future of possibilities, imagination, leadership, radical incentives, and new paradigms. It cannot be created by using the same patterns of thinking and expectations that maintain the currently fragmented and fractured health delivery system. Patients deserve a system that promotes health and access to high-value care options. High-value care options can only be borne by limitations on self-interests, a willingness to risk new ventures, highly educated provider teams composed of diverse and flexibly skilled personnel, and a market that tolerates social capital as part of the market advantage. To truly change our expectations that the U.S. healthcare system is "good enough," passionate providers, politicians, markets, and communities must demand better and be willing to leverage a spirit of adventure combined with applied science. DNP leaders must demonstrate knowledge, courage, innovation, and adaptability to complexity while avoiding the noise of detractors who stand to lose when the status quo is dismantled. Developing DNP practice in the U.S. healthcare system is not for the faint of heart—indeed it will be made whole through the appropriate utilization of the DNP professional.

■ REFERENCES

Aiken, L. H., Cheung, R. B., & Olds, D. M. (2009). Education policy initiatives to address the nurse shortage in the United States. *Health Affairs, 28*, w646–w656.

Altman, S. H., Butler, A. S., & Shern, L. (Eds.). (2016). *Assessing progress on the Institute of Medicine report* The Future of Nursing. Washington, DC: National Academies Press.

American Association of Colleges of Nursing. (2006). *Essentials of doctoral education for advanced practice nursing.* Washington, DC: Author.

American Association of Colleges of Nursing. (2010). *The research-focused doctoral program in nursing.* Retrieved from http://www.aacnnursing.org/Portals/42/Publications/PhDPosition.pdf

American Association of Colleges of Nursing. (2016). *Advancing healthcare transformation: A new era for academic nursing.* Washington, DC: Author. Retrieved from http://www.aacnnursing.org/Portals/42/Publications/AACN-New-Era-Report.pdf

American Hospital Association. (2014). *2014 National health care governance survey report.* Chicago, IL: AHA Center for Healthcare Governance.

APRN Joint Dialogue Group (2008). *Consensus model for APRN regulation: Licensure, accreditation, certification & education.* Retrieved from https://www.ncsbn.org/consensus_model_for_APRN_Regulation_July_2008.pdf

Barr, H. (2002). *Interprofessional education today, yesterday and tomorrow: A review.* London, UK: Learning and Teaching Support Network for Health Sciences & Practice.

Barr, H., Koppel, I., Reeves, S., Hammick, M., & Freeth, D. (2005). *Effective interprofessional education: Argument, assumption and evidence.* Oxford, UK: Blackwell.

Benner, P., Sutphen, M., Leonard, V., & Day, L. (2009). *Educating nurses: A call for radical transformation.* San Francisco, CA: Jossey-Bass.

Bolton, L., & Aronow, H. (2009). The business case for TCAB: Estimates of cost savings with sustained improvement. *American Journal of Nursing, 109*, 77–80.

D'Amour, D., & Oandasan, I. (2005). Interprofessionality as the field of interprofessional practice and interprofessional education: An emerging concept. *Journal of Interprofessional Care, 19*, 8–20.

DesRoches, C., Donelan, K., Buerhaus, P., & Zhonghe, L. (2008). Registered nurses' use of electronic health records: Findings from a national survey. *Medscape Journal of Medicine, 10*, 164.

Dreifuerst, K. T., McNelis, A. M., Weaver, M. T., Broome, M. E., Draucker, C. B., & Fedko, A. S. (2016). Exploring the pursuits of doctoral education by nurses seeking or intending to stay in faculty roles. *Journal of Professional Nursing, 32*(3), 202–212.

Drucker, P. F., & Maciariello, J. A. (2006). *The effective executive in action: A journal for getting the right things done.* New York, NY: Harper Collins.

Duchovny, N., Trachtman, S., & Werble, E. (2017, May). Projecting demand for the services of primary care doctors: Working Paper 2017-03. *Congressional Budget Office*. Retrieved from https://www.cbo.gov/publication/52748

Fang, D., & Kesten, K. (2017, January). *Retirements and succession of nursing faculty in next 10 years 2016-2025*. Oral Presentation at the AACN Doctoral Conference, Naples, Florida.

Fauteux, N., Brand, R., Fink, J. L. W., Frelick, M., & Werrlein, D. (2017, March). The case for removing barriers to APRN practice. In M. J. Ladden, S. Hassmiller, & N. Fauteux (Eds.), *Charting nursing's future*. Issue 30.

Fineberg, H. V. (2011). Foreword. In Institute of Medicine, *The future of nursing: Leading change, advancing health*. Washington, DC: National Academies Press.

Institute of Medicine. (2010). Report brief. Washington, DC: National Academies Press. Retrieved from http://www.nationalacademies.org/hmd/~/media/Files/Report%20 Files/2010/The-Future-of-Nursing/Future%20of%20Nursing%202010%20 Report%20Brief.pdf

Institute of Medicine. (2011). *The future of nursing: Leading change, advancing health*. Washington, DC: National Academies Press.

Interprofessional Education Collaborative Expert Panel. (2011). *Core competencies for interprofessional collaborative practice: Report of an expert panel*. Washington, DC: Interprofessional Education Collaborative.

Interprofessional Education Collaborative. (2016). *Core competencies for interprofessional collaborative practice: 2016 update*. Washington, DC: Author.

Kovner, C. T., Fairchild, S., & Jacobson, L. (2006). *Nurse educators 2006: A report of the faculty census survey of RN and graduate programs*. Washington, DC: National League for Nursing.

National Association of Community Health Centers, The Robert Graham Center and Capital Link. (2007). *Access granted: The primary care payoff*. Washington, DC: Author.

National Nurse-Led Care Consortium. (n.d.). About us. Retrieved from https://nurseledcare .org/about.html

Newhouse, R. P., Stanik-Hutt, J., White, K. M., Johantgen, M., Bass, E. B., Zangaro, G., . . . Weiner, J. F. (2011). Advanced practice nurse outcomes 1990–2008: A systematic review. *Nursing Economics, 29*(5), 230–250.

Patient Protection and Affordable Care Act (PL 111–148) and Health Care and Education Affordability Reconciliation Act (PL 111–52) (2010).

Reeves, S., Zwarenstein, M., Goldman, J., Barr, H., Freeth, D., Hammick, M., & Koppel, I. (2008). Interprofessional education: Effects on professional practice and health care outcomes. *Cochrane Database of Systematic Reviews*, (1), CD002213. doi:10.1002/14651858. CD002213.pub2

Robert Wood Johnson Foundation. (2010). *Nursing leadership from bedside to boardroom: Opinion leaders' perceptions*. Retrieved from https://www.rwjf.org/en/library/ research/2010/01/nursing-leadership-from-bedside-to-boardroom.html

Task Force on the Implementation of the DNP. (2015). *The doctor of nursing practice: Current issues and clarifying recommendations*. Retrieved from http://www.aacnnursing.org/ Portals/42/DNP/DNP-Implementation.pdf?ver=2017-08-01-105830-517

Thompson, D., Johnston, P., & Spurr, C. (2009). The impact of electronic medical records on nursing efficiency. *Journal of Nursing Administration, 39*, 444–451.

Waneka, R., & Spetz, J. (2009). *2007–2008 annual school report: Data summary and historical trend analysis*. Sacramento: California Board of Registered Nurses.

Beyond Outcomes: Understanding and Impacting the Patient Experience

CHRISTINA DEMPSEY

National drivers to reform the healthcare system include increased cost and a mandate for improved quality. The United States spends more money per capita on healthcare, when compared to other high-income nations; however, our outcomes are ranked among the worst (The Commonwealth Fund, 2015). With a transformation of the national healthcare system underway, we are presented with an opportunity to seek to understand the complexities of care with a wider lens, a broader focus that leads us to a question upon which a truly patient-centered transformation of the U.S. healthcare system might occur—*what is patient experience?* How do you measure something so abstract? More importantly, how do we address the patient's experience in today's ever-changing healthcare environment? Let us first understand how we came to measure the patient perception of care.

In 1985, Notre Dame professors Irwin Press, PhD, and Rod Ganey, PhD, founded Press Ganey. They sought to understand and measure patient's perceptions of the care they received in the hospital. Developing a patient satisfaction survey, they asked about the care experience, such as "Nurses' attitude toward your requests" or "Physicians concern for your questions and worries." A five-item Likert scale quantified response based on patients' perceptions of care quality: very poor, poor, fair, good, or very good.

As scientists, Dr. Press and Dr. Ganey designed the survey items to be psychometrically sound. Questions were carefully worded to prevent influencing answers, and further, sequenced to provide insights without leading or prompting a certain response. During the 1990s and 2000s, hospitals across the United States used the Press Ganey patient satisfaction survey and the data collected provided new insight into patients' experiences and a tool for benchmarking performance (Dempsey, 2017).

In 2006, the Centers for Medicare and Medicaid Services (CMS) partnered with the Agency for Healthcare Research and Quality (AHRQ) to develop the Hospital Consumer Assessment of Healthcare Providers and Systems (HCAHPS) survey as part of a larger CAHPS program. The federal agency wanted to better understand patient's perceptions of their care and sought an instrument that would provide a uniform source of measurement for public reporting. In 2012, under the CMS Hospital Inpatient Quality Reporting (Hospital IQR) program, implementation of the HCAHPS survey became mandatory for all hospitals nationwide. Further, to increase hospital accountability and create incentives for improving quality, CMS tied Medicare reimbursements to survey scores.

The HCAHPS survey was designed to complement, not compete with, quality improvement instruments such as the Press Ganey survey that many hospitals were already using. In addition to administering its own survey, Press Ganey became approved by CMS to administer HCAHPS for clients. The HCAHPS survey contains 21 measures of patient perspectives and rating items that encompass the following topics: communication with doctors, communication with nurses, responsiveness of hospital staff, pain management, communication about medicines, discharge information, cleanliness of the hospital environment, quietness of the hospital environment, and transition of care (HCAHPS, n.d.). The survey also includes four screening questions and seven demographic items used for patient-mix adjustment across hospitals and for analyses. As a way to achieve the goal of fair comparisons across all hospitals that participate in HCAHPS, AHRQ adjusts for factors not directly related to hospital performance but that affect patients' responses to the HCAHPS survey items. Factors may include the way the survey was administered, also called the mode; characteristics of the patients in participating hospitals; and differences between patients who participate and those that do not. AHRQ adjustments were intended to eliminate any advantage or disadvantage in scores that are beyond a hospital's control (HCAHPS, 2008). In contrast to the qualitative response scale of the Press Ganey survey, the HCAHPS survey uses a frequency scale, which asks patients how often they observe specific behaviors. For example, HCAHPS asks: "During this hospital stay, how often did nurses treat you with courtesy and respect?" The possible responses include never, sometimes, usually, and always.

Although helpful, the frequency information is insufficient for fully understanding patients' perceptions about the care they received. For example, asking a patient how often a nurse was in the room to check on him or her might confirm that the nurse was physically present every hour, but what if the nurse was inattentive or distracted every time he or she came in the room? For the data to have meaning and to best understand the patient's experience of care, it is simply not enough to ask how often something happened. We must also know, from the perspective of the patient, how well it was done.

Unfortunately, CMS has deemed that asking patients the HCAHPS questions while they are receiving care in the hospital is prohibited (HCAHPS, n.d). More importantly, when patients are admitted for healthcare, they are vulnerable and must depend upon the people caring for them. Often, they are reluctant to provide honest answers while in care because they are afraid that negative responses may impact their care. So, often patients wait to provide that information until they feel safe after care has been provided. Further, measuring patient's perceptions of care is not limited to the hospital setting. The number of patient visits in the ambulatory setting is increasing markedly, as is the acuity level of care in such settings. More frequently, patients are being asked to provide their perceptions of the care they received in ambulatory environments such as the provider practice, ambulatory surgery, and outpatient clinics.

Increasingly, as the patient's perceptions of care are measured, there is recognition that patient "satisfaction" is not synonymous with patient experience. Patient satisfaction may be considered a superficial measure of the care delivered— something akin to making people happy and being nice. In contrast, patient experience reflects the totality of that care experience—clinically, operationally, culturally, and behaviorally.

The truth is that very few, if any, patients are happy about being in the hospital or seeking care. It can feel chaotic, unwieldy, and overwhelming, especially because they are sick or in pain or, perhaps, they have a family member who is sick or in pain. In this regard, efforts to merely increase their "happiness" would be misdirected, nor would they appreciably improve their experience of care. People who are trying to navigate a healthcare system that may be foreign to them and confusing while they are sick or in pain are, in a word, *suffering*. The reduction of suffering, therefore, is the way to improve the patient experience (Dempsey & Mylod, 2016).

The degree to which patients suffer is quantifiable, and can be measured through patient experience surveys, which provide an understanding of both how often and how well care was provided. Survey responses provide caregivers insight into patients' met and unmet needs, which can be further characterized as the results of inherent suffering or avoidable suffering. Figure 3.1 illustrates how these needs fall into inherent and avoidable suffering as identified through HCAHPS and the Press Ganey proprietary surveys (Dempsey & Mylod, 2016).

Inherent suffering occurs even if healthcare was provided in a perfect way. The diagnoses and treatment of patients cause suffering. Consider a diagnosis of breast cancer; the mere diagnosis and the treatment alone cause suffering such as fear and discomfort. As caregivers, we may mitigate this suffering by providing good

Respond to Inherent Patient Needs	Prevent Avoidable Suffering
Promote Confidence in **Skill**	Improve **Teamwork**
Manage **Pain**	Deliver Care with **Courtesy**
Ensure **Safety**	Be **Helpful**
Inform/Prepare	Avoid Unnecessary **Wait**
Personalize Care	Make **Processes** Efficient/Easy
Reduce **Fear/Anxiety**	Clean/Quiet **Environment**
Protect **Privacy**	Adequate **Amenities**
Include in Decisions/Choice	Appropriate **Service Recovery**
Demonstrate **Empathy**	

FIGURE 3.1 Behaviors charted by the Press Ganey and HCAHPS surveys that relate to inherent and avoidable suffering.

HCAHPS, Hospital Consumer Assessment of Healthcare Providers and Systems.

information, including the patients in decisions about their care, reducing their fear, and providing medications to reduce pain, but, the fact is, we cannot eliminate this kind of suffering.

However, there is a great deal of suffering that we, as caregivers, unnecessarily impose upon the people who come to us for care: when we make people wait, when we do not provide clean and quiet environments, when processes are inefficient, or when we do not work well together as a team to care for them. All of these things cause suffering, and occur repetitively in hospitals and ambulatory clinics across the healthcare delivery system. If we are to improve the patient experience, it is the avoidable suffering that we must seek to influence. And the good news is that it is within our control to eliminate this kind of suffering.

American psychologist Abraham Maslow represented human development and motivation as a pyramid, with the most foundational physiologic needs, such as food, water, warmth, and rest, at the base of the hierarchy, topped first by safety needs, then belongingness and love, esteem, and, at the pinnacle, self-actualization (Maslow, 1943).

Importantly, Maslow posited that each component of the pyramid represents a hierarchy of needs that require fulfillment before additional needs can be addressed. So, people must *feel* safe before they feel belonging, self-esteem, or self-actualization (Maslow, 1943). When people are in care, dependent upon caregivers for their survival in care, this feeling of safety becomes paramount. As healthcare providers, we use a variety of methods to preserve patient safety; practicing good hand hygiene, using universal precautions, demonstrating superior technical skill, and an understanding of disease processes—all things that patients assume are already in place. However, when we do not work well together as a team to care for them, when we allow the bathrooms to be dirty, when we do not perform hand hygiene before and after delivering care, or when we provide conflicting information between caregivers—we essentially deprive patients of the *feeling* of safety. In this way, even when perhaps inadvertent, we cause patient suffering by failing to provide for these basic needs.

Such a deficit is quantifiable through patient experience surveys. Patients are not likely to provide an "always" answer or rate a caregiver highly if they did not feel safe in their care. For example, as a clinician, you may assure that a patient is turned frequently to prevent pressure injuries and you may place bed alarms on the bed to prevent falls, thus ensuring safety. However, if the patient does not *feel* safe because the care team provides conflicting information or perhaps discusses each other in negative ways in front of the patient, that lack of perceived safety influences the patient's response on every other question.

Understanding the patient experience has significant value. The evidence supports that patients who perceive a reliably better experience have lower readmission rates, lower lengths of stay, higher PSI-90 safety scores, and lower hospital acquired conditions (Press Ganey, 2015c). In this regard, it becomes clear that clinical quality, patient safety, and the patient experience are not really separate attributes. They are tightly intertwined.

To address the challenges in optimizing the healthcare experience for all patients, it is important to understand that patients perceive a different experience based on things such as age, gender, ethnicity, education level, and, not surprisingly, diagnosis. Segmenting patient populations permits an assessment of survey data relative to specific conditions. The data are segmented in order to provide a mechanism to evaluate specific met and unmet needs. Through segmentation of the data, improvement efforts may be more targeted thus ensuring the greatest impact.

Survey questions reveal met and unmet patient needs for information, discharge preparation, responsiveness to call lights, environment of care, and others so that, rather than implementing blanket or generalized improvement efforts, those efforts may be targeted directly to those high-risk or problem-prone areas of improvement for the population of patients in a particular unit or practice.

The horizontal bar graph in Figure 3.2 reflects patient experience scores for individuals with congestive heart failure compared with the general population of medical patients. The lines to the left reflect items in which patients with congestive heart failure have a greater unmet need than other medical patients, such as those with pneumonia. The lines to the right demonstrate the needs of congestive heart failure patients that have been met better than those of other medical patients. These types of data—the segmentation and the analyses—provide important insight. doctors of nursing practice (DNPs) who are prepared with a foundation of translation science can assess the data, appraise the evidence, and identify an appropriate intervention for the specific population. For example, based on these data, it can be said that patients with congestive heart failure require more information about their illness, their medications, and the side effects of their medications in order to stay out of the hospital. They need more help with toileting, and they need a prompter response to call lights. If healthcare organizations do not segment patient populations in order to address met and unmet needs, they may work to improve the patient experience in more general ways that may or may not achieve the improvement for high-volume and challenging patient populations (Dempsey & Mylod, 2016).

Patient loyalty and willingness to recommend an institution or a specific provider becomes increasingly important as the patients who bear greater responsibility for the costs for their care are transformed into "consumers." Consumerism means that these patients are more knowledgeable about their care and actually seek out information on social media and the Internet regarding experiences of care with particular providers or organizations. An analysis of data from nearly 1 million ambulatory care patients suggests that when healthcare organizations better meet the needs of specific patient populations, patients become more loyal and more willing to recommend the organization to others. With a focus on population health management and a push to cover more lives and thus better revenue, loyalty and willingness to recommend a provider, practice, or healthcare organization becomes not only the right thing to do but also necessary to sustain and grow revenue (Mahoney, 2016).

Press Ganey researchers (2017) analyzed key drivers of "recommendation failure rate," or the percentage of patients that did not give a top box rating on a five-point scale indicating their likelihood to recommend either the provider or the practice to others. Of the respondents, 15.7% of patients were "not very likely" to recommend their provider or their practice to others. Researchers determined that the single most important variable driving "likelihood to recommend" was the patient's confidence in the skill of his or her clinician, followed by the patient's perception that the care team worked well together, and finally, the perception that caregivers demonstrated

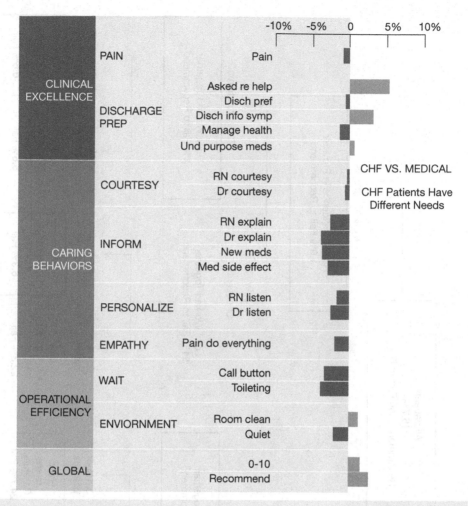

FIGURE 3.2 **A comparison of met and unmet needs between congestive heart failure and other patients.**

CHF, congestive heart failure.

concern for the patient's worries. Surprisingly, issues that are commonly thought to drive loyalty, such as wait times and amenities (private rooms, food, parking), did not significantly influence "likelihood to recommend" scores and thus, did not contribute to enhanced patient loyalty to the practice.

What these data support is that, fundamentally, patients want good clinicians who work well together and who listen to them. Even patients who reported confidence in clinicians, 11% of them declined to recommend them if a lack of teamwork was perceived in their care team, and further, another 22.3% would not recommend providers if they felt that caregivers did not demonstrate concern about the issues the patients were concerned about (Press Ganey, 2017) (Figure 3.3).

Similar themes were found after analyses of patient experience data from hospitalized patients. Based on HCAHPS data, the key drivers of top HCAHPS ratings for hospitals across all service lines were examined. Across medical, surgical, and maternity services, the perception that staff worked well together was the key driver for

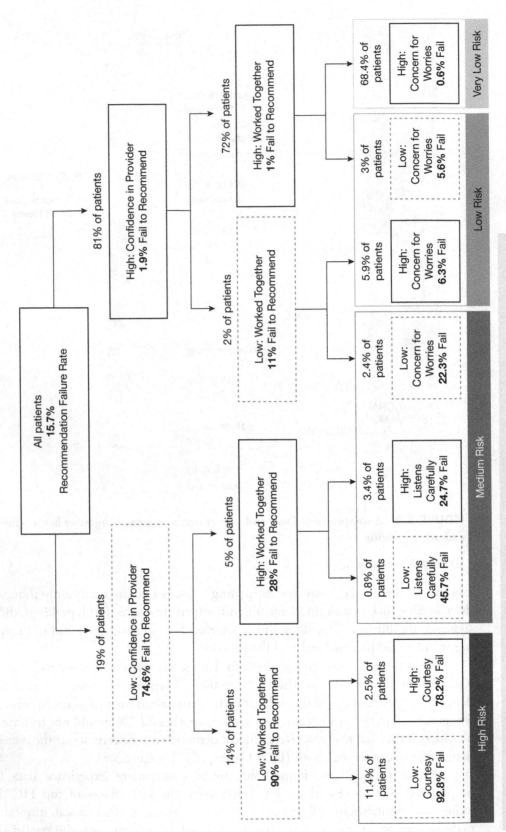

FIGURE 3.3 Factors that affected patient's willingness to recommend clinicians, in order of their impact.

patient likelihood to recommend the hospital. Of those patients who perceived that staff worked well together, 87.1% gave the hospital high overall ratings. When patients felt that teamwork was lacking, only 36.7% gave the hospital top ratings. Room cleanliness and nurse courtesy only drove patients' willingness to recommend hospitals *after* care coordination expectations were met (Press Ganey, 2017) (Figure 3.4).

These needs of teamwork, room cleanliness, and nurse courtesy do have a common theme. Reflecting on Maslow's Hierarchy of Needs, when patients perceive that the people taking care of them are working well together as a team, coordinating and collaborating based on a shared plan of care, *patients feel safe*. When caregivers talk to patients about their care and encourage their involvement in decisions about their care, *patients feel safe*. When the patient's room and bathroom are clean, patients perceive that the entire organization is clean and that they will not get an infection—*they feel safe*. Again, the feeling of safety is fundamental to the patient experience (Dempsey, 2017).

Further analyses in the emergency department (ED) demonstrate those items most correlated with a patient's "likelihood to recommend" the ED have little or nothing to do with wait times or amenities. On the contrary, those things most correlated are about personalization, information, pain control, connection, and empathy (Press Ganey, 2015b). Without this understanding, organizations may focus on improving service standards like eye contact or comfortable waiting rooms or chairs. This focus on the more superficial aspects of care would not influence the patient experience in a significant or sustainable way. Rather, in this practice setting, assisting caregivers to understand how to make connections, personalize care, and provide meaningful information about the patient's care and success after discharge, clear and accurate instructions about pain, and providing medication for its management establish a foundation upon which a successful patient experience can be achieved in the ED (Press Ganey, 2015).

In order to provide an optimal patient experience across the continuum of care, caregivers must be committed, educated, and supported, in short, they must be engaged. Strategies for improvement of the care experience hinge significantly upon the engagement of the people who provide care. As shown in Figure 3.5, analyses of patient experience have demonstrated that when caregivers are engaged, patients are more likely to perceive a better experience across every domain of HCAHPS (Dempsey & Reilly, 2016).

Specifically evaluating the nursing workforce and further acknowledging the importance of nurse perceptions of the professional practice environment, researchers found that when nurses are likely to recommend an organization for employment, patients are more likely to recommend the organization as a patient as depicted in Figure 3.6 (Press Ganey, 2015c).

Unfortunately, challenges in the provision of care, such as declining reimbursement, patient complexity, technological advances, staffing, and education, directly influence both the patient and the caregiver experience. When the Patient Protection and Affordable Care Act (ACA) was enacted in 2010, it required a transition from traditional payment models and established that, moving forward, hospitals would be reimbursed based on scores that measured processes of clinical care *and* importantly, the patient's experience of care. At its inception, most of a hospital's reimbursement

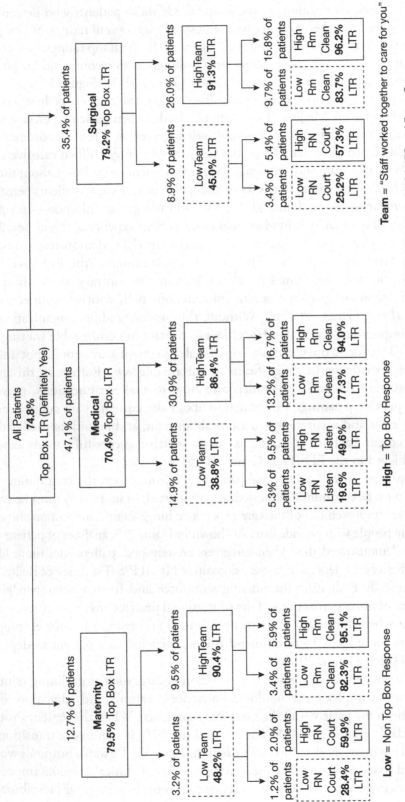

FIGURE 3.4 Key drivers of top HCAHPS ratings for hospitals across all service lines.

HCAHPS, Hospital Consumer Assessment of Healthcare Providers and Systems.

Source: Key Drivers of Top HCAHPS Ratings for Hospitals Across All Service Lines © 2006 Institute for Innovation. Reprinted with permission.

Analyses reflect more than 1.5 million responses to Inpatient surveys returned during the calendar year of 2013 that included HCAHPS and Press Ganey measures.
© 2016 Institute for Innovation

High = Top Box Response

Low = Non Top Box Response

Team = "Staff worked together to care for you"

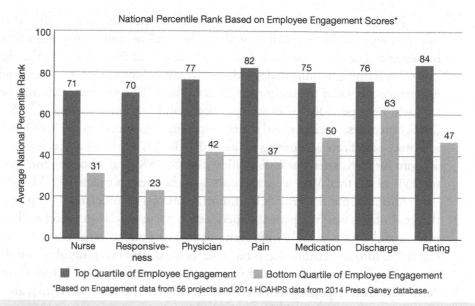

FIGURE 3.5 Relationship between engagement and experience.

HCAHPS, Hospital Consumer Assessment of Healthcare Providers and Systems.

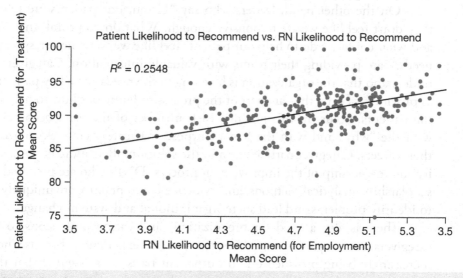

FIGURE 3.6 Patient loyalty and nurse loyalty.

still reflected measures that were more clinically focused and this change has created significant uncertainty within the healthcare market. As value-based purchasing (VBP) scores began to drive reimbursement, 70% of VBP points were based on clinical processes of care, with patient experience accounting for the remaining 30%. However, that paradigm is shifting. More of VBP is now focused on outcomes, including safety and quality, and the patient experience.

The ACA is under intense scrutiny, but the movement away from volume and toward value will likely continue with quality and outcomes driving healthcare reimbursement. The consensus both inside and outside of the industry is that focusing on care value is the right thing to do, and it is too compelling to ignore. Patient and caregiver experience are slated to account for 25% of the VBP score, while clinical processes of care will be superseded by outcomes, safety, and efficiency metrics (CMS, 2017.) In 2016, outcomes, efficiency, and patient experience encompassed 90% of VBP with clinical processes of care accounting for just 10%. In 2018, patient and caregiver experience account for 25%, safety for 25%, clinical care for 25%, and efficiency and cost reduction for 25% of the total VBP score and corresponding reimbursement (CMS, 2017).

Although metrics provide an important means to understand the progress toward the goal of the optimal patient experience, a focus solely on scores will not provide meaningful or sustainable improvement in the patient experience. Scores must be translated into something that is tangible, tactical, and meaningful to people who care for patients and families. At staff meetings, leaders often stand before teams and say: "Our scores on responsiveness are terrible! We're in the 30th percentile, and corporate has given us a goal of the 80th percentile. We have to do better!" In this scenario, caregivers hear that they must improve a score but are not provided with information that reflects what the score actually means to patients or the organization, and further, are not offered specific strategies that might be applied to improve it.

On the other hand, leaders who say "Listen, our patients are telling us that they don't feel like we are responsive enough. What do you think that might mean and what could we do to help our patients feel like we were more responsive to their needs?" are providing their teams with valuable information. Caregivers must now understand that the organization is listening to the needs voiced by patients and that, as providers of care, they are part of the process to figure out how to help better meet the patients' needs. In this manner, each member of the team becomes connected with the "why" and with the larger purpose that caregivers seek to accomplish in their careers. Caregiver participation in the solution offers more buy in, accountability, and ownership of the improvement process. DNPs who are prepared for clinical scholarship, analytical methods, and evidence-based practice are uniquely positioned to identify problems and lead such organizational and systems change.

There is also a need for organizations and caring professions to assure that caregivers are prepared to address the patient experience. Because healthcare is increasingly being provided on an outpatient basis, it is essential that those caring for patients understand how to connect with patients across the continuum of care. Caregivers may lack personal experience as a patient in either an ambulatory or inpatient setting. Consequently, there is a risk that telling caregivers to be empathic and compassionate may come without context as they may lack a personal frame of reference for these emotions, fears, and pain. Further, some seasoned caregivers have become less resilient, which leads to burnout and detachment.

The strategies for improving the patient experience require continuous education and commitment, which, if lacking, will be reflected in the publicly reported quality data, VBP scores, and ultimately in the institutional and provider reimbursement which is based, in part, on the patient experience. With a CAHPS program either in place or on the Centers for Medicaid and Medicare Services road map for implementation in virtually every setting and patient population, the patient experience must be considered much like any other important quality program undertaken by healthcare organizations. For example, healthcare organizations and many regulatory standards require education and testing around CPR at least every 2 years so that caregivers can assure not only that they are able to perform the skill well, but also that it comes naturally when the caregiver must use it. Addressing the patient experience is no different and those related skills must be taught and reinforced in order to achieve performance excellence and sustainable improvement in the patient experience of care.

Many academic organizations have begun to use simulation to transform practice and to support the learning of new skills. This is undoubtedly a safe way to practice procedures before performing them on a patient. However, with simulation, even the most technologically advanced mannequins, do not cry, get angry, or try to hit the caregiver. Caregivers must be provided an opportunity to practice connecting with patients just as they practice processes and procedures. One innovative organization, University of Delaware, has developed a program in conjunction with the Theater Department of the University. "Health Care Theater" engages nursing students in simulations on theater students trained to behave like sick patients and family members. Immediately after the simulations, faculty members from the Theater Department debrief the theater students and help them develop feedback for the nursing students. This innovative program has grown to become two fully approved university courses that are cross-listed in the theater and nursing departments. Students are incorporated into all nursing simulations, run by the staff in the simulation lab. According to Cowperthwait et al. (2015), a clinical faculty member at the University of Delaware and the nurse responsible for this innovation, nursing students benefit from "over 650 hours of quality simulation and patient-centered feedback each semester."

More importantly, students are provided with a powerful opportunity to learn the human dimensions of caring for patients, which helps them connect not only to the patient but also to why they became caregivers in the first place. Consistent with interprofessional learning standards, Healthcare Theater now includes physical therapy, medical anthropology, behavioral health, and nutrition programs at the University of Delaware (Dempsey, 2017). This kind of innovation is what is needed to provide tangible and tactical ways to improve how caregivers deliver compassionate and connected care in an environment that is increasingly task driven and checklist oriented.

To further address the epidemic of suffering in healthcare today, a framework that addresses the totality of the patient experience was developed in 2013 by Press Ganey's chief nursing officer and colleagues and informed by clinicians, administrators, and patients from across the country. The Compassionate Connected Care® framework addresses the clinical, operational, cultural, and behavioral aspects of the care experience (Dempsey, 2014; Press Ganey, 2014) (Figure 3.7).

Clinical excellence only matters when it is connected with outcomes. Given public reporting of data, outcomes are increasingly important. However, beyond the numbers, great healthcare providers are really only great if the outcomes of their care

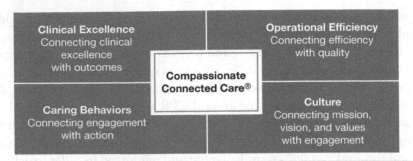

FIGURE 3.7 The Compassionate Connected Care® model.

matter to patients. If a patient with total knee arthroplasty is not able to walk 20 feet unassisted a month after surgery, the outcome is what is important, not the surgeon's technical expertise in the operating room (OR). Similarly, quality must be connected to efficiency. If quality costs too much, it becomes harder to provide the optimal experience—efficiency matters to patients. Engaged employees demonstrate the behaviors needed for the optimal experience. Finally, an organization's mission, vision, and values provide the culture for engaged employees to thrive. That mission, vision, and values are the shared purpose by which the organization will achieve its goals.

To define the themes of the Compassionate Connected Care model and translate them into compelling actions caregivers can provide, more than 100 clinicians, nonclinicians, and patients were asked to provide one-sentence "image statements" reflecting their notions of compassionate and connected care. The statements were collected to create an affinity diagram that would provide the full picture and clear definition of compassionate and connected care (Press Ganey, 2014).

A total of 117 image statements were collected and analyzed and resulted in six themes of the Compassionate Connected Care framework (Dempsey et al., 2014).

- **Acknowledge suffering:** We should acknowledge that our patients are suffering and show them that we understand.
- **Body language matters:** Nonverbal communication skills are as important as the words we use.
- **Anxiety is suffering:** Anxiety and uncertainty are negative outcomes that must be addressed.
- **Coordinate care:** We should show patients that their care is coordinated and continuous, and that "we" are always there for them.
- **Caring transcends diagnosis:** Real caring goes beyond delivery of medical interventions to the patient.
- **Autonomy reduces suffering:** Autonomy helps preserve dignity for patients.

The strategies related to these themes do not require more money or more staff. They are actions that when deployed consistently by caregivers, result in improvement in the patient experience (Table 3.1).

TABLE 3.1 Image Statements and Actions by Caregivers

We should acknowledge that our patients are suffering and show them that we understand

Actions	Images
Bearing witness to their suffering shows patients that we care	A physician says, "I'm sorry," to a patient who said she did not sleep well the night before.
	A doctor who has just told a daughter that her mother is terminally ill sits with her to console her.
	When care does not go as planned, staff apologize, acknowledge the impact on the patient, and engage the patient in exploring options.
Asking the patient what they are worried about allows them to be a person rather than a disease	The clinician asks the patients what concerns they may address.
	The clinician asks the patients what they are most concerned about.
	While caring for a patient, the clinician discovers something personal about the patient that establishes a connection to make a positive, memorable moment for future interactions with the care team.
	The clinician asks how the patient would prefer to be addressed.
	The clinician notes a patient's greatest concern on the communication board so all caregivers are aware.
Anticipating and mitigating the patient's discomfort shows concern for their suffering	The nurse applies EMLA cream to the patient's hand before starting the IV.
	Staff members update the patient and family of delays at least every 30 minutes.
	Staff members inform the patient and family of what to expect prior to beginning any procedure or test.

Nonverbal communication skills are as important as the words we use

Actions	Images
Eye contact matters	The clinician sits at eye level and looks the patient in the eye during the conversation.
	The front desk caregiver looks up from the computer to establish eye contact.
	As the patient begins to say what is really on his mind, the caregiver pushes his or her laptop aside, leans forward, and listens attentively.
	The caregiver explains to a patient that he or she is listening and is fully engaged with the patient while documenting on the computer.
Physically touching the patient closes distance	The nurse gently holds the patient's shoulder while obtaining blood pressure.
	The physician sits down and holds the patient's hand while explaining tests and treatments.
	The clinician takes a seat and holds the patient's hand when the patient starts to cry.
	The physician makes a point of shaking hands with patients and visitors when introducing himself or herself.

(continued)

TABLE 3.1 Image Statements and Actions by Caregivers (*continued*)

Body position matters	The physician sits face to face with the patient while talking with him or her.
	The caregiver does not turn his or her back to the patient until the interaction is over and the caregiver leaves the room.

Anxiety and uncertainty are negative outcomes that must be addressed

Actions	Images
Reducing uncertainty and anxiety for patients and families acknowledges that they are in a stressful situation	Caregivers round on patients frequently in a way that is purposeful and meaningful to the patient—inquiring about pain, positioning, toileting, and at least one nondisease/treatment-oriented discussion topic.
	The employee notices a "lost guest" and personally escorts the person to his destination. Staff members describe what will happen next when the patient arrives at the exam room. Clinicians tell patients when they will be in to see them.
Reducing waits shows we understand patients' suffering and respect their time	There is no lag time in response when a patient presses the call light. Staff members provide an estimate of wait times.
	Staff members do not pass call lights without inquiring if they can help.

We should show patients that their care is coordinated and continuous, and that we are always there for them

Actions	Images
Showing patients that the relationship does not end when they are not directly in contact deepens the relationship	The clinician calls the patient for follow-up within 48 hours.
	Clinicians' follow-up appropriately when information is received on the discharge phone call.
	Clinicians show that they are concerned about what will happen when the patient goes home and provide instructions to make them successful in their recovery.
	Caregivers "manage up" each other, complementing the caregivers on the care.

Real caring goes beyond delivery of medical interventions to the patient

Actions	Images
Personal touches outside medical care strengthen relationships	The nursing assistant brings a patient his or her favorite dish from the cafeteria as he or she awakens from surgery.
	The director of service excellence walks a patient's service dog outside the hospital to give a stressed family member time to grab lunch.
Caring for the patient means caring for the family	The nurse gives a warm blanket to a family member who is cold.
	On a nightly basis, the nurse holds the phone to the ear of a terminally ill patient, so his daughter can say goodnight.

(*continued*)

TABLE 3.1 Image Statements and Actions by Caregivers (*continued*)

Autonomy helps preserve dignity for patients

Actions	Images
The patient is a full participant in guiding his or her care	The clinician asks patient and family members about their preferences in care issues lying ahead.
	The clinician asks the patient for his or her preferences on even minor issues, such as the preferred hand for an IV.
	The clinician provides a full range of care options when discussing diagnosis and treatment plans.
	Caregivers involve the patient in beside shift reports.

IV, intravenous.

As an example of how the Compassionate Connected Care framework might influence care, a provider might walk into an exam room and consider the three major actions of nonverbal communication: making eye contact, touching the patient, and sitting down, which is a body position that encourages communication and preserves the patient's sense of dignity.

Considering autonomy, the provider would provide the patient with options about his or her care and condition and then encourage the patient to choose the option that he or she thinks best meets his or her needs at that time. Providing the patient with the ability to make decisions about his or her care not only preserves dignity, it also allows the patient to be a full participant in care. Often, providers express concern that they do not have enough time to make a meaningful connection with their patients. They say that there are too many patients, not enough staff, and too much to do. However, research has shown over thousands of encounters, it takes, on average, just 56 seconds to make a meaningful connection (Dempsey, 2017). Applying the 56-second exercise to every encounter demonstrates that the provider cares about the person for whom he or she is caring and who happens to be a patient at the moment. For example, this can be achieved by simply asking the patient something about himself or herself that has nothing to do with the reason he or she has been admitted or come to a provider for care. The patient will likely talk about family, his or her job, hobbies, or pets. Whatever is said, the caregiver should find something to connect with that patient by discussing what the patient is passionate about. Every time the caregiver talks with the patient from that moment forward, something can be discussed related to that information that has nothing to do with the reason he or she is in care and everything to do with who he or she is as a person. It changes not only the patient's perception of the care experience and the caregiver, but also the caregiver's perception. The patient feels safe because she is known as Mary, a mother of twin girls who is also a teacher, and not just the "mastectomy in 902."

None of these strategies will significantly or sustainably improve the patient experience unless they are applied consistently and with sincerity. Consistency over time delivers on the promise of the highly reliable organization (HRO) to reduce suffering and provide the optimal experience (Dempsey, 2017). As Figure 3.8

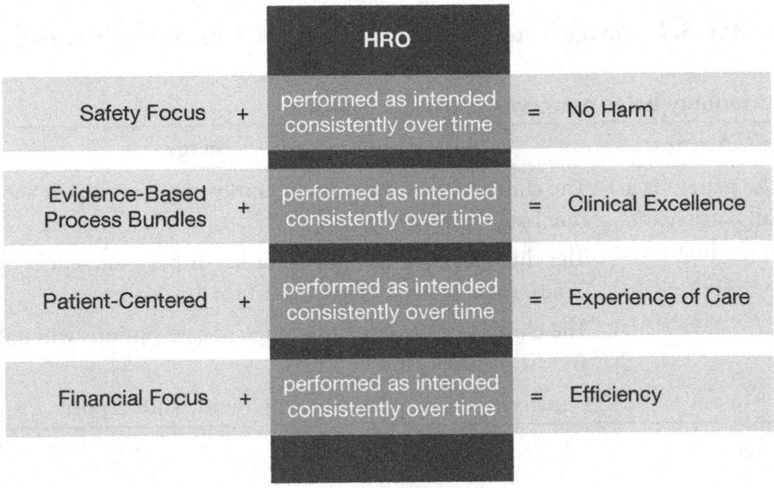

FIGURE 3.8 The importance of consistent performance over time.

HRO, highly reliable organization.

demonstrates, the outcomes of excellent clinical care and patient experience delivered in a safe environment with zero harm and in an efficient manner are achieved only when there is focus and consistency of practice.

Strategies such as hourly rounding, bedside shift report, and huddles have been shown to improve the patient experience. These and other tactics, provided within the context of the Compassionate Connected Care framework, when delivered consistently improve the totality of the patient experience clinically, operationally, culturally, and behaviorally. When the experience of the patient and the people who care for them improves, it also improves for the organization and, ultimately, for the healthcare industry as a whole. There is no question that health reform has driven an agenda where healthcare providers and organizations are under intense pressure and scrutiny to provide exceptional care and experience while also lowering cost. The focus on quality and safety outcomes will not and should not go backwards regardless of legislation and debates in Washington, DC. Quite simply, it is the right thing to do. As experts in nursing practice, the DNP is uniquely positioned to lead this transformation of the healthcare system toward true person centered care.

■ REFERENCES

Centers for Medicare and Medicaid Services. (2017). *Hospital value-based purchasing*. Retrieved from https://www.cms.gov/Outreach-and-Education/Medicare-Learning-Network-MLN/MLNProducts/downloads/Hospital_VBPurchasing_Fact_Sheet_ICN907664.pdf

The Commonwealth Fund. (2015). U.S. spends more on health care than other high-income nations but has lower life expectancy, worse health [Press release]. Retrieved from http://www.commonwealthfund.org/publications/press-releases/2015/oct/us-spends-more-on-health-care-than-other-nations

Cowperthwait, A., Saylor, J., Carlsen, A., Schmitt, L. A., Salam, T., Melby, M. K., & Baker, S. D. (2015). Healthcare theatre and simulation: Maximizing interprofessional partnerships. *Clinical Simulation in Nursing*, *11*(9), 411–420. doi:10.1016/j .ecns.2015.05.005

Dempsey, C. (2017). *The antidote to suffering: How compassionate connected care improves safety, quality, and experience.* Columbus, OH: McGraw-Hill.

Dempsey, C., & Mylod, D. (2016). Addressing patient and caregiver suffering. *American Nurse Today*, *11*(11). Retrieved from https://www.americannursetoday.com/ addressing-patient-caregiver-suffering

Dempsey, C., & Reilly, B. A.(2016). Nurse engagement: What are the contributing factors for success? *Online Journal of Issues in Nursing*, *21*(1). doi:10.3912/OJIN.Vol21No01Man02

Dempsey, C., Wojciechowski, S., McConville, E., & Drain, M. (2014). Reducing patient suffering through compassionate connected care. *Journal of Nursing Administration*, *44*(10), 517–524. doi:10.1097/NNA.0000000000000110

Hospital Consumer Assessment of Healthcare Providers and Systems. (n.d.). *The HCAHPS survey: Frequently asked questions.* Retrieved from https://www.cms.gov/medicare/ quality-initiatives-patient-assessment-instruments/hospitalqualityinits/downloads/ hospitalhcahpsfactsheet201007.pdf

Hospital Consumer Assessment of Healthcare Providers and Systems. (2008). Mode and patient-mix adjustment of the CAHPS® hospital survey (HCAHPS). Retrieved from http://www.hcahpsonline.org/globalassets/hcahps/mode-patient-mix-adjustment/ final-draft-description-of-hcahps-mode-and-pma-with-bottom-box-modedoc -april-30-2008.pdf

Mahoney, D. (2016). Breaking new ground in the era of healthcare consumerism. Retrieved from http://www.pressganey.com/docs/default-source/industry-edge/issue-3/breaking -new-ground-in-the-era-of-health-care-consumerism.pdf?sfvrsn=2

Maslow, A. H. (1943). A theory of human motivation. *Psychological Review*, *50*(4), 370–396.

Press Ganey. (2014). *Compassionate Connected Care: A care model to reduce patient suffering.* Retrieved from http://www.pressganey.com/docs/default-source/default-document -library/compassionate_connected_care.pdf

Press Ganey. (2015a). Consumerism: Earning patient loyalty and market share. Retrieved from http://www.pressganey.com/resources/research-notes/consumerism-earning-patient-loyalty -and-market-share

Press Ganey. (2015b). Increasing value in the emergency department: Using data to drive improvement. Retrieved from http://www.pressganey.com/resources/white-papers/ increasing-value-in-the-emergency-department-using-data-to-drive

Press Ganey. (2015c). *Nursing special report: The influence of nurse work environment on patient, payment and nurse outcomes in acute care settings.* Retrieved from http://www.pressganey .com/about/news/nursing-special-report-the-influence-of-nurse-work-environment-on -patient-payment-and-nurse-outcomes

SECTION TWO

Scholarship and the DNP

LINDA C. ANDRIST

Doctor of nursing practice (DNP) degree programs prepare nurse leaders who will be instrumental in transforming the profession to meet the challenges of the burgeoning healthcare system of our nation. Clinical scholarship is at the heart of doctoral education and practice. This section takes the reader through the process of clinical scholarship, beginning with Andrist's and Crabtree's definition of clinical scholarship and the evolution of students into scholars. They discuss how the role of the DNP is to generate nursing knowledge from practice (Chapter 4).

Sipe continues this section with the process of carrying out the culminating piece of scholarship in DNP education programs—the DNP project. She begins with the research or *burning question* from clinical practice and then guides the reader through the development, implementation, evaluation, and dissemination of the project (Chapter 5).

The authors in Chapter 6, all nurse executives or administrators, discuss some kinds of projects that DNPs carry out such as practice change initiatives and quality improvement projects. These are all examples of nurse executive scholarship that contribute to changing nursing practice.

Chapter 7 is written by recent graduates of DNP programs across the country and contains their stories in their own voices of the DNP project experience. They share how they came to develop their *burning question* into a project and some of the challenges and opportunities they met along the path. Their stories will help other DNP students to be mindful of the issues and challenges in carrying out their scholarship and can be a lesson to practicing DNPs as well.

The Formation of Clinical Scholars: The Generation of Nursing Knowledge From Practice

LINDA C. ANDRIST AND KATHERINE CRABTREE

The focus of doctor of nursing practice (DNP) degree programs is to prepare nurse leaders who can transform nursing to meet the burgeoning healthcare challenges of our nation. The curriculum leading to the DNP degree emphasizes a clear vision of nursing's future to alleviate the healthcare crisis in our nation. Transforming nursing practice requires the preparation of leaders who can articulate nursing science and integrate knowledge and practice. A DNP-prepared nurse is expected to create new models of care, change practice, and improve health outcomes. The premise of this chapter is that clinical nurse scholars prepared in DNP programs acquire an inquiry approach to their practice that enables them to generate knowledge from practice. Expert clinicians are prepared to give voice to the need for change, and design and evaluate practice improvements through collaboration. Working with patients, families, and communities to implement population health goals and reduce disparities requires collaborating with other professionals and it requires policy change. The DNP program offers a curriculum that engages nurses in these activities to ensure that graduates are capable of envisioning the exciting possibilities for the profession and actualizing them. Doctors of nursing practice find themselves well positioned to meet the challenges of the 21st century. One of the contributions of the DNP is to produce knowledge from practice—this is clinical scholarship.

▨ SCHOLARSHIP TRADITIONS

As the profession strove to legitimize its science, practitioners neglected the scholarship of practice and the knowledge that can be acquired through practice. In 1999, Fawcett called for all nurses to become nurse scholars to save the professional discipline from extinction by merging research and practice and closing the research–practice gap.

She advocated for the post-baccalaureate nurse doctorate (ND), the early precursor of the DNP, as an entry to nursing practice. Although the ND did not survive, the concept of doctoral preparation of nurses who can bridge the gap between research and practice to achieve better outcomes for patients is alive and well, as demonstrated by the growing number of schools offering the DNP.

The focus on the discovery of new knowledge via accepted quantitative research has garnered respect for the discipline and enhanced its standing in the scientific community, as evidenced by the development and funding of the National Institute of Nursing Research. Furthermore, nurse theorists have developed broad theories addressing person, environment, health, and nursing to define the scope and substance of the discipline. While these theories and nursing philosophies have been used to guide research and advance the profession, we have lagged in valuing knowledge generated from practice. The grand theories of pioneering nurse philosophers such as Martha Rogers gave way to theories narrower in scope. These mid-range theories provided frameworks for investigating clinical phenomena such as pain and uncertainty. Mid-range theories linked concepts more closely to practice phenomena (Fawcett & Alligood, 2005; Peterson & Bredow, 2017) and better outcomes of care. Because these mid-range theories were more closely tied to practice phenomena, they also fostered the development of quantitative measures to capture human responses to health and illness states for further research. Social science theories such as role theory, self-efficacy, resilience, and hardiness were imported into nursing to further study and explain phenomena of interest to nurses. Nurse researchers, using quantitative research methods, adapted or devised new tools to study these concepts.

The development of postmodern philosophies of science and the use of qualitative methods has also shaped our view of nursing science. Research methods such as ethnography, phenomenology, grounded theory, critical social theory, and feminist theory were adopted by nurse researchers to better understand the patient's experience of health and illness through more holistic approaches (Polit & Beck, 2017). These researchers expanded the use of qualitative methods to explore phenomena and processes that describe and explain the lived experience of patients and families adapting to life-changing experiences that impact health outcomes.

Nurses are drawn to qualitative approaches to research in part because of the connection they feel to patients and families as they seek to understand how best to provide support for health, healing, recovery, and resilience. Nurses encounter patients during times of transition, when there are rich opportunities for teaching, coaching, and for changing patients' perspectives and health behaviors. Qualitative research methods bring together the researcher and patient informant in a type of relationship that is not sought or possible with quantitative research. Narrative methods enhance story telling arising from interaction with patients. Knowledge arising from practice may be used to create interventions and new models of care.

The accelerating popularity of naturalistic research and mixed-method studies blending quantitative and qualitative methods stems from the desire for a more comprehensive understanding of the human experience of health and illness. Recognizing that a combination of quantitative and qualitative methods provides a more complete picture; nurse researchers are using mixed methods to ensure greater understanding of clinical phenomena. Often, this comprehensive approach to discovery would be best served through partnerships between researchers and clinical nurse scholars as they uncover practice knowledge. Using an inquiry approach to practice, nurse scholars conceptualize clinical phenomena needing further investigation, thus providing a fruitful basis for partnering with nurse researchers that enriches the discipline.

■ DEFINITIONS OF CLINICAL SCHOLARSHIP AND DEVELOPMENT OF PRACTICE KNOWLEDGE

Recognition of the need for clinical scholarship is evident throughout the literature. Clinical scholarship contributes to the knowledge of the discipline through conceptualization, investigation, evaluation, and dissemination of knowledge to inform practice, education, policy, and research. Although clinical scholarship includes research and theory development, it is not limited to these two forms of scholarship. The advancement of nursing science requires nurses to contribute through research, theory, and *practice.* Accordingly, Diers (1995) placed clinical scholarship within a context of discovery which involves "observation of patients or practice including one's own participation or reaction to patients or situations" (p. 24).

The University of Washington School of Nursing coined the title *practice inquiry* in 2004 to capture the investigative focus of the DNP:

> Practice inquiry is an ongoing, systematic investigation of questions about nursing therapeutics and clinical phenomena with the intent to appraise and translate all forms of "best evidence" to practice, and to evaluate the translational impact on the quality of healthcare and health outcomes. Through the process of translating science to practice, APRNs observe, describe, understand, and appraise clinical phenomena and their interface with empirically and theoretically based knowledge. The investigative focus integrates scientific curiosity and inquiry with the realities of everyday practice. (Magyary, Whitney, & Brown, 2006, p. 143)

Many have proposed that the DNP is a clinical scholar who does practice inquiry to produce practice knowledge. Dahnke and Dreher (2016) propose that the DNP produces practice-based evidence and they discuss a "practice epistemology for the practice doctorate: *practice knowledge development*" (p. xxi). They describe practice *knowledge* as the "by-product of *practice research*" (p. 365).

We concur and proposed in the first edition of this text that the definition of practice knowledge is *the knowledge gained through examination of experience and study that leads to mastery of (or expertise in) a defined area of practice that is shared with others for evaluation, validation, and application.* In this manner, practice knowledge improves the health of patients, families, and communities, and contributes to knowledge within the profession.

EXHIBIT 4.1   An Iterative Process for Development and Dissemination of Practice Knowledge

1. Advanced practice knowledge and skills (competencies) within a population focus
   a. Clinical literature
   b. Research literature
2. Passion for caring, excellence, and learning
3. Reflection on practice experiences (e.g., micro: health processes, healing behaviors, illness trajectories, interventions that promote recovery and resilience; macro: collaborations and continuity across boundaries, systems, care processes)
4. Dialogue with peers and colleagues to evaluate, validate, and refine
   a. Conceptualization and recognition of clinical problems
   b. Data on patterns, variations, outcomes of care
   c. Development of interventions that address clinical problems, improve processes, reduce cost
5. Pilot testing (care models, creative approaches, etc.)
6. Evaluation of results with practice application
7. Dissemination of outcomes

Practice-derived knowledge leads to clinical scholarship when it is exposed to further evaluation, validation, and eventually to dissemination. Schon's (1983) *The Reflective Practitioner* is an example of a clinical scholar who is able to use practice encounters to reflect on and to conceptualize practice experiences that guide future encounters. However, the knowledge acquired by the nurse remains private knowledge until it is vetted through peer review, then disseminated and evaluated by the profession. Once articulated and validated, this knowledge can be developed into systematic approaches to care delivery and used to promote the development of professional standards and guidelines (Exhibit 4.1).

■ THE INQUIRY CONTINUUM: RESEARCH AND OTHER FORMS OF INQUIRY

The inquiry projects conducted by DNP-prepared nurses span a broad continuum. At one end, inquiry overlaps with research. The continuum also includes translation of research into practice, quality improvement and program evaluation, and practice improvement projects. The purpose, scope, methods, and resources used to mount inquiry projects also vary considerably. As quality improvement standards become more rigorous, the data generated may have use beyond local application.

Dahnke and Dreher (2016) ask important questions about the type of knowledge produced in a DNP program and inquiry processes used to produce it. Action research is appropriate for students engaged in inquiry projects within their work environment as it is designed to simultaneously study and make changes in practice.

They also describe another approach to clinical inquiry that is conducted within a "context of application," that emphasizes generation of knowledge from clinical interactions taking place outside of traditional controlled research. Originally proposed by Gibbons (1994) as distinct from traditional research, this alternate mode of inquiry produces knowledge that crosses disciplinary boundaries with multiple participants contributing to the generation, appraisal, and diffusion of the knowledge and evidence acquired.

Dahnke and Dreher consider the forms of inquiry in a DNP program as still evolving and varying across the research–inquiry continuum with potential transdisciplinary application and advocate for keeping a full range of options open as dialogue about clinical knowledge generation continues. However, they raise important challenges for nursing: "DNP scholars ought to be clarifying now what the nature of DNP-generated knowledge is, and what the domain of practice inquiry should be" (p. 381).

If a school has both a PhD and a DNP program, there may be separation of clinical inquiry from pure research based on the faculty's philosophies, research skills, and resources. In other universities, graduate studies require all doctoral degree programs to meet certain standards of research and designate the type of product acceptable for awarding a doctoral degree. It is hoped that the future of clinical inquiry will involve partnerships between clinical experts and researchers who bring their expertise in methods to bear on the study of the problem. In the past, dissertations from PhD programs often generated knowledge that had little or no impact as they were shelved and forgotten after the degree was awarded. To avoid this outcome, both PhD and DNP programs are requiring different types of formats for products of inquiry. If the goal is for clinically based inquiry projects to impact care delivery, policy, future research, and nursing education, the requirement may be to submit a document in a format suitable for publication in a peer-reviewed journal. Just as practice continues to change and evolve over time, it is incumbent upon faculty and educational institutions to adopt strategies that communicate this knowledge widely. Dissemination is also a way to examine outcomes, for example, products of the scholarly endeavor, potential impact, and productivity of DNP program scholars.

Rolfe and Davies (2009) point out that Gibbons is challenging our traditional assumptions about how knowledge is generated and how its value is judged. The answers to the questions that were raised offer a vision of future transdisciplinary doctoral programs where contextualized knowledge is generated and applied immediately. The conceptualization of knowledge generation from practice and application in practice has implications for transforming doctoral education. Transdisciplinary practice doctoral programs might produce rich dividends for nursing and society to augment the contribution to knowledge from traditional research doctorates. Recognition of the contribution of nurses with practice doctorates to knowledge generation and practice improvement is needed to counter the insistence that only traditional research doctorates are rigorous enough to produce knowledge.

There has been a dramatic increase in the number of DNP-prepared faculty teaching in DNP programs. With this infusion and the publication of the American Association of

Colleges of Nursing (AACN) White Paper in 2015, the scholarship expected of the DNP has become clearer. Rolfe and Davies reiterate this point: "It is increasingly understood that DNP knowledge production is measured according to its contribution to improved outcomes rather than its contribution to generalizable knowledge" (Task Force on the Implementation of the DNP, 2015, p. 2). However, Dahnke and Dreher warn us that restricting DNPs to only translate and disseminate evidence may hurt the profession because the number of DNP graduates far outnumbers PhD graduates (2016).

■ DEVELOPING CLINICAL SCHOLARS

Walker, Golde, Jones, Buesche, and Hutchins (2008) reported the results of a 5-year Carnegie Foundation study of doctoral education in over 100 programs spanning six disciplines in *The Formation of Scholars*. Personal identity as a scholar who is committed to professional integrity and accountability for the future of the discipline is internalized during doctoral study. Similarly, the DNP curriculum shapes the identity of the clinical scholar by nurturing curiosity, passion for learning, commitment to excellence, and ethics in order to make a meaningful difference in the health of patients.

Expert nurses illustrate the development of practice knowledge. Riley, Beal, and Lancaster (2007) studied 36 nurse clinicians from four acute care Magnet® hospitals. Peers within their practice environments recognized these nurses as expert nurses. When asked about scholarly nursing practice, these experienced nurses described themselves as "active learners, out-of-the-box thinkers, passionate about nursing, available and confident" (p. 429). They described a tolerance for ambiguity and uncertainty in practice settings that were often chaotic. They were flexible adapters and innovators "committed to the highest professional standards" who at times were also "rule bender(s)" and "risk taker(s)" who "buck the system" (pp. 427–431). They accepted challenges and took responsibility as leaders to achieve excellence in care. Their self-descriptions of their nursing identity as they engaged in practice represented the values of the profession. They were eager to share their practice knowledge and instill a passion for practice in others. They described their nursing practice not as a list of skills they had mastered or tasks to be performed. They described themselves as "being leaders, caring, sharing knowledge with others, evolving and reflecting on practice" (Riley et al., 2007, p. 425). These are the characteristics of clinical scholars.

Nursing's social contract with society obligates clinical scholars to develop unfolding practice knowledge fully, to validate it, and to use it to benefit society. To accomplish this, the DNP program provides transformative experiences via immersion in practice. Through personal and vicarious encounters, DNP students learn to identify practice knowledge and its potential for application.

■ SCHOLARLY ROLE MODELS

Faculty in DNP programs who are actively engaged in practice knowledge generation and dissemination provide role models for emerging clinical scholars. Clinical experts who are immersed in the practice area can serve as mentors to promote professional development of clinical nurse scholars as well. These experts may be nurses or colleagues outside of nursing (physicians, epidemiologists, behavioral or nonbehavioral scientists, methodologists, policy makers, etc.). Mentors open doors to professional networks and provide access to patient populations for scholarly projects. As mentors engage DNP nurses in dialogue about substantive issues in the area of practice, those nurses learn to appraise the clinical and research literature. The mentoring relationship also helps students cope with anxieties as they take on greater responsibility for decision making in complex situations and as they act as agents for change in practice or policy. Mentors help students acquire the competencies, experience, and assurance needed to be a leader.

Delivery of quality care requires interprofessional communication and collaboration. Team approaches are needed to integrate contributions from multiple disciplines. However, we have not determined when, where, and how collaboration with other disciplines is best learned. Clearly, this too often takes place on the "firing line," which is too late to attain the quality of cooperative care needed. Clinical nurse scholars who become involved in interprofessional journal clubs learn to share their perspectives and expertise as they evaluate the literature for practice application. Their colleagues learn what DNP nurses can contribute to the dialogue and what perspective they bring to understanding health problems and health services. When DNP-prepared nurses provide grand rounds on cases that demonstrate complex decision making, they showcase their clinical expertise. As they conduct practice improvement projects to improve quality of care, evaluate clinical programs, and translate research into practice, they demonstrate the value they bring to the table in clinical arenas, whether that influence affects practice, research, policy, or nursing education.

As clinical nurse scholars describe the expanding boundaries of the discipline, they also promote understanding of areas where these boundaries overlap with other disciplines. Diers (1995) acknowledged that nurse scholars, through education and practice experiences, are prepared to make a "creative leap" to move the discipline forward. Thus, they enlarge the discipline by pushing its borders and collaborating with colleagues from other disciplines to redefine knowledge in their specialty. Integration of knowledge derived from the field of genetics is an example of how nurses are working collaboratively to advance the application of new knowledge in advanced practice nursing. Joint educational opportunities that provide learning together are needed to enable the highest level of interprofessional collaboration. Quality practice does not occur in isolation from other disciplines. Mentors of DNP students can facilitate interprofessional collaboration through peer review, quality improvement projects, and serving together on standards, ethics, or policy committees. The communication of knowledge to a variety of audiences promotes and reinforces successful interprofessional collaboration. Opportunities for joint inquiry and publication abound.

Accountability is key to leadership roles. To paraphrase Melanie Dreher (1999), clinical scholars are leaders prepared to own the outcomes of their actions. The clinical scholar holds him or herself accountable for learning and growth and is open to feedback. Doctoral programs that encourage peer review processes, constructive collegial exchange, and scholarly feedback provide opportunities for professional development.

Engaging faculty and students in open dialogue models a community of scholars to appraise practice knowledge and examine implications for practice application.

The challenge before us as nursing faculty and mentors is how to prepare nurse scholars who value practice knowledge and recognize and regularly reflect on it. Clinical nurse scholars give voice to this knowledge and share with others the outcomes achieved. Clinical nurse scholars are setting new benchmarks for practice as they evaluate care against the national standards and devise new clinical guidelines to improve practice.

■ CLINICAL SCHOLARS AS LEADERS IN HEALTHCARE DELIVERY

Healthcare reform was supposed to drastically change the landscape of healthcare delivery. The Affordable Care Act (ACA) aimed to change how the government pays for healthcare, the organization of delivery of healthcare, workforce policy, and make the government more adept and inventive in pursuing future reform. One of the ways to change how the government pays for healthcare was to enforce penalties for hospital readmissions for Medicare beneficiaries. Since this was implemented in 2012, readmission rates have declined from more than 19% to less than 18%. Another measure was to offer incentives to reduce hospital-acquired conditions. And indeed, data from the Department of Health and Human Services (DHHS) demonstrated a decrease in hospital-acquired conditions of 17% from 2010 to 2013 (Blumenthal, Abrams, & Nuzum, 2015).

DNPs have played a valuable role in these changes—see Chapters 5 and 6 for examples of DNP projects that impacted both reducing hospital-acquired infections and reducing readmission rates.

The commitment of clinical nurse scholars to improving health and access to quality care also includes devising strategies through health promotion programs, education, and screening. Providing care for populations who have been left out of the mainstream requires leadership, commitment, planning, and new models of care involving community outreach efforts. The move from master's preparation to DNP preparation of the advanced practice nurse emphasizes the move to a population perspective for delivery of care, and partnering with communities to make services available to more individuals and their families. Nurses have a strong sense of social justice. As nurses advocate for health equity with access to affordable quality healthcare, DNP-prepared nurse scholars are providing leadership in forming interprofessional coalitions to advance the agenda of equitable, cost-effective healthcare.

As DNP programs have grown, there is more focus on translating research and evidenced-based practice (EBP). The DNP is in a prime position to use practice inquiry to translate and apply EBP to practice that will improve outcomes. According to Tymkow, "the translation and dissemination of clinical knowledge is the core of clinical scholarship" (2017, p. 66).

The DNP-prepared nurse learns to access information, evaluate it, and integrate that knowledge in practice. Preparation of clinical scholars who take an inquiry approach to practice requires learning new skills and using knowledge management technologies to improve health outcomes. Knowledge management technologies are transforming the clinical environment. Using best practices, the DNP-prepared nurse maximizes implementation of those strategies known to be effective. As research grows, scholarly systematic reviews and other strategies are needed for synthesis of research results. Working in collaboration with other healthcare providers, the clinical nurse scholar can introduce evidence-based practices through innovative models of care to improve care quality. As clinical scholars learn to use sophisticated search strategies and new technologies for knowledge management, they become better puzzle solvers. They discover patterns in practice problems and develop possible solutions. Skills in using the latest evidence to solve clinical problems require efficient retrieval of relevant information and its appraisal. Clinical nurse scholars with doctoral preparation and expertise in the health of populations will be at the table with other decision makers because they will know how to appraise research findings and can contribute to the development, implementation, and evaluation of evidence-based practice guidelines.

Drawing on practice expertise, the clinical nurse scholar integrates practice knowledge with the formal knowledge derived from research and the clinical literature to develop new approaches to care. As leaders of change, scholars also use these technologies to monitor rapidly expanding knowledge bases from which to retrieve relevant research and practice information for quality improvement and translation of research into practice. Technology can alert them to the publication of new guidelines or research in specified areas of practice, allowing them to remain updated. Ongoing review of practice and the latest evidence continually offers potential improvements to be evaluated. As clinical scholars analyze and interpret new knowledge for its practice implications, they integrate and adapt knowledge from expanding scientific fields such as genomics, ethics, and the humanities.

Technology is also changing the patient/provider interface. Patients can retrieve information on the Internet and query their care provider about it or supply regular updates on physiological data and their response to treatments. Learning how to fully use this technology to communicate with patients allows the clinical scholar multiple opportunities to expand electronic feedback to patients and to elicit further information when symptoms recur. Telehealth is making care possible across geographical distances that would otherwise limit or even deny access to care. Sharing of data and consultation with specialists electronically allows improved access to care and more patients to be served. Clinical nurse scholars need to examine and describe how technology and telehealth influence the knowledge arising from practice.

The electronic health record is also changing the way that clinical information is stored, retrieved, and made accessible to multiple care providers in multiple sites. Involvement of clinical nurse scholars in the development of these systems ensures that the data captured can be used for generating nursing practice knowledge. Previously, the technology was organized for business purposes rather than for use by clinicians to evaluate and change practice. In harnessing the power of these technologies for practice, clinical scholars are able to identify patterns, track trends, monitor their population, notify themselves and patients of the need for periodic screening, follow up interventions, evaluate outcomes against national benchmarks, and appraise the quality of practice. DNP-prepared nurses and their practice partners can evaluate the sustainability of evidence-based changes made in practice. Furthermore, clinical inquiry is facilitated as databases describing practice allow retrieval, analysis, and evaluation of care and its outcomes.

As astute observers, clinical nurse scholars discern knowledge from practice encounters, whether from databases or through reflection on a sentinel patient encounter. Through examination of unanticipated outcomes of care processes, the clinical nurse scholar may gain insights for validation and pursue additional data gleaned from the database for the larger patient population. These technologies allow the clinical nurse scholar to explore whether variations are health promoting or health limiting. Using technology to retrieve data, clinical scholars can examine processes and evaluate responses to various types of interventions. Observing patterns of care outcomes over time will allow clinical scholars to advance practice more quickly and to share their practice-based data as evidence that care is meeting national standards.

The clinical scholar conveys practice knowledge and clinical wisdom to others through clinical case reports, explicates lessons learned when launching innovative care models, and discontinues practices that are ineffective. As these scholars merge practice knowledge formed through experience and expertise with scientific knowledge to inform decision making, they are advancing practice to its highest level.

Nurse researchers, nurse theorists, and nurse clinicians value nursing knowledge, but they approach discovery of knowledge in different ways. The discipline of nursing will benefit most through recognition of each of their unique contributions. Their talents and skills enrich the profession and ultimately benefit the recipients of our care and teaching.

■ REFERENCES

Blumenthal, D., Abrams, M., & Nuzum, R. (2015). The Affordable Care Act at 5 years. *New England Journal of Medicine, 372,* 2451–2458. doi:10.1056/NEJMhpr1503614

Dahnke, M. D., & Dreher, H. M. (2016). Next steps toward practice knowledge development: An emerging epistemology in nursing. In M. Dahnke & H. M. Dreher (Eds.), *Philosophy of science for nursing practice: Concepts and application* (2nd ed., pp. 355–391). New York, NY: Springer Publishing.

Diers, D. (1995). Clinical scholarship. *Journal of Professional Nursing, 11*(1), 24–30.

Dreher, M. (1999). Clinical scholarship: Nursing practice as an intellectual endeavor. In Clinical Scholarship Task Force Resource Paper. *Sigma Theta Tau International,* 26–33. Retrieved from https://www.sigmanursing.org/docs/default-source/position-papers/clinical_scholarship_paper.pdf?sfvrsn=4

Fawcett, J. (1999). The state of nursing science: Hallmarks of the 20th and 21st centuries. *Nursing Science Quarterly, 12* (4), 311–315. doi:10.1177/089431849901200411

Fawcett, J., & Alligood, M. (2005). Influences on the advancement of nursing knowledge. *Nursing Science Quarterly, 18*(3), 227–232. doi:10.1177/0894318405277523

Gibbons, M. (1994). Preface. In M. Gibbons, C. Lomoges, H. Nowotny, S. Schwartzman, P. Scott, & M. Trow (Eds.), *The new production of knowledge* (pp. vii–ix). London, UK: Sage.

Magyary, D., Whitney, J. D., & Brown, D. M. (2006). Advancing practice inquiry: Research foundations of the practice doctorate in nursing. *Nursing Outlook, 54*, 139–151.

Peterson, S. J., & Bredow, T. S. (2017). *Middle range theories: Application to nursing research* (4th ed.). New York, NY: Lippincott Williams & Wilkins.

Polit, D. F., & Beck, C. T. (2017). *Nursing research: Generating and assessing evidence for practice* (10th ed.). Philadelphia, PA: Wolters Kluwer.

Riley, J., Beal, J. A., & Lancaster, D. (2007). Scholarly nursing practice from the perspectives of experienced nurses. *Journal of Advanced Nursing, 61*(4), 425–435. doi:10.1111/j.1365-2648.2007.04499.x

Rolfe, G., & Davies, R. (2009). Second generation professional doctorates in nursing. *International Journal of Nursing Studies, 46*(9), 1265–1273.

Schon, D. (1983). *The reflective practitioner: How professionals think in action*. London, UK: Basic Books.

Task Force on the Implementation of the DNP. (2015). *The doctor of nursing practice: Current issues and clarifying recommendations*. Washington, DC: American Association of Colleges of Nursing. Retrieved from http://www.aacnnursing.org/Portals/42/DNP/DNP-Implementation.pdf?ver=2017-08-01-105830-517

Tymkow, C. (2017). Clinical scholarship and evidenced-based practice. In M. Zaccagnini & K. White (Eds.), *The doctor of nursing practice essentials* (3rd ed., pp. 67–144). Sudbury, MA: Jones & Bartlett.

Walker, G. E., Golde, C. M., Jones, L., Bueschel, A., & Hutchins, P. (2008). *The formation of scholars: Rethinking doctoral education for the twenty-first century*. Stanford, CA: Carnegie Foundation for the Advancement of Teaching.

DNP Project: Development, Implementation, Evaluation, and Dissemination

MARGIE H. SIPE AND LINDA C. ANDRIST

■ THE EVOLUTION OF SCHOLARSHIP IN DNP PROGRAMS

The doctor of nursing practice (DNP) project is a scholarly work that is often a requirement of DNP programs. There are other terminologies that have been used for this work, most frequently the *capstone project*, but following the 2015 position paper from American Association of Colleges of Nursing (AACN), many programs have moved to change the title of this scholarly project to the DNP Project (Task Force on the Implementation of the DNP, 2015). This helps distinguish the title from projects in other programs or disciplines, at different educational levels, which sometimes use the term *capstone* or *dissertation* (National Organization of Nurse Practitioner Faculties [NONPF], 2013). The expectations for the project vary across institutions depending upon the focus. New formats and designs of projects are being proposed and tested, although there is little in the literature describing the outcomes from these new models. Some examples of these new models include group projects (Task Force on the Implementation of the DNP, 2015) or expansion of master's level projects increasing the scope to a larger population. The nature of the project still evokes strong debate, which will likely continue until more DNP projects are disseminated in the literature. One way around the controversy is to encourage more DNP and PhD partnerships (Murphy, Steffileno, & Carlson, 2015), as working together will highlight the key strengths of both types of scholarly work in a way that is collaborative and not hierarchical. It will also be important to continue discussion among DNP program faculty, still predominately PhD prepared, to help appropriately guide students to projects that can contribute to nursing knowledge that is translational and impactful (Dols, Hernandez, & Miles, 2017). There are still some schools of nursing that may require more in-depth assignments that appear similar to a thesis or practice dissertation. There is general agreement, however, that the focus of the students' scholarly work should be projects that translate evidence into practice (Dols et al., 2017).

There continues to be more recent support for DNP students to complete projects that focus on quality improvement to establish evidence-based practice (Melnyk, 2016). Some authors offer pros and cons on the debate of one type of project versus another (research vs. quality improvement) (Gardenier, Stanik-Hutt, & Selway, 2010). Others distinguish between quality improvement projects, evidence-based practice, and research (E. Carter, Mastro, Vose, Rivera, & Larson, 2017). Arguments for research projects are that the DNP-prepared graduate will contribute to nursing knowledge by focusing on research grounded in practice. Those against research for DNP projects state that the curricula of DNP programs do not prepare the students for this competency. Additionally, the focus on research may distract from the attainment of the *DNP Essentials* developed by AACN in 2006. Textbooks on DNP and numerous articles and blogs still discuss this topic. Through improvement science methodologies, there may be new discoveries that at times need to be tested with more rigorous standard research methods, using control groups where appropriate. The approach taken by DNP students in discovery, even within an improvement science framework, should be grounded in thorough inquiry and assessment (Nelson, Cook, & Raterink, 2013). This is often called scholarship of application. The AACN (Task Force on the Implementation of the DNP, 2015) states clinical scholarship is demonstrated when the DNP student focuses on improved outcomes, combining nursing scholarship with the eight *DNP Essentials of Doctoral Education*. AACN goes on to clarify distinctions between research and practice focused scholarship.

Graduates of both terminal nursing degree programs (PhD and DNP) can generate new knowledge. Because of the difference in focus in PhD programs (more focused research methods and statistical analysis courses), the graduates of these programs may engage in studies that can be more diversely generalizable. In DNP programs, the focus is on generation of new knowledge that is gained from practice changes or implementation of new innovative processes (see Chapter 4). This knowledge application may be helpful to similar practice settings but is not generalizable in wider applications (Task Force on the Implementation of the DNP, 2015).

The proposal to require a DNP degree as entry into practice for advanced practice nurses by 2015 did not come to fruition. Many new DNP programs were developed with DNP being the terminal degree for advanced practice nurses. Other programs used a stepped approach where students completed the master's level nurse practitioner courses and upon completion of this level received a MSN degree with eligibility to sit for certification exams. The students can then proceed to upper level or second tier DNP level courses. These programs typically also accept postmaster's applicants. All students must meet the same advanced practice DNP competencies, but the scope of their DNP projects might be different (Melnyk, Gallagher-Ford, Long, & Fineout-Overholt, 2014). The implications of this mix of students with different levels of experience has also helped to create some confusion for both students and faculty.

Some DNP programs have transitioned to preparing entry-into-practice advanced practice nurses. This changes the way clinical and didactic content is presented over the course of the program. These types of programs mean that the student has less clinical experience preentry and must use time in the program to gain advanced knowledge and skills. One way to help with this focus is to eliminate the requirement for one DNP project but instead require a portfolio of examples of scholarly work that demonstrate competencies in the framework of smaller quality improvement exercises (M. Carter et al., 2016).

The DNP project is focused on an advanced nursing practice specialty or interprofessional intervention that may benefit a group, population, or community (NONPF, 2007). This work is usually based on clinical practice and involves partnerships with other entities such as healthcare organizations, schools, community agencies, or groups. The DNP project can take different forms, including practice change initiatives, evidence-based protocols, clinical guidelines, and health policy. Other DNP projects may focus on the development, implementation, and evaluation of interprofessional strategies to improve healthcare. This focus on projects that affect all disciplines is timely and demonstrates the leadership role that nurses can exhibit within interprofessional teams. The completion of the DNP project also is one assignment that helps to demonstrate the attainment of the DNP practice competencies that will be needed by the DNP graduates as they assume leadership roles within organizations (Malloch, 2017).

The development of this scholarly work is a step-by-step process that includes a systematic approach and translation of evidence into practice. These processes include (a) description of the innovation or clinical inquiry, (b) application of the best evidence from the literature, (c) collection of data using methods or tools that are standard and acceptable, and (d) definition of outcomes to be measured. Additionally, the project should be conducted according to ethical principles and the dissemination methods peer reviewed, whether public and/or professional presentations (NONPF, 2007).

■ PROJECT DEVELOPMENT

THE BURNING QUESTION FROM PRACTICE

Sister Callista Roy wrote that "practice . . . is the unifying factor for all of knowledge development. For example, nurses often enter doctoral education with burning questions from advanced practice" (Roy & Jones, 2007, p. 4). This is the premise that underlies DNP project development; it is grounded in practice and designed to add to practice knowledge. The burning question may arise from a practice situation in which the student wonders if an observation is evidence-based or coincidental, or from reading the research literature and thinking about replicating a study with a different population (Terry, 2018).

Students should plan to develop their question in each doctoral course starting early in their educational program, concentrating on building their literature to fine-tune the question. For example, in an outcomes measurement course, a student might examine patient dissatisfaction in the emergency department due to compassion fatigue on the part of staff. In an epidemiology/population health course, this student then could look at aggregate populations regarding the same subject.

Several cautionary words are needed regarding the DNP project question. Students should consider the following:

1. Will they have sufficient time to carry out the project within the scope of the DNP program? (Terry, 2018)
2. Is the project within the scope of the DNP?
3. Do they have sufficient resources—such as financial resources (Terry, 2018) and available faculty expertise in the area?

A faculty advisor should be involved in each step of the process to ensure that the student is on target and is proceeding in a reasonable fashion. Students may come with a general area of interest, but may need help in refining it and determining what part of this interest has scope for a DNP project that can be completed within the structure of the curriculum. In one of the authors' knowledge and inquiry courses, faculty have students discuss their *burning* questions, critique each other, and search the literature for theoretical models to apply to their question. In the research analysis and critique course, they search for the best evidence, analyze and critique the literature, and begin a review of the literature. These two courses form the foundation for the proposal. Many programs also have affiliations with academic medical centers or larger health systems where nurse scientists may have research initiatives that could be further developed in a translational improvement project. These partnerships can be useful for students who have a broad area of interest but struggle defining a clinical question.

FORMULATING A PICO(T) QUESTION

After the identification of a topic from clinical practice, the student uses the literature to guide the development of the initial question or practice inquiry to develop the PICO(T) question. PICO(T) is a framework that can be used to develop clinical questions in a systematic manner (Stillwell, Fineout-Overholt, Melnyk, & Williamson, 2010). Some questions lend themselves to this format better than others. The use of the PICO(T) framework facilitates the development of questions with the scientific underpinnings of evidence-based practice to diagnose, treat, and facilitate patient understanding of their prognosis (Melnyk & Fineout-Overholt, 2015). This framework is useful for developing clinical questions to examine the best evidence to answer these questions and is associated with improved quality reporting from randomized controlled trials (RCTs) (Rios, Ye, & Thabane, 2010). It is important that these RCTs are well designed so that the evidence is generalizable. For a DNP student, the PICO(T) question can be used in an evidence-based practice search or for a systematic review of the literature. With a more focused PICO(T) question, the search will yield appropriate studies targeted to the practice inquiry.

The acronym PICO(T) stands for *P*, the population of interest; *I*, intervention or issue of interest; *C*, comparison of interest or intervention/issue; *O*, the outcome of interest or what will be improved for the population of interest; and *T*, for time, which is optional for the PICO(T) question (Stillwell et al., 2010). These are explained as follows.

P is the specific population of interest. What is the population of interest that is the focus of the practice inquiry? There should be specific details identifying the population, including age, ethnicity, gender, or diagnosis. This information can be used to focus the scope of the practice inquiry while not excluding other relevant groups from the question. The population can also be a specific position category such as nurse practitioners, registered nurses, nurse executives, informaticists, and the like. These can further be delineated by population foci for advanced practice nurses, for example, as identified in the *Consensus Model for APRN Regulation: Licensure, Accreditation, Certification, and Education* (APRN Consensus Work Group & National Council of State Boards of Nursing APN Advisory Committee, 2008).

I is focused on the intervention or issue of interest, or what the investigator will do for the patient or population of interest. It is important to depict a clear and concise statement of the intervention or issue of interest. This strategy will focus the question so that the project or study may evaluate a new clinical practice guideline, model, protocol, or therapy.

C stands for the comparison of interest or intervention/issue. What are the alternatives to the identified intervention? This section is relevant for those populations of interest that may have treatment alternatives or different interventions that may influence the outcomes.

O is focused on the outcome of interest or what will be improved for the population of interest. DNP projects are frequently initiated to improve the quality of patient care or to enhance organizational processes. The project or study will evaluate the effect of the intervention on the outcomes of the population to determine if they were improved, had no effect, or resulted in adverse or negative results.

T is for time and is optional for the PICO(T) question. Time is referenced in relation to the scholarly project. This approach is particularly helpful for work that is either time limited or if there is data collection at specific periods that are examining changes over time. The use of time is also helpful for determining the starting and ending points of the intervention. An explanation of PICO(T) and recommended items for each component of the framework are identified in Table 5.1.

TABLE 5.1 Components of a PICO(T) Question

PICO(T)	Question	Examples
Population	What is the population of interest that is the focus of the practice inquiry?	Age
		Ethnicity
		Gender
		Health status
		Diagnoses
Intervention	What will the investigator do for the patient or population of interest?	Clinical practice guideline
		Model
		Protocol
		Therapy

(continued)

TABLE 5.1 Components of a PICO(T) Question (*continued*)

PICO(T)	Question	Examples
Comparison	What are the alternatives to the identified intervention?	Alternative intervention
		No intervention
		Placebo
		No diagnosis
		No risk factor
Outcome	What will be improved for the population of interest?	Improvement results from intervention
		Intervention results in more positive outcomes than no intervention
		Placebo has no effect on outcome
		Intervention results in decreased diagnoses
		Intervention results in decreased risk factors
Time	What amount of time will it take to demonstrate the outcome?	Time for the intervention to achieve an outcome
		Time subjects observed for the outcome

PICO(T), the population of interest, intervention or issue of interest, comparison of interest or intervention/issue, the outcome of interest or what will be improved for the population of interest, and time.

Using a standardized format such as the PICO(T) will guide the inquiry to develop questions that are searchable using the best evidence. The data to answer the question may vary depending upon the question and the information in the literature. Some questions are best answered by systematic reviews or meta-analyses, while others may be developed so that qualitative studies are the source of the evidence. The question will then guide the design of the project or study. Examples of PICO(T) questions are in Table 5.2.

EXPLORING THEORETICAL FRAMEWORKS

Theory-based nursing is central to advanced nursing practice and defines the DNP. Nursing theory distinguishes the DNP from the medical model because, rather than working with decontextualized pieces of data, nursing practice occurs in the exchanges between patient and nurse. The advanced practice nurse has a relationship with the patient and their unique values and goals, not with the disease (Eldridge, 2017). Nursing theories help guide practice by providing a foundation to understand patients, their problems, and to formulate interventions to help them. Eldridge noted:

> Nursing theory improves our care by giving it structure and unity, by providing more efficient continuity of care, by achieving congruence between process and product, by defining the boundaries and goals of nursing actions, and by giving us a framework in which to examine the effectiveness of our interventions. (p. 14)

TABLE 5.2 Examples of PICO(T) Questions

PICO(T)	Question 1	Question 2
Population	In opiate dependence users completing a detoxification program who are risk for relapse . . .	In elders being transferred to a long-term care facility after hospitalization for pneumonia who are at risk for medication errors ...
Intervention	How does receiving intensive outpatient therapy . . .	How does a new medication reconciliation form . . .
Comparison	Compared to the standard of care (weekly support groups) . . .	Compared to the hospital's standard discharge form . . .
Outcome	Affect their relapse rate . . .	Affect the number of medication errors on admission . . .
Time	3 months after treatment?	2 weeks after discharge?

PICO(T), the population of interest, intervention or issue of interest, comparison of interest or intervention/issue, the outcome of interest or what will be improved for the population of interest, and time.

We recognize that DNP students are also nurse administrators, health policy experts, informaticists, and educators. There are many social science, organizational, and educational theories and models to bring to the DNP project.

Theory-based nursing practice applies theories, principles, and models from a variety of sources to practice. Conceptual models and grand theories are broad in scope and focused on the large nursing arena, while middle range theories are more specific, focused, and narrow. They concentrate on specific health experiences, health or illness problems, or a particular patient population (Eldridge, 2017).

McEwen and Wills, in their fourth edition of *Theoretical Basis for Nursing* (2014), commented that nursing theory books have failed to keep up with trends in theory, specifically with middle range theories, application to practice, and evidence-based practice. In the past few years, more attention has been placed on this trend, and each year there are new books and book revisions, providing a more extensive selection of texts and resources for students to use. Theory experts believe that middle range theory is the preferred direction for knowledge development (Peterson, 2017).

Middle range theory is defined as a "set of related ideas that are focused on a limited dimension of the reality of nursing" (Smith & Liehr, 2014, p. xiii). They grow and develop at the intersection of research and practice and provide guidelines for nursing practice (Smith & Liehr, 2014). Examples of middle range theories are in Table 5.3.

TABLE 5.3 Examples of Middle Range Theories

Middle Range Theory	Reference
Uncertainty in illness (uncertainty during diagnosis and treatment of illness)	Mishel (1988)
Comfort (needs for ease, relief, and transcendence)	Kolcaba (1994)
Community empowerment (improving health in communities)	Hildebrandt (1996)

(*continued*)

TABLE 5.3 Examples of Middle Range Theories (*continued*)

Middle Range Theory	Reference
Story theory (story as the context for a nurse-person health-promoting process)	Smith and Liehr (1999)
The synergy model (critical care)	Hardin (2005)
Unpleasant symptoms (symptom management)	Lenz, Pugh, Milligan, Gift, and Suppe (1997)
The tidal model of mental health recovery (psychiatric mental health nursing)	Barker (2001)
Postpartum depression theory (psychiatric mental health nursing, obstetrical nursing, women's healthcare)	Beck (1993)

SYNTHESIS OF THE LITERATURE

A thorough review of the literature provides the best evidence to support the development, implementation, and evaluation of the DNP project. Each component of the PICO(T) question can be used to guide the process of gathering evidence from the literature.

After the development of the PICO(T) question, there are many databases that can be used to determine the best evidence. An initial inquiry may be with resources such as CINAHL, MEDLINE, and/or PsycINFO, depending upon the type of question. These information resources often have a large repository of articles on a variety of topics. The use of one or more of these databases will be dependent upon the focus of the PICO(T) question (see Table 5.4).

TABLE 5.4 Sources of Best Evidence

American College of Physicians (ACP) Journal Club

CINHAL

Cochrane Database of Systematic Review

Database of Abstracts of Reviews of Effects (DARE)

DynaMed

Joanna Briggs Institute

U.S. Preventive Services Task Force

National Guideline Clearinghouse

PubMed Clinical Queries

TRIP Database

UpToDate

Virginia Henderson International Nursing Library

BUILDING THE DNP PROJECT TEAM

The development of the project team is an important part of the DNP project process. The team should have representation of doctorally prepared advanced practice nurses and/or interprofessional providers, depending upon the scope of the project. The number of project team members is usually set by the program or the complexity of the clinical question; sometimes several content experts may be required. Many schools recommend at least one faculty and one clinical site member be part of the team. If the study is being done in an academic facility, and a nurse scientist is available, this person may be a great choice. Besides supporting a PhD/DNP partnership, these individuals often can be helpful in navigating the institutional review board (IRB) in the organization. There should be a content expert on the committee who is knowledgeable about the evidence-based topic and/or clinical expert in the general content area. Some schools may also require a DNP project team member who is knowledgeable about the project methods, for example, faculty researcher experienced in improvement science formats. Often faculty support is provided for assistance with statistical procedures or analyses.

Typically, the proposal may be developed, implemented, and evaluated in a staged process in various courses that support the development and implementation of the DNP project. Programs are beginning to have project discussions with students earlier. Students often choose particular DNP programs based on interests of faculty scholars who might be helpful in mentoring. The DNP project team should be identified prior to writing the proposal and as the PICO(T) question is being developed. The team will oversee all aspects of the project, including the submission for approval by the IRB. In some programs, the faculty "first reader" not only provides guidance for the development of the proposal and review of final analysis but also serves as the principal investigator (PI). There are often formal documents signed during this process, including the agreement to serve on the DNP project team along with the final approval of the completed project.

The student and the project team will work together for at least two to three semesters until completion of the project. The earlier this relationship can be formed, the more beneficial it can be for both faculty member and student. The intense mentoring relationship is a reciprocal one and enables the faculty member to be most helpful to the student and for the student to achieve at an optimal level. The expectations for this relationship need to be established prior to the formulation of the DNP project committee. The relationship between committee members and the student needs to be collaborative. Students should be encouraged to establish a detailed timeline with frequent deliverables that enables the project to be added on to and otherwise refined prior to total project review. The strength of this mentoring relationship will be key in facilitating the development of the proposal, implementation of the project, and the evaluation of the outcomes.

WRITING THE PROPOSAL

The development and completion of the proposal are complex processes that include input from each of the project team members. Attention must be given to the format and structure of the proposal, along with the writing style. Each DNP program sets the criteria for the development of the proposal, depending upon the purpose of the scholarly work. This information should be made available to the student prior to the development of the proposal. Some programs suggest the format of the proposal follows the general guidelines of the journal for which the student is considering submission. The other consideration in proposal development is the type of project.

Once the PICO(T) question has been developed, systematic review has been completed, and the plan for the project finalized, work can begin on the proposal. In many programs, the development and approval of the proposal is accomplished in the first project course. Important points for the student to consider are (a) read and follow carefully the proposal guidelines; (b) seek the recommendations of the DNP project team and content experts; (c) incorporate the correct components of the style of writing such as the American Psychological Association (APA) so that headings and reference formats are correct; (d) review the proposal for ethical issues or evidence of bias; and (e) meticulously prepare for the review by knowing the content well and anticipating any questions. Students should anticipate several revisions of their proposal based on the committee's feedback.

According to Nebiu (2000), a project proposal is a description of activities that are focused on solving a specific problem. Components of the proposal should include (a) rationale for the project, (b) activities or plan for the project with a timeline, (c) methodology, and (d) resources needed to complete project such as participants, materials, and costs. Phases of a project cycle are (a) assess the literature or research studies, (b) identify the focus of the project, (c) design the project, (d) consider costs and resources to implement the project, (e) implement the project activities, and (f) evaluate the results of the project. These elements should be considered when developing the proposal according to the guidelines established by the school. The proposal guidelines may differ according to whether the focus is a clinical practice guideline, practice protocol, health policy change, or practice inquiry. Exhibit 5.1 provides an example of one school's outline for the proposal.

EXHIBIT 5.1   DNP Project Proposal Paper

I. Introduction and Outline of the Proposed Project
- Introduction should contain two or three paragraphs at the most
- Tells the reader what is being proposed and why
- Clearly states the purpose of the project

II. Background
- This section provides the reader with the set and setting of the project, as well as the rationale for why it is important. Often included in this section

(continued)

EXHIBIT 5.1   DNP Project Proposal Paper (*continued*)

are related articles, professional opinions, statistics, supporting data, and the theoretical construct of the project (introducing your nursing theory)
- The Background section may be substantial—especially if there has been little empirical research

III. Synthesis of the Literature
- Discuss which databases were searched, terms and descriptors used in the search, studies yielded (number, types)
- Group the articles by categories

Refer to: Machi, L., & McEvoy, B. (2016). *The literature review: Six steps to success* (3rd ed.). Thousand Oaks, CA: Corwin Press. ISBN 978-1506336244.

IV. Theoretical Framework
- All papers need a theoretical grounding
- The theoretical piece needs to be identified by name (middle range or other)
- The theoretical piece needs to be integrated throughout the paper—not just mentioned and then forgotten; show how the theory fits in, the theory drives your issue, guides your examination of the varied questions, and helps to develop any intervention and evaluation you are doing

V. The Project Description
- Outline the project (the actual project is part of the Appendix)
- Discuss the methods, tools, and techniques that will guide implementation
- Identify your project team members, how they were chosen, and the roles they have agreed to play
- Formulate a plan for eliciting system involvement in implementing the project
- Describe the fiscal, ethical, political, legal, and legislative facets related to implementation of the project in a selected clinical/organizational context
- Address any potential constraints for facilitating a successful project
- Develop a plan for critically evaluating the project using a multidimensional framework (see evaluation rubric)

Project Evaluation Rubric

Objectives	What evidence-based measures/instruments will be applied to the evaluation plan?	What method of analysis will you use for each objective?	In what ways will you evaluate the success of your project?

(*continued*)

EXHIBIT 5.1   DNP Project Proposal Paper (*continued*)

VI. Discussion
  - Written discussion due with final paper
  - Relate the project's purpose to the background and literature review
  - Discuss what is missing in the area you are addressing and how your project will contribute to the reader's knowledge development about this topic
  - Discuss the development of the project
  - Often the actual project is part of the Appendix (such as a teaching tool) and will be referred to in this section

VII. Conclusion
  - Due with final proposal
  - Tell the reader what was done
  - Apply project to nursing by referring to any nursing theory used or by discussing application to nursing practice

VIII. References
  IX. Appendices

INSTITUTIONAL REVIEW BOARD

The IRB is convened to protect human subjects. The IRB is composed of at least five members representing experience and expertise in research and diversity in race, gender, and culture. The IRB will also have members knowledgeable in and experienced with subjects in vulnerable categories, including children, prisoners, pregnant women, and the handicapped or mentally disabled. The IRB may also require documentation of informed consent or may waive this requirement.

Quality improvement projects usually do not require IRB approval but research studies do. Since human subjects may be involved in quality improvement, it is prudent to consult with the IRB to confirm whether or not a review is needed. The functions of the IRB are to review and approve, make recommendations for modifications, or disapprove an IRB application. The IRB is also responsible for the continuing review of approved research at least once annually.

There are three different categories of review for research. Full review is required of research, including those subjects in the vulnerable category. Research involving minimal risk or with minor changes to approved studies may be in the category of expedited review. This review may be conducted by the IRB chairperson or by one or more IRB members appointed by the chairperson. The IRB will have a procedure for notifying all members of the status of approval for research in this category. Research in the exempt review category is identified in Exhibit 5.2.

EXHIBIT 5.2   Categories of Exempt Research

Research conducted in established educational settings that may include regular or special education instruction

Research using educational tests such as cognitive, diagnostic, aptitude, and achievement tests. The research may also use surveys, interviews, or observations of public behavior

The subjects cannot be identified or linked to the research

The subjects cannot be public officials or candidates for public offices and confidentiality of subjects must be maintained

Research consisting of existing data, documents, records, or specimens

Research or projects investigated by or requiring approval of department or agency administrators which are designed to evaluate or examine public benefit or service programs, procedures for having benefits or services from these programs, changes or alternatives to these services, and changes in methods or levels of reimbursement for benefits or services

Research involving taste and food quality and evaluation of consumer acceptance

Source: U.S. Department of Health and Human Services. (2009). Code of Federal Regulations, Table 45 public welfare, Part 4 protection of human subjects. Retrieved from http://www.hhs.gov/ohrp/humansubjects/guidance/45cfr46.html#46.108

Students, in concert with their DNP project team, need to discuss whether they will need to have IRB approval early on. Most institutions have a contact person who can review the student's ideas and help negotiate the process, whether the project is exempt, expedited, or full review. Many schools have an organizational IRB that may be affiliated with a university or academic medical center that reviews student proposals, which is helpful when the student's project is not being conducted in a particular practice organization. Attention must be paid to IRB submission deadlines and meeting dates in order not to extend the timeline that the student anticipates. One important consideration of a student's project plan is allowing time for additional review by the school's leadership team, for example, program director or dean, who may be required to review the submission before it goes to the formal IRB committee. When two institutions are involved (e.g., the school and a hospital), the first reader can help the student identify how the process will work. In some institutions, first readers need to be the PI.

DNP Project Implementation and Evaluation

Once the DNP project team has approved the DNP project proposal, the next important step is the implementation of the project within the specified time frames and evaluation of the results. The final step is the dissemination of the information collected during the implementation of the DNP project.

■ DNP PROJECT IMPLEMENTATION

The DNP project implementation involves a detailed plan that is a component of the proposal. The more detailed the plan with approval of stakeholders, the more likely the direction of the proposal will have minimal variations. Important competencies for the student that lead to the successful completion of the project include the ability to manage and collaborate with the team, manage the integral tasks of the project, and implement leadership skills for the team and key stakeholders (Balch, John, Reynolds, & Rick, 2015). Expertise at achieving these competencies is honed during the development, implementation, and evaluation of the project.

The institutional stakeholders within the organization where the project is being carried out should be consulted at this point about the process that the student plans in the implementation of the project, collection of data, or other methods of conducting the project. Their endorsement is important to limit any challenges and facilitate the implementation of the project. The key stakeholders can also facilitate the implementation of the DNP project through endorsement of the project and setting the stage for approval by the employees. Spending time meeting with department leaders and staff early in the proposal process can facilitate enthusiasm and investment in seeing the project proceeds without setbacks. Additionally, they should receive updated progress reports, and have the opportunity to address concerns throughout the implementation (McElmurry et al., 2009).

Once approval is received from the Institutional Review Board, if needed, the implementation of the DNP project may commence. Since not all DNP projects require IRB approval, for example, quality improvement projects, it is important to request a letter from the IRB stating that DNP project was on quality improvement. Many journal editors require documentation that the DNP project either has IRB approval or that it is a quality improvement project. The DNP project implementation must follow the plan as identified in the proposal. Any changes to the plan will require the filing and approval of an amendment for those DNP projects having oversight of the IRB. If the project underwent a full or expedited review process, as the DNP project was implemented, there may be changes to the plan that require approval of the IRB through the submission of an amendment form.

It is important to develop the team prior to the implementation of the DNP project. According to Tuckman (2001), the stages of team development include forming, storming, norming, performing, and adjourning. Forming includes orientation to the task, storming includes intragroup conflict, norming is openness to other group members, performing is constructive action, and adjourning is disengagement. The evolution of the team may progress through these stages depending upon their communication and cohesiveness. The student should focus on using their leadership and management skills to guide the team through these stages.

PROJECT MANAGEMENT

The implementation of the DNP project should follow the detailed plan. The project team, including the faculty, should have regularly scheduled meetings. The key stakeholders should also have periodic updates about the status of the DNP project. Communications at all levels are important to the success of the project.

Project management is the use of knowledge, skills, instruments, and personnel to plan and implement a project within identified timelines and specified budgets while addressing stakeholders' expectations (Nicholas, 2001). Any risks or challenges encountered should have a plan in place to address these issues and keep the DNP project on track.

The student is in a role similar to a project manager. This role involves planning, organizing, and completing the project within the identified time frame and costs. The risks and issues associated with the DNP project should also be a consideration for the student who is managing the project. This role is also important to guide or lead the members and stakeholders through the different stages of team development so that the project will be successful (Williams & Murphy, 2005).

■ DNP PROJECT EVALUATION

Upon project completion, there are several approaches to evaluating the success of the DNP project. Some programs may have ongoing processes, or formative evaluation, whereas others may evaluate the outcomes once the project is complete (summative evaluation), while others use both.

DATA ANALYSIS

The anticipated data analysis approach is identified in the plan for the project. Taking into account any modifications in the information collected, there may be some changes on how the outcomes are evaluated. Once data are analyzed, the results can be compared to the aims or objectives of the DNP project.

The ability to evaluate the implications of the results of the data analysis requires knowledge of statistical processes. The student may need guidance from the DNP project team and/or consultants. It is important that the conclusions of the findings are accurate. Some of this expertise comes from knowledge gained in the DNP program and the experience of conducting a DNP project. It is important to base conclusions on the evidence rather than making erroneous recommendations.

BENCHMARKING THE OUTCOMES

After the data are analyzed, the outcomes of the project are compared with current benchmarks or outcomes. It is important to link back to the literature, comparing and contrasting results to outcomes reported. These benchmarks may be based on standards of practice or best practices identified by institutions and national professional organizations. The outcomes of the project may be compared with these other standards to determine the success of the project in translating evidence. If the project experienced outcomes different from other benchmarks or information in the literature, an exploration of the reasons for these results is indicated. There may have been a problem with the design of the DNP project methodology, data analysis procedures, or interpretation of the outcomes. If the project is successful in improving practice and patient safety, then strategies should be developed to incorporate this change into other microsystems within the organization or other organizations. This process would entail the development of a new plan and potentially a new group of team members and key stakeholders. In the meantime, the student should share the outcomes with team members, key stakeholders, and organizations at local, regional, state, national, and international levels.

VENUES FOR DISSEMINATION

The old adage *if it's not written down it didn't happen* can be applied to knowledge development in nursing. It is our professional responsibility to share knowledge—knowledge generated from practice. Publishing in peer-reviewed journals has the highest prestige in the hierarchy of scholarship dissemination. DNP students and graduates who plan on teaching in academia will want to build their scholarship portfolio. Therefore, aiming for peer-reviewed venues is encouraged. Conferences generally do peer review for podium presentations or poster sessions and are a much faster way to get project outcomes out to professional colleagues. Many DNP programs also require a public sharing of the student's work in a forum of faculty, students, and invited guests. While this is not considered a project defense, it is an excellent opportunity for students to get feedback as well as gain added confidence in presentation skills. Alternatively, poster presentations can be part of a local dissemination required at the college or university.

Poster Presentations

Presenting the DNP project as a poster is an effective venue for the dissemination of the project outcomes. A poster presentation is a widely accepted strategy used for conferences sponsored by nursing and other disciplines. Scholarship can be shared in a more timely fashion, although with a more limited audience than when published in a journal.

Conference committee members often post notices of the meeting with a request for abstract submissions for poster and/or podium presentations. There are usually specific instructions for the abstract submissions, including format, blinded or not blinded, and total word count. The focus of the abstract should be congruent with the goals of the conference and/or professional organization. This relationship to conference goals is crucial, and the student should consider this prior to submission. It is not unusual for excellent submissions to be rejected when there is insufficient alignment with conference goals. The abstract submission is usually due by a specific date, with the decision to accept or not accept made by a committee that usually does a blinded peer review.

The software program often used for developing posters is PowerPoint (Microsoft Corporation, Redmond, Washington). There are several Internet sites that have suggestions for making good poster presentations.

Many presenters include handouts of their abstract during the poster session. This session gives the audience the opportunity to review the posters at the conference. Some individuals will speak with the presenter to discuss their similar projects or ask advice on future projects. These sessions provide presenters and the audience time to network during the conference. If you have the opportunity to present at a conference, make sure you are available at the poster to answer questions. Discussion with interested viewers may lead to further collaboration or opportunities to replicate your work in other organizations or settings. Finally, some conferences recognize posters in specific categories such as projects or research and offer awards for being voted "best" poster in a selected category.

Podium Presentations

There are two major elements to a podium presentation: the content and how it is presented (Larkin, 2015). The setting of the presentations, such as a unit-based meeting, a roundtable conference, or a formal local, national, or international conference, will set the tone for the kind of presentation and the amount of audience participation. Consider whether you need to use slides for a presentation. Sometimes the impact of your topic, similar to a TED talk, can be best shared without the use of slides. If slides are used, consider using these as you would note cards, with a few points that you want to emphasize. Many DNP organizations have specific requirements, (see www.doctorsofnursingpractice.org/podium-presentation-requirements, as an example).

Understanding the audience is critical in any presentation and will make or break the session. Content should be aimed in a voice that the participants will understand. For example, using heavy theoretical content without tying it to practice will put nonlicensed nursing personnel to sleep! Practicing staff nurses or advanced practice nurses expect the latest information and that the presenter is knowledgeable and current in practice. Take into consideration the size of the audience, the composition (generalists vs. specialists), and the demographics (age, ethnicity, and level of education); these are important factors in order to reach the level of the audience. Larkin suggests telling the audience why they should care about your topic and what's in it for them, convey your excitement of the subject matter, tell your story, and keep it short (Larkin, 2015).

The use of body language is also important; many speakers practice in front of a mirror or with colleagues to help critique their presentation style. Simple rules apply: do face the audience, look individuals in the eye as if you are talking to them, smile, use different kinds of vocal inflection, use your hand gestures judiciously; do not read your notes or pace back and forth across the podium. At the end of the session, summarize your talk if it is a long one, and if short, give a clinical "bottom line" to allow the audience to focus on the purpose of the talk (Schmaltz & Enstrom, 2014).

Preparing Manuscripts for Publication

Consult your author guidelines for your selected journal. In some cases, a letter of inquiry to the editor can assist in establishing whether that particular journal is a good venue for your work. It is useful to read similar articles published in journals to which you are considering submission. This exercise can provide guidance in determining common outlines used. Texts such as *Writing for Publication in Nursing* by Oermann and Hays (2015) walk an author through the steps from selecting a journal to the publishing process. The format for submission of quality improvement work may require the use of SQUIRE guidelines (Goodman et al., 2016). If the proposal and final project paper are designed using this format, it can facilitate easier editing for article submission. Software applications such as EndNote are very helpful in formatting various journal styles and creating a reference list. There are also free software applications that work well, such as Mendeley or Zotero. Schools may provide a particular resource for students to use; this can be helpful if peers are using the same program and librarians are very familiar with the program and can provide extra support. Not all programs work the same and it is helpful to review a few and choose one that works well for you. Massachusetts Institute of Technology (MIT) provides a comprehensive comparison grid of a few of the common programs and may assist you in your selection (http://libguides.mit.edu/references).

Publishers of peer-reviewed journals will send your manuscript for peer review, which can take a matter of a few months to complete. Do not be disheartened by the publishing process; it can take months and many revisions before your manuscript is actually published. The final product is worth the wait!

■ REFERENCES

APRN Consensus Work Group & National Council of State Boards of Nursing APN Advisory Committee. (2008). *Consensus Model for APRN Regulation: Licensure, accreditation, certification, and education.* Chicago, IL: National Council of State Boards.

Balch, M., John, R., Reynolds, M., & Rick, C. (2015). Requisite competencies and skills for effective project planning and program management. In J. Harris, L. Roussel, S. E. Walters, C. Dearman, & P. Thomas (Eds.), *Project planning and management: A guide for nurses and interprofessional teams* (2nd ed.) Sudbury, MA: Jones & Bartlett.

Barker, P. J. (2001). The Tidal Model: Developing an empowering, person-centered approach to recovery within psychiatric and mental health nursing. *Journal of Psychiatric and Mental Health Nursing, 8,* 233–240.

Beck, C. T. (1993). Teetering on the edge: A substantive theory of postpartum depression. *Nursing Research, 42*, 42–48.

Carter, E., Mastro, K., Vose, C., Rivera, R., & Larson, E. (2017). Clarifying the conundrum: Evidence-based practice, quality improvement, or research? The clinical scholarship continuum. *Journal of Nursing Administration, 47*(5), 266–270. doi:10.1097/NNA.0000000000000477

Carter, M., Accardo, D., Cooper T., Cowan, P., Likes, W., Lynch-Smith, D., & Melaro L. (2016). Recommendations from an early adopter of a doctor of nursing practice program. *Journal of Nursing Education, 55*(10), 563–567. doi:10.3928/01484834-20160914-04

Dols, J. D., Hernández, C., & Miles, H. (2017). The DNP project: Quandaries for nursing scholars. *Nursing Outlook, 65*(1), 84–93. doi:10.1016/j.outlook.2016.07.009

Eldridge, C. R. (2017). Nursing science and theory: Scientific underpinnings for practice. In M. E. Zaccagnini & K. White (Eds.), *The doctor of nursing practice essentials: A new model for advanced practice nursing* (3rd ed., pp. 3–38). Sudbury, MA: Jones & Bartlett.

Gardenier, D., Stanik-Hutt, J., & Selway, J. (2010). Point counter-point. Should DNP students conduct original research as their Capstone projects? *Journal for Nurse Practitioners, 6*(5), 364–365.

Goodman D., Ogrinc G., Davies L., Baker G. R., Barnsteiner J., Foster, T., . . . Thor, J. (2016). Explanation and elaboration of the SQUIRE (Standards for Quality Improvement Reporting Excellence) guidelines, V.2.0: Examples of SQUIRE elements in the healthcare improvement literature. *British Medical Journal of Quality and Safety,* 1–24. doi:10.1136/bmjqs-2015-004480

Hardin, S. R. (2005). Introduction to the AACN Synergy Model for patient care. In S. R. Hardin & R. Carlow (Eds.), *Synergy for clinical excellence: The AACN Synergy Model for Patient Care.* Sudbury, MA: Jones & Bartlett.

Hildebrandt, E. (1996). Building community participation in health care: A model and example from South Africa. *Image: Journal of Nursing Scholarship, 28*, 155–159.

Kolcaba, K. (1994). A theory of holistic comfort for nursing. *Journal of Advanced Nursing, 19*, 1178–1184.

Larkin, M. (2015). How to give a dynamic scientific presentation. Retrieved from https://www.elsevier.com/connect/how-to-give-a-dynamic-scientific-presentation

Lenz, E. R., Pugh, L. C., Milligan, R. A., Gift, A., & Suppe, F. (1997). The middle-range theory of unpleasant symptoms: An update. *Advances in Nursing Science, 19*(3), 14–27.

Malloch, K. (2017). Leading DNP professionals: Practice competencies for organizational excellence and advancement. *Nursing Administration Quarterly, 41*(1), 29–38. doi:10.1097/NAQ.0000000000000200

McElmurry, B. J., McCreary, L. L., Parke, C. G., Ramos, L., Martinex, E., Parikh, R . . . Fogelfeld, L. (2009). Implementation, outcomes, and lessons learned from a collaborative primary care health program to improve diabetes care among urban Latino populations. *Health Promotion Practice, 10*(2), 293–302. doi:10.1177/1524839907306406

McEwen, M. W., & Wills, E. M. (2014). *Theoretical basis for nursing* (4th ed.). Philadelphia, PA: Lippincott Williams & Wilkins.

Melnyk, B. M. (2016). The doctor of nursing practice degree-evidence-based practice expert. *Worldviews on Evidence-Based Nursing, 13*(3), 183–184. doi:10.1111/wvn.12164

Melnyk, B. M., & Fineout-Overholt, E. (2015). *Evidence-based practice in nursing & healthcare: A guide to best practice* (3rd ed.). Philadelphia, PA: Wolters Kluwer Health/Lippincott Williams & Wilkins.

Melnyk, B. M., Gallagher-Ford, L., Long, L. E., & Fineout-Overholt, E. (2014). The establishment of evidence-based practice competencies for practicing registered nurses and advanced practice nurses in real-world clinical settings: Proficiencies to improve healthcare quality, reliability, patient outcomes, and costs. *Worldviews on Evidence-Based Nursing, 11*(1), 5–15.

Mishel, M. H. (1988). Uncertainty in illness. *Image: Journal of Nursing Scholarship, 20*, 225–231.

Murphy, M., Staffileno, B., & Carlson, E. (2015) Collaboration among DNP-and PhD-prepared nurses: Opportunity to drive positive change. *Journal of Professional Nursing, 31*(5), 388–394. doi:10.1016/j.profnurs.2015.03.001

National Organization of Nurse Practitioner Faculties. (2007). *NONPF recommended criteria for NP scholarly projects in the practice doctorate program.* Washington DC: Author. Retrieved from http://c.ymcdn.com/sites/www.nonpf.org/resource/resmgr/imported/scholarlyprojectcriteria.pdf.

National Organization of Nurse Practitioner Faculties. (2013). *Titling of the doctor of nursing practice project.* Retrieved from http://www.nonpf.org/resource/resmgr/dnp/dnpprojectstitlingpaperjune2.pdf

Nebiu, B. (2000). *Project proposal writing.* Szenendre, Hungary: The Regional Environmental Center for Central and Eastern Europe.

Nelson, J., Cook, P., & Raterink, G. (2013). The evolution of a doctor of nursing practice capstone process: Programmatic revisions to improve the quality of student projects. *Journal of Professional Nursing, 29*(6), 370–380. doi:10.1016/j.profnurs.2012.05.018

Nicholas, J. (2001). *Project management for business and technology: Principles and practice* (2nd ed.). Upper Saddle River, NJ: Prentice Hall.

Oermann, M. H., & Hays, J. C. (2015). *Writing for publication in nursing* (3rd ed.). New York, NY: Springer Publishing.

Peterson, S. B. (2017). *Middle range theories: Application to nursing research* (4th ed.). Philadelphia, PA: Walters Kluer Health/Lippincott Williams & Wilkins.

Rios, P. L., Ye, C., & Thabane, L. (2010). Association between framing of the research question using the PICOT format and reporting quality of randomized control trials. *Biomedical Central Medical Research Methodology, 10*(1), 2010. doi:10.1186/1471-2288-10-11

Roy, C., &. Jones, D. (2007). *Nursing knowledge development and clinical practice.* New York, NY: Springer Publishing.

Schmaltz, R. M., & Enström, R. (2014). Death to weak PowerPoint: Strategies to create effective visual presentations. *Frontiers in Psychology, 5*, 1138. doi:10.3389/fpsyg.2014.01138

Smith, M., & Liehr, P. (1999). Attentively embracing story: A middle range theory with practice and research implications. *Scholarly Inquiry for Nursing Practice: An International Journal, 13*, 187–204.

Smith, M., &. Liehr, P. R. (2014). *Middle range theory for nursing* (3rd ed.). New York, NY: Springer Publishing.

Stillwell, S., Fineout-Overholt, E., Melnick, B., & Williamson, K. (2010). Evidence-based practice, step by step: Asking the clinical question, a key step in evidence-based practice. *The American Journal of Nursing, 110*(3), 58–61. doi:10.1097/01.NAJ.0000368959.11129.79

Task Force on the Implementation of the DNP. (2015). *The doctor of nursing practice: Current issues and clarifying recommendations.* Retrieved from http://www.aacnnursing.org/Portals/42/DNP/DNP-Implementation.pdf?ver=2017-08-01-105830-517

Terry, A. J. (2018). *Clinical research for the doctor of nursing practice* (3rd ed.) Sudbury, MA: Jones & Bartlett.

Tuckman, B. W. (2001). Developmental sequence in small groups. *Group Facilitation: A Research and Applications Journal, 3*, 66–81.

U.S. Department of Health and Human Services. (2009). *Code of Federal Regulations*, Table 45 public welfare, Part 4 protection of human subjects. Retrieved from http://www.hhs.gov/ohrp/humansubjects/guidance/45cfr46.html#46.108

Williams, J., & Murphy, P. (2005). Better project management: Better patient outcomes. *Nursing Management, 36*(11), 41–47.

Nurse Executive and Administration Views of DNP Scholarly Projects: System Change

IMPROVING SEPSIS MORTALITY WITH THE COMPREHENSIVE UNIT-BASED SAFETY PROGRAM

THERESA TRIVETTE

Hospitals worldwide continue to focus efforts to improve overall compliance with delivering evidence-based care for patients with sepsis; however, system failures continue to challenge hospitals in their pursuit to deliver timely effective care in today's healthcare system (Damiani et al., 2015; Djurkovic, Baracaldo, Guerra, Sartorius, & Haupt, 2010). The Institute of Medicine's (IOM) landmark report, *To Err Is Human: Building a Safer Health System* (1999), first highlighted the ongoing difficulty of healthcare systems to deliver consistent safe care, and was the first to focus its report on the need for healthcare organizations to measure, review, and learn from patient safety events and to change the system to deliver safer healthcare (Kohn, Corrigan, & Donaldson, 2000).

Healthcare institutions have demonstrated improved patient outcomes when there is a strong organizational culture of safety that supports teamwork and transparency, encourages learning from mistakes without blame, and rewards employees for success (Goh, Chan, & Kuziemsky, 2013; Hinde, Gale, Anderson, Roberts, & Sice, 2016). Organizations that design performance improvement using a systematic approach that includes teamwork, learning from failures, and robust performance improvement have demonstrated increased compliance with evidence-based care, improved patient outcomes, and a better overall culture of safety (Damiani et al., 2015). The Comprehensive Unit-Based Safety Program (CUSP) provides a structured program to improve the culture of safety as a framework for improving patient outcomes with focused effort to address both adaptive work centered on teamwork and culture as well as technical work specific to standard work of delivering evidence-based practice (Agency for Healthcare Research and Quality [AHRQ], 2016).

The doctor of nursing practice (DNP)-prepared nurse leader is well suited to lead quality improvement (QI) initiatives using the CUSP program to improve evidence-based care. For example, this QI project focused on applying the adaptive work of the CUSP program, coupled with the technical work of the evidence-based sepsis bundle delivered on time, to aid in reducing mortality in patients with a primary diagnosis of severe sepsis or septic shock. The purpose of the project was to evaluate the effectiveness of implementing the key program objectives of the CUSP program to help improve the culture of safety in the ICU and improve sepsis bundle delivery as a strategy to reduce severe sepsis and septic shock mortality. The project team, led by the DNP-prepared nurse leader, used the CUSP as a method to empower frontline staff to participate actively in process improvement to achieve improved communication, teamwork, and evidence-based practice delivery (AHRQ, 2016).

The project team followed these CUSP key components:

- Project leader gathered safety climate, sepsis bundle compliance, and septic shock mortality data to establish baseline performance.
- Quality representative engaged unit staff in the application of the science of safety, performance improvement tools, and effective teamwork principles.
- Project leader engaged executive leadership to support the project and establish behavior accountability with emergency room and ICU providers and staff.
- Team validated current evidence-based protocol for delivery of the sepsis bundle and identified gaps in the guidelines for focus of ongoing improvement.
- Staff applied performance improvement concepts and tools to improve targeted gaps identified in current performance.
- Staff evaluated the success of those performance improvement activities.
- Staff conducted postintervention measurement of the safety culture, process, and outcome measures using same data definitions as baseline measurement (AHRQ, 2016).

Engaging a multidisciplinary team to work together within the CUSP framework resulted in improved safety culture and improved compliance with the delivery of evidence-based care for sepsis patients. This framework allowed open participation and transparency in barriers to consistent delivery of care. The work of the unit not only increased awareness and accountability, but also improved the communication and teamwork between staff and across units with the emergency department and laboratory and pharmacy services. The ICU team focused on improving patient care and building a teamwork and staff engagement to enable reliable evidence-based care delivery. The work of the unit not only increased in awareness and accountability, but also improved the communication and teamwork among staff and across units such as the emergency department and laboratory and pharmacy services. Nursing and physician leaders led monthly discussions regarding science of safety, patient-centered outcomes, and accountability for ensuring the highest quality of care. Senior leadership communicated its commitment to supporting the team's grassroots efforts to reduce mortality. Physician engagement in both the ICU and emergency department settings was also crucial in ensuring improved delivery of the sepsis bundle.

The ICU and emergency department teams also participated in patient safety and process improvement training with a formal rapid improvement event to address gaps identified in the care of the septic patient. A sepsis steering team was chartered and included executive champions, physician champions, nursing leaders from both units, frontline nurses from both units, clinical pharmacists, nurse techs, educators, and infection prevention staff. This team conducted a full analysis of current performance during the first process improvement training week. Frontline staff were engaged in the identification of gaps, solution ideas, and development of grassroots projects intended to address the identified evidence-based practice performance gaps in each unit. The ICU used the structure of its clinical practice committee to address ongoing gaps in continuing the sepsis bundle in the ICU setting. One example of a small test of change included the ICU staff's design of a large poster hung in the patient's room to provide a visual display of the timing of each element of the bundled care continuum for the patient. As the bundle elements were delivered, the time and date were recorded on the visual display as a communication vehicle for the rest of the team. The emergency department team used its grassroots team to develop solutions to address variation in the triage process to ensure all staff understood the standard process to ensure patients that met sepsis alert criteria received the critical elements as quickly as possible. The physicians and pharmacists worked together to ensure timely antibiotic delivery and fluid resuscitation from arrival to and including the ICU stay. To sustain the improvements achieved in those projects, leaders, staff, and physicians reviewed each variance in performance, weekly, to understand the root cause of the variation and identify additional process improvements to implement based on the findings of those weekly reviews.

Using transformational leadership to drive systematic, data-driven organizational change is one of the most important key success factors for a DNP-prepared leader. Therefore, DNP project areas that focus on patient safety, culture of safety, and teamwork are essential fields of study for the DNP student preparing to lead patient care delivery systems in a fast-changing healthcare delivery system fraught with significant complexity and risk for serious harm if care is not delivered in a safe and reliable manner.

INTRODUCING MINDFULNESS AS A TOOL TO REDUCE NURSE LEADERS' STRESS

CHRISTINE BUCKLEY

Today's healthcare environment is a complex, rapidly changing landscape, strewn with competing demands and conflict, often creating a stressful workplace for clinical teams. These stressors may particularly impact nursing leaders. Whether in the role of frontline manager or senior-level executive, all levels of nursing leadership are accountable for clinical imperatives such as meeting extensive regulatory requirements, improving clinical quality, providing access to care, and improving the patient's experience, while concurrently reducing healthcare costs. Nurse leaders oversee the largest workforce in healthcare and are positioned to significantly influence the care environment. These roles set the stage not only for excellence in clinical practice, but also the less tangible aspects of the institution's or unit's culture of care. It is no surprise then that nurse leaders have been identified as particularly vulnerable to the negative effects of excess stress (Judkins, 2004; Pipe & Bortz, 2009; Pipe et al., 2009; Shirey, Ebright, & McDaniel, 2008, 2013; Shirey, McDaniel, Ebright, Fisher, & Doebbeling, 2010). Possible negative impacts of stress have been identified as burnout, poor job performance, or physical ailments (Figley, 1995; Pipe & Bortz, 2009; Pipe et al., 2009; Shirey, 2007; Shirey et al., 2008; Shirey et al., 2013).

Increasingly, mindfulness strategies have been highlighted as an important tool for reducing nursing stress reduction in a variety of healthcare settings (Cohen-Katz, Wiley, Capuano, Baker, & Shapiro, 2004, 2005; McKay, Rajacich, & Rosenbaum, 2002; Pipe & Bortz, 2009; Pipe et al., 2009; Potter et al., 2013; Shirey, 2007; Sitzman & Watson, 2014; Watson, 1999; Watson, 2008). Mindfulness focuses on an awareness of the present moment and a letting go of the past or future concerns. The centering and acceptance afforded through mindfulness practices offers an opportunity to alter one's response to stressful events, thereby attenuating the potential negative effects (Kabat-Zinn, 1994; Pipe et al., 2009; Sitzman & Watson, 2014; Watson, 2008). Several pilot programs reported in the literature focus on introducing mindfulness practices as a stress-reduction or resiliency strategy for staff nurses (Cohen-Katz et al., 2004, 2005; Potter et al., 2013), as well as nurse leaders (Pipe & Bortz, 2009; Pipe et al., 2009). Although there was significant variability in both the structure and measurement tools used in these pilot programs, all demonstrated some measure of success in the reduction of participants' report of symptoms related to stress following an introduction to mindfulness practices (Cohen-Katz et al., 2004, 2005; Pipe & Bortz, 2009; Pipe et al., 2009; Potter et al., 2013).

Encouraging nurse leaders' focus on the present moment through mindfulness provides a stress-reduction tool that may enhance leadership engagement and satisfaction. Learning self-care tools, such as mindfulness, to better manage stress may reduce nurse leaders' perceived stress and help alleviate its negative potential effects. Reducing stress is an important component of a plan to recruit, retain, and engage talented nurse leaders.

This DNP project offered an approach to mindfulness in the workplace intended to explore ways to overcome the barrier of time, as well as the educational or perhaps even cultural gap that overlooks the essential need for self-care. Giving each other and ourselves permission to attend to some basic self-care throughout the day is an important first step to a more present and mindful team. With an already overburdened schedule, the challenge begins with incorporating concepts of mindfulness into our routine. We all breathe, yet we may often be unaware of the potential for our breath to provide much needed centering throughout the day. Simple awareness of our breath before entering a patient's room, breathing together as a group before beginning a meeting, or taking a moment to focus our attention before eating, all have the potential to reduce perceived stress and transform those activities. These simple acts require only the time it takes to inhale and exhale. It is the quality of approach to breathing that may offer an opportunity for a moment of self-care or a stress-release valve throughout the day. Mindfulness practices are just that; a practice and a lifelong endeavor. There are many options to bring mindfulness into our day and each individual must explore and identify what works best. Breath awareness is a basic, universal option that may be offered and incorporated into even the most hectic schedule of the healthcare provider.

I was interested in exploring ways to incorporate mindfulness practices into the workday within the hospital setting as a strategy to mitigate the negative effects of stress. Specifically, I sought to assess whether or not simple mindfulness activities would reduce nurse leaders' experience of perceived stress. Nurse leaders set the stage for the practice environment within their areas and serve as role models for their team. Nurse leaders adept at practicing self-care may be positioned to improve the care environment by their personal attention to being fully present, in addition to creating fertile ground for the entire team to practice self-care.

Jean Watson's Theory of Human Caring provided the theoretical framework for this project. Transpersonal caring relationships beginning with self and then extending outward to others provide the opportunity for caring practices. Embracing altruistic values and practicing loving kindness with self and others are core concepts of this theory. The imperative of self-care is the foundation from where caring for others becomes possible (Watson, 1999, 2008).

During this pilot, I studied the impact of a voluntary 1-hour educational program, followed by the incorporation of 5-minute mindfulness practices into existing nurse leader meetings. The educational session reviewed the importance of self-care and introduced mindfulness practices to the group. Using the Perceived Stress Scale (Cohen, Kamarck, & Mermelstein, 1983) as a simple pre- and posttest, I assessed perceived stress levels of nurse leader participants before and after this simple intervention. Results from this pilot demonstrated a significant reduction in reported stress postintervention among volunteer participants. Additionally, respondents expressed interest in additional interventions and reported a perceived benefit of the program. These results encourage further study to explore mindfulness or other self-care activities that may be incorporated into the clinical setting, positively impacting nurse leaders and consequently, the healthcare environment.

EXPLICATING THEORY-BASED CARE COORDINATION NURSING PRACTICE

JOANNE HOGAN

Several organizations identify care coordination as an essential component to solving the U.S. healthcare crisis (AHRQ, 2010; American Nurses Association, 2012;

National Quality Forum, 2010). Even the Affordable Care Act of 2010 promulgated establishment of care coordination programs to curb costs and improve quality of care (Ferris et al., 2010; Torres, 2012). In 2014, the Advisory Board reported that 97% of the healthcare leaders planned to invest in care coordination personnel (Advisory Board Company, 2014). Care coordination efforts focus on patients with multiple chronic diseases who are at high risk for adverse outcomes, incur high costs of care, and have difficulty accessing care. While new roles and care delivery models emerge to fill the gaps in healthcare, it is increasingly important to leverage the knowledge and skill of nurses. Much is written about nurses as care coordinators. The preponderance of evidence reduces it to tasks in the process of care placing sustainable improvements in jeopardy.

To gain understanding of nurse–patient relationships and caring practices of nurses providing care coordination across the continuum, a mixed methods (MMs) study was undertaken. The nurses practiced within a successful care coordination program, were embedded in primary care sites, and assigned to complex patients who were members of an accountable care organization (ACO). Ethnography was used to observe and identify caring nursing behaviors during telephonic and face-to-face nurse–patient encounters. Directed content analysis enabled categorizing observations to caring theory concepts. In addition, nurses completed the Caring Factor Survey–Care Provider Version (CFS–CPV) to determine their perceptions of caring in clinical practice. Comparative results from observational and survey components of the study provided in-depth understanding of caring practices of nurse care coordinators. Findings informed future roles for nurses, practice development, care delivery models, and health policy in an evolving healthcare system.

■ CHOOSING A THEORY

Expert professional nursing requires theory. Without theory, nursing practice and its outcomes cannot be fully understood, developed, replicated, or expanded. Theory exploration considers the context, values, and essence of expert nursing practice. Investigating successful nursing care coordination uncovers several key components. Nurses' abilities to develop personalized care plans, mobilize and coordinate resources and cross-continuum care, engage patients and families in healthy behaviors, conduct patient education, activate patients and families, and manage resource utilization repeatedly emerge as critical success factors. Direct contact with patients and families and the care team is equally important. Despite the presence of care coordination models and frameworks, descriptors of nursing practice fail to include human caring processes and relationship-based care. To understand caring and relationships in nursing care coordination, Jean Watson's Caring Science Theory serves as a framework to explicate nursing practice (Watson 2008, 2012).

Nurses' abilities to establish caring relationships with their patients and families and extended healthcare teams support continued engagement and motivation in health-promoting behaviors. A brief description of Watson's Ten Caritas Processes provides a glimpse into the concepts required for truly caring relationships.

The Caritas processes describe a worldview of oneness, phenomenology, transpersonal caring relationship, caring occasions, and caring moments. Through the practice of loving-kindness nurses demonstrate compassion, empathy, concern, and equanimity with self and others. Self-care becomes a living exemplar of health and healing. Authentic presence of the nurse instills faith and hope while honoring patients' beliefs and worldviews. Recognition of feelings requires nurses' self-introspection and exploration. Psychological growth leads to sensitivity and acceptance of others' feelings. Nurses and their patients form unions built on trust that transcends the physical environment and honors human dignity and preservation. Encouraging patients' expressions of positive and negative feelings supports healing. Nurses engage in all ways of knowing/being/doing to creatively and systematically provide patient care, thus demonstrating the artistry and science of caring. Wholistic teaching–learning builds upon past experiences, their meaning, and significance to gauge patients' readiness to learn. Healing environments extend beyond the physical to include healing and harmony with the nurse as the integral component. Nurses in caring practice meet patients' unified physical and spiritual needs which are interdependent and equally important to healing. Belief in spiritual mystery opens the nurse and patient to the possibility of miracles (Watson, 2008).

■ DETERMINING METHODOLOGY

MIXED METHOD DESIGN

An MM design requires the planned integration of qualitative and quantitative data and findings. Careful triangulation of qualitative and quantitative data has several advantages. Words and numbers provide for complementary information allowing each to stand on its own or "complement" the other. It may be practical in that one method may answer or address what another cannot. MM can be productive by providing incremental findings simultaneously, exploring and confirming answers to complex questions. Investigators can be more confident in the validity of results when they are supported by more than one type of data. MM encourages further collaboration between qualitative and quantitative researchers with similar interests (Polit & Beck, 2012).

MMs research has practical issues. First and foremost is the skill of the investigator. Competence in both methods is required. Assembling a team with knowledge and understanding of qualitative and quantitative approaches is useful. The cost of collecting, analyzing, and integrating two or more types of data should be considered. MM may also be more time consuming. Developing an accurate timeline before beginning is a wise idea (Polit & Beck, 2012).

CONTENT ANALYSIS

Content analysis is primarily a qualitative research method used to analyze textual data. The text may be verbal, print, or electronic form and obtained by various means: surveys, interviews, observations, focus groups, or print media. The large amount of text is examined intensely for the purpose of systematically classifying into categories that represent similar meaning. Communications can be explicit or inferred for the purpose of categorization (Hsieh & Shannon, 2005). The goal of content analysis is "to provide knowledge and understanding of the phenomenon under study" (Downe-Wamboldt, 1992, p. 313).

Hsieh and Shannon (2005) describe three types of content analysis. Conventional content analysis starts with observation and is most often used to describe a phenomenon with limited theory or literature. Codes and categories are derived and defined from the data and analysis. Summative content analysis begins with keywords that are identified prior to or during analysis. Key words are derived from the literature or investigators' interest.

The third type, directed content analysis, validates, disputes, or extends a theoretical framework or theory (Hsieh & Shannon, 2005). Key theoretical concepts serve as initial coding categories, in this study they are Watson's Ten Caritas Processes. Operational definitions of each concept are determined from the literature. Ethnographic observations of nursing practice are transcribed, intensively reviewed, and categorized or assigned new codes if they could not be categorized. Exemplars serve as explicit descriptive evidence. A content expert as auditor improves accuracy of categorization and trustworthiness and reduces bias.

SURVEY

Literature can reveal valid and reliably tested surveys as one means of quantitative measurement of nursing theory. In this study, the CFS–CPV (J. Nelson & Watson, 2012) was administered to RN care coordinators via RedCap (Harris et al., 2009). The survey was amended to include demographic information. The CFS–CPV is a 10-item Likert scale instrument soliciting providers' (nurses') perceptions of caring in clinical practice. Each item corresponds with one of the Ten Caritas Processes (J. Nelson, Thiel, Hozak, & Thomas, 2016). Mean scores for each item and summative scores were calculated; no items were deleted as the alpha Cronbach was acceptable (alpha = .80) and sample size was small.

TRIANGULATION

Both methods demonstrated support for caring practices of RN care coordinators in relationship with patients. Some Caritas processes were more strongly supported than others. There were minor differences in perceived and observed findings. With regard to extending a theory, there were tangible things such as linking to resources and procuring medications and supplies that nurses did routinely and did not "fit" into one of the Caritas processes. Therefore, an additional pragmatic Caritas process was suggested: Creating intentional connections on behalf of persons for their well-being. These results inform nursing theory, future academic preparation nurses, ongoing education of RN care coordinators, and recruitment and retention.

■ IMPLICATIONS FOR DNP NURSE EXECUTIVES

Explicating theory-based nursing practice has far-reaching implications for DNP nurse executives. The essence and impact of expert nursing practice on cost, quality, patient experience, and clinician work life can have profound influence on policy and new models of care, particularly related to population health and chronic disease management. Understanding nursing practice informs education and development of current and future nurses, and prepares them to successfully assume emerging roles in a new healthcare environment. Finally, directed content analysis is an important method to confirm or extend a theory, thereby adding new nursing knowledge and understanding at the intersection of theory and practice.

ENHANCED HUDDLES: A TRANSLATIONAL TOOL TO BRING EVIDENCE-BASED INFORMATION TO CLINICAL PRACTICE

ROLLIE PEREA

The healthcare industry, as compared to other business enterprises such as banking, manufacturing, computer, finance, and engineering, has lagged behind in QI enhancements. Hospitals have been unable to achieve the highest standard as have most high-reliability, high-risk industries, such as the aviation and nuclear power industries (Chassin & Loeb, 2013). In recent times, healthcare has started to adopt concepts and practices from other industries to attain optimal quality standards. As an example, LEAN Six Sigma manufacturing concepts have been integrated from the automobile industry to healthcare as a means to reduce waste and enhance the overall delivery of care (Koning, Verver, Heuvel, Bisgard, & Does, 2006). Despite the ongoing, protracted efforts by hospitals nationwide, serious clinical events continue to reoccur, such as patient falls, hospital-acquired infection, and medication errors. The fundamental reason hospitals continually fail is the lack of proven change management tools, steadfast leadership, and process changes that reach the true core of the problem (Chassin & Loeb, 2013 p. 469).

One prime example of a major process enhancement in nursing was the creation of the communication tool called "clinical huddles." The concept of huddles has been prevalent in healthcare for nearly a decade and the process continues to evolve (Goldenhar, Brady, Sutcliffe, & Muething, 2013). Originally, the huddle process was created as part of a module within the TEAM STEPPS system created by the AHRQ. The huddle was a team-building tool to increase effective communication through information sharing (Glymph et al., 2015). By utilizing huddles, the act of open dialogue promoted teamwork, increased productivity, improved quality, reduced cost, and ultimately helped achieve desired clinical outcomes (Ajeibe, McNeese-Smith, Phillips, & Leach, 2014). The purpose of early huddles was to promote collaboration, exchange vital information, and increase awareness of patients' concerns (Glymph et al., 2015).

Many nursing articles have discussed the function of safety huddles and the potential benefits to quality care metrics and process issues. One study in particular looked at huddles from a unique perspective. The researchers wanted to learn and dissect the mechanism of change promoted by safety huddles. Instead of simply evaluating the outcomes and end results, they were interested in looking at "how" huddles exacted change. Researchers identified a dearth of literature on how an integrated huddle system is able to improve quality care, reduce patient harm, and diminish patient care errors (Goldenhar et al., 2013). The majority of studies are based on the relationship between huddles and clinical outcomes such as falls and infection reduction, but little on how huddles directly addressed and influenced root cause problems. We have seen the early benefits of huddles, but nursing needs to explore the next evolutionary path of huddles to determine their full influence and long-term value in improving quality care (Goldenhar et al., 2013) Future projects aiming to address the quality deficits of hospitals must involve one of these categories. One such endeavor is described as follows.

■ ENHANCED HUDDLE GENESIS AND MECHANISM OF ACTION

Enhanced Huddles (EH) was a novel tool created by this author as the next evolutionary stage of clinical huddles. EH was trialed and developed through years of observation and analysis in various hospital settings. The EH conceptual model was based on the 1962 Rogers's Innovation Decision Mode. He observed that farmers were delayed in adopting new agriculture concepts, although these ideas could have easily led to profitable and beneficial compensation. As a result, he formulated the Model of the Innovation–Decision Process (Rogers, 2003). He postulated that adopting an innovation was not an impulsive or single overt act, but rather a mental process that occurred in a set pattern or in stages.

Building on Rogers's Innovation-Decision process and combining it with communication benefits of huddles, the EH is a process of adoption designed for the clinical setting. EH has its own unique relevant phases of development specific to frontline clinical staff who utilize clinical huddles. In this model, there are four "phases of actualization." The phases can be both sequential or individuals may leap over phases depending on prior exposure to the concept. The progression through the phases is unpredictable, varied, and, in some cases, it is not necessary for the person to go through the later phases to bring about the desired outcome. A summary of the EH model definition and explanation is detailed next.

■ FOUR PHASES OF ACTUALIZATION

Phase 1: *Functional awareness*—Gaining basic knowledge or "functional awareness." The word functional implies a rudimentary understanding of basic facts with minimal context.

Phase 2: *Practical awareness and application*—Taking the basic information and cognitively processing the information to determine its value to clinical practice.

Phase 3: *Conscious engagement*—Finding meaningful connection and relevance of information and how it affects the patient.

Phase 4: *Deliberate and progressive action*—Transcending focus from a task-based activity to the incorporation of evidence-based practice at all levels of care (Figure 6.1).

■ IMPLEMENTING EH FOR CLINICAL IMPACT

Implementation of the EH model alone does not ensure translational conversion of evidence-based theory to clinical practice. The EH model must be combined with The Joint Commission's recommended change process called Rapid Process Improvement (RPI). RPI advocates the utilization of LEAN Six Sigma and change

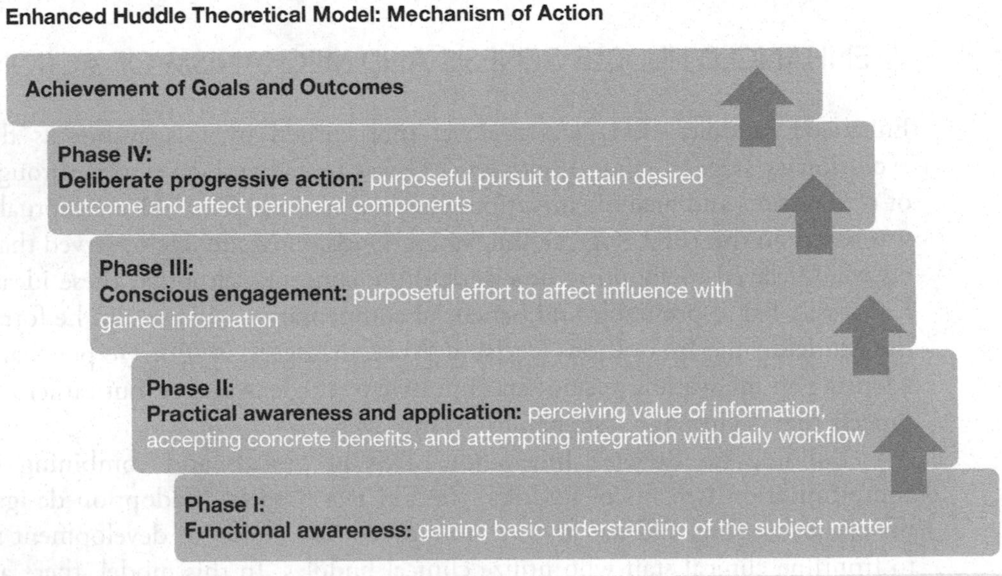

Enhanced Huddle Theoretical Model: Mechanism of Action

Achievement of Goals and Outcomes

Phase IV:
Deliberate progressive action: purposeful pursuit to attain desired outcome and affect peripheral components

Phase III:
Conscious engagement: purposeful effort to affect influence with gained information

Phase II:
Practical awareness and application: perceiving value of information, accepting concrete benefits, and attempting integration with daily workflow

Phase I:
Functional awareness: gaining basic understanding of the subject matter

FIGURE 6.1 **Four phases of actualization.**

Adapted from Rogers, E. (2003). *Diffusion of innovations* (5th ed.). New York, NY: Free Press.

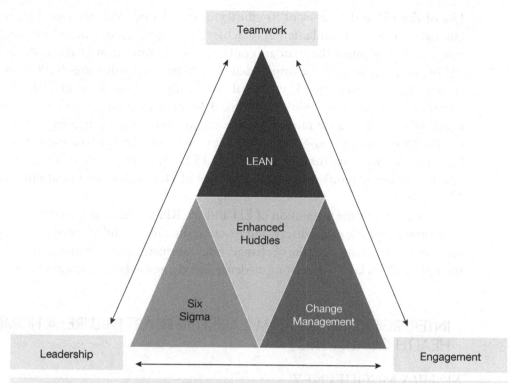

FIGURE 6.2 **RPI and Enhanced Huddle translational conceptual model.**

RPI, Rapid Process Improvement.

management concepts with any quality or process improvement initiative (Chassin & Loeb, 2013). This author postulates that the RPI process requires a vehicle to communicate the enhancements and EH serves that purpose. It is theorized that by combining RPI and EH processes most theory-based protocols can be put into practice and achieve meaningful outcomes. In addition, the EH process promotes the two-way communication between administration and frontline clinical staff to create a culture of change, increase staff engagement, and promote empowerment and teamwork. The combined RPI and EH model best depicts how the combined concepts integrate and create the optimum practice culture (Figure 6.2).

■ EH PROJECT IMPLEMENTATION

The combined EH and RPI change model was implemented at a 125-bed community hospital. Daily huddles were held on both a medical–surgical and telemetry units over a 1-year period. The purpose of the project was to identify practice deficits, process breakdowns, and ultimately create a comprehensive plan to improve inpatient diabetes management as part of the organizational goal to become a Diabetes Center of Excellence as stipulated by The Joint Commission.

Use of the EH and analysis of its efficacy in translating evidence-based research to clinical practice was fundamental to achieving project goals. The subject hospital's aim was to implement the standards outlined by the American Diabetes Association (ADA) and adhere to its recommended clinical practice guidelines (CPG) for inpatient care. There were two key clinical goals measured on the units. The first was administering mealtime insulin within 30 minutes of a finger-stick blood glucose check (85% compliance rate goal). The second was treating hypoglycemic events within 15 minutes (85%–90% compliance rate goal). Initial baseline measures for both metrics were approximately 10% to 15%. The end result of the project was The Joint Commission's award for Certificate of Distinction for In-patient Diabetes Management.

In summary, the integration of EH and the RPI model is an effective process tool in improving quality care delivery, and theoretically can be implemented for any quality care project. Creating a culture of change, empowerment, and communication through the EH model is key to translating evidence-based knowledge to clinical practice.

INTERPROFESSIONAL TEAM CARE FOR HEART FAILURE: A HOME HEALTH QUALITY PILOT

MAURA MCQUEENEY

DNP-prepared nurse executives contribute to nursing knowledge and inquiry when they reframe the phenomena observed in their day-to-day practice using conceptual models and theories that may explain the phenomena, and then test those concepts and theories through sound methods of research, evidence-based practice, and QI in their workplace. A "burning question" for the executive nurse DNP candidate seeking a DNP project focus might be, "If I could improve just one outcome for my unit of responsibility, what would it be?" In this case, my one outcome of concern was a higher than desired rate of hospitalization for patients in the home health setting. The DNP project that reframed this frustrating leadership challenge and tamed it to become a workplace solution was both exciting and gratifying.

Patients with a primary diagnosis of heart failure represent 15.9% of the total Medicare beneficiary population, which is one of the most frequently referred populations for skilled home healthcare services in the United States. Nationally, 30-day rehospitalization rates from the skilled home healthcare setting for all diagnoses average 13.3%. The objective of this QI study was to determine the feasibility and effectiveness of an interprofessional team's synchronous planning, coordination, and evaluation of care for patients with heart failure in the home health setting. This model represents an enhancement to the traditional home healthcare delivery model whereby a single nurse asynchronously plans, coordinates, and evaluates care with other disciplines involved, communicating details of the plan via phone, email, voice mail, or medical record notation.

■ BACKGROUND

A paucity of evidence exists for studies on effective models of care for patients with heart failure in the home healthcare setting. The medical literature points to certain single interventions such as home telemonitoring, home nursing visits, patient education programs, and telephonic follow-up studies; however, no studies examine a team approach that coordinates and targets the resources of multiple professional disciplines in the home health setting covered under the current Medicare Home Health benefit. Care coordination is defined as the organization of patient care between the patient, caregivers, and healthcare providers to improve the delivery of care (McDonald et al., 2007).

Few care coordination models have been developed specifically for home healthcare (Parker et al., 2014), and methods of care coordination are not specifically mandated. Therefore, most Medicare-certified home health agencies deliver care thus: an RN opens a case and then may request that other professionals see the patient once the RN attains a physician order for additional therapy. Ruggiano (2012), who has studied effective clinical communication in home care comments, "One specific area that should be explored is how interprovider communication and collaboration in homecare is affecting patient outcomes. More research is needed to determine the effectiveness of potential interventions aimed at improving interprovider communication" (p. 292).

This feasibility study applied an interprofessional team approach to 35 patients with heart failure admitted to a Medicare-certified home health agency over a 3-month period. The team hypothesized that meeting three times weekly to discuss patient goals and decide by consensus on visit type and frequency for each patient would improve communication, care coordination, and reduce patient rehospitalization rates.

■ CONCEPTUAL FRAMEWORK

I used Donabedian's (1988) framework for appraising healthcare quality and E. C. Nelson and colleague's (2002) concept of QI within healthcare microsystems. Donabedian's (1988) framework emphasizes three factors in evaluating healthcare services: structures, processes, and outcomes. E. C. Nelson et al. (2002) proposed that improving healthcare quality requires system redesign on two levels—large system and small system—and that conditions for improvement include learning, measuring improvement, and accountability. Nelson and colleagues espoused a theory that the small systems or clinical microsystems are the small, functional, frontline units that provide the most healthcare to the most people can attain peak performance by methodically approaching problems and that specific processes blend together to improve quality and job enjoyment. They also contended that measurement becomes a friend of change.

■ METHODS

The entire agency where I am the executive leader was informed about the pilot goals so that intake and support staff could properly identify patients eligible for the pilot study. Ten professional and support staff volunteered for the pilot study to apply an enhanced care coordination model to patients with a primary diagnosis of heart failure.

The interprofessional team structure consisted of me as the administrative leader, one advanced practice RN, one RN with extensive experience in care of patients with heart disease, one physical therapist, one occupational therapist, one home health aide, one registered dietician, one registered pharmacist (joined by phone conference call), and two medical social workers. Additional RN and physical therapists joined as needed to substitute for core team members during vacation days. Patients and families were considered team members, as were the community physicians of record. These latter team members did not join the team coordination sessions though they were invited to do so in an introductory letter.

Team goals were to incorporate the principles and values of effective team healthcare into a home healthcare team pilot that targeted patients with a primary diagnosis of heart failure and to measure the time, cost, and 30-day rehospitalization rates for the study participants. All patients with a primary diagnosis of heart failure were directed to the pilot RN caseload for a period of 3 months. The interprofessional team met every Monday, Wednesday, and Friday for 1 hour in the morning to review the cases admitted and to coordinate the interprofessional schedules for each patient to assure that the patient received a full complement of professional visits from the team.

■ RESULTS

The pilot group 30-day rehospitalization rate was 11.4%. This compared favorably to the 30-day rehospitalization rate of 18.62% in the same agency for 524 patients with heart failure (ICD 9 428) treated in the 12-month period prior to the pilot project. Cost per episode for the pilot patients reflected a higher use of visits overall; particularly, the more costly occupational therapy visits. In contrast, the pilot used the team home health aide at a lower frequency than was found in the prior year. The pilot cost per episode was $2,090.42 compared to the prior year group episode average of $1,761.00. In a global payment model, this added cost of less than $400.00 represents 10% of the average hospitalization cost of $4,000.00 and demonstrates for the agency's ACO partner that it can be a *value* partner. The agency can save the high cost of hospitalization and can assemble an interprofessional team in short order to cocreate new pathways in home health delivery.

■ REFERENCES

Advisory Board Company. (2014). High-risk patient care management. Retrieved from http://www.advisory.com/research/health-care-advisory-board/studies/2012/high-risk-patient-care-management

Agency for Healthcare Research and Quality. (2010). *The roles of patient-centered medical homes and accountable care organizations in coordinating patient care.* Retrieved from https://pcmh.ahrq.gov/page/roles-patient-centered-medical-homes-and-accountable-care-organizations-coordinating-patient

Agency for Healthcare Research and Quality. (2016). Comprehensive unit-based safety program (CUSP). Retrieved from http://www.ahrq.gov/professionals/quality-patient-safety/cusp/index.html

Ajeibe, D., McNeese-Smith, D., Phillips, D., & Leach, L. (2014). Effect of nurse-physician teamwork in the emergency department: Nurse-physician perception of job satisfaction. *Journal of Nursing & Care, 3*, 1–8. doi:10.4172/2167–1168.1000141

American Nurses Association. (2012). *The value of nursing care coordination: A white paper of the American Nurses Association.* Retrieved from http://www.nursingworld.org/carecoordinationwhitepaper

Chassin, M., & Loeb, J. (2013). *High-reliability health care: Getting there from here.* Retrieved from http://www.jointcommission.org/assets/1/6/Chassin_and_Loeb_0913_final.pdf

Cohen, S., Kamarck, T., & Mermelstein, R. (1983). A global measure of perceived stress. *Journal of Health and Social Behavior, 24*(4), 385–396.

Cohen-Katz, J., Wiley, S. D., Capuano, T., Baker, D. M., & Shapiro, S. (2004). The effects of mindfulness-based stress reduction on nurse stress and burnout: A quantitative and qualitative study. *Holistic Nursing Practice, 18*(6), 302–308.

Cohen-Katz, J., Wiley, S. D., Capuano, T., Baker, D. M., & Shapiro, S. (2005). The effects of mindfulness-based stress reduction on nurse stress and burnout, part II: A quantitative and qualitative study. *Holistic Nursing Practice, 19*(1), 26–35.

Cohen-Katz, J., Wiley, S. D., Capuano, T., Baker, D. M., Deitrick, L., & Shapiro, S. (2005). The effects of mindfulness-based stress reduction on nurse stress and burnout: A quantitative and qualitative study, part III. *Holistic Nursing Practice, 19*(2), 78–86.

Damiani, E., Donati, A., Serafini, G., Rinaldi, L., Adrario, E., Pelaia, P., . . . Girardis, M. (2015). Effect of performance improvement programs on compliance with sepsis bundles and mortality: A systematic review and meta-analysis of observational studies. *PLOS ONE, 10*(5), e0125827. doi:10.1371/journal.pone.0125827

Djurkovic, S., Baracaldo, J. C., Guerra, J. A., Sartorius, J., & Haupt, M. T. (2010). A survey of clinicians addressing the approach to the management of severe sepsis and septic shock in the United States. *Journal of Critical Care, 25*(4), 658.e1–658.e6. doi:10.1016/j.jcrc.2010.04.005

Donabedian, A. (1988). The quality of care: How can it be assessed? *Journal of the American Medical Association, 260*, 1743–1748.

Downe-Wamboldt, B. (1992). Content analysis: Method, application, and issues. *Health Care for Women International, 13*(3), 313–321.

Ferris, T., Weil, E., Meyer, G., Neagle, M., Heffernan, J. L., & Torchiana, D. F. (2010). Cost savings from managing high-risk patients. In National Research Council, *The healthcare imperative: Lowering costs and improving outcomes: Workshop series summary* (pp. 301–310). Washington, DC: National Academies Press.

Figley, C. R. (1995). Compassion fatigue: Toward a new understanding of the cost of caring. in B. H. Stamm (Ed.), *Secondary Traumatic Stress: Self-care issues for clinicians, researchers and educators* (2nd ed., pp. 3–28). Lutherville, MD: Sidran.

Gabow, P. & Conway P.H. (2015). Lean: *a comprehensive approach to the transformation our health care system needs.* Retrieved from http://healthaffairs.org/blog/2015/08/13/lean-a-comprehensive-approach-to-the-transformation-our-health-care-system-needs

Glymph, D., Olenick, M., Barbera, S., Brown, E., Prestianni, L., & Miller, C. (2015). Healthcare utilizing deliberate discussion linking events (huddles): A systematic review. *AANA Journal, 83*(3), 183–188.

Goh, S. C., Chan, C., & Kuziemsky, C. (2013). Teamwork, organizational learning, patient safety and job outcomes. *International Journal of Health Care Quality Assurance, 26*(5), 420–432. doi:10.1108/IJHCQA-05-2011-0032

Goldenhar, L., Brady, P., Sutcliffe, K., & Muething, S. (2013). Huddling for high reliability and situation awareness. *BMJ Quality Safety, 22*, 899–906. doi:10.1136/bmjqs-2012–001467

Harris, P. A., Taylor, R., Thielke, R., Payne, J., Gonzalez, N., & Conde, J. G. (2009). Research electronic data capture (REDCap)—A metadata-driven methodology and workflow process for providing translational research informatics support. *Journal of Biomedical Informatics, 42*(2), 377–381.

Hinde, T., Gale, T., Anderson, I., Roberts, M., & Sice, P. (2016). A study to assess the influence of interprofessional point of care simulation training on safety culture in the operating theatre environment of a university teaching hospital. *Journal of interprofessional care, 30*(2), 251–253. doi:103109/13561820.2015.1084277

Hsieh, H. F., & Shannon, S. E. (2005). Three approaches to qualitative content analysis. *Qualitative Health Research, 15*(9), 1277–1288. doi:10.1177/1049732305276687

Judkins, S. K. (2004). Stress among nurse managers: Can anything help? *Nurse Researcher, 12*(2), 58–70. doi:10.7748/nr2004.10.12.2.58.c5939

Kabat-Zinn, J. (1994). *Wherever you go there you are: Mindfulness meditation in everyday life.* New York, NY: Hyperion.

Kohn, L. T., Corrigan, J. M., & Donaldson, M. S. (Eds.). (2000). *To err is human: Building a safer health system.* Washington, DC: National Academy Press. doi:10.17226/9728

Koning, H., Verver, J., van den Heuvel, J., Bisgard, S., & Does, R. (2006). Lean six sigma in healthcare. *Journal of Healthcare Quality, 28*(2), 4–11.

McDonald, K. M., Sundaram, V., Bravata, D. M., Lewis, R., Lin, N., Kraft, S., . . . Owens, D. K. (2007). *Closing the quality gap: A critical analysis of quality improvement strategies* (Vol. 7: Care Coordination, pp. 33–50). Rockville, MD: Agency for Healthcare Research and Quality. Retrieved from https://www.ncbi.nlm.nih.gov/books/NBK44012

McKay, P., Rajacich, D., & Rosenbaum, J. (2002). Enhancing palliative care through Watson's carative factors. *Canadian Oncology Nursing Journal, 12*(1), 34–44.

National Quality Forum. (2010). *Measurement framework: Evaluating efficiency across patient-focused episodes of care.* Retrieved from http://www.qualityforum.org/Publications/2010/01/Measurement_Framework__Evaluating_Efficiency_Across_Patient-Focused_Episodes_of_Care.aspx

Nelson, E. C., Batalden, P. B., Huber, T. P., Mohr, J. J., Godfrey, M. M., Headrick, L. A., & Wasson, J. H. (2002). Microsystems in health care: Part 1. Learning from high-performing front-line clinical units. *The Joint Commission Journal on Quality Improvement. 28*(9), 472–493.

Nelson, J., Thiel, L., Hozak, M. A., & Thomas, T. (2016). Item reduction of the Caring Factor Survey-Care Provider Version, an instrument specified to measure Watson's 10 processes of caring. *International Journal for Human Caring, 20*, 123–128. doi:10.20467/1091-5710-20.3.123

Nelson, J., & Watson, J. (2012). *Measuring caring international research on caritas as healing.* New York, NY: Springer Publishing.

Parker, E., Zimmerman, B. A., Rodriquez, S., & Lee, T. (2014). Exploring best practices in home health care: A review of available evidence on select innovations. *Home Health Care Management & Practice, 26*(1), 17–33. doi:10.1177/1084822313499916

Pipe, T. B., & Bortz, J. (2009). Mindful leadership as healing practice: Nurturing self to serve others. *International Journal for Human Caring, 13*(2), 34–38.

Pipe, T. B., Bortz, J. J., Dueck, A., Pendergast, D., Buchda, V., & Summers, J. (2009). Nurse leader mindfulness meditation program for stress management. *The Journal of Nursing Administration, 39*(3), 130–137. doi:10.1097/NNA.0b013e31819894a0

Polit, D. F., & Beck, C. T. (2012). *Nursing research* (9th ed.). New York, NY: Wolters Kluwer/ Lippincott Williams & Wilkins.

Potter, P., Deshields, T., Berger, J. A., Clarke, M., Olsen, S., & Chen, L. (2013). Evaluation of a compassion fatigue resiliency program for oncology nurses. *Oncology Nursing Forum, 40*, 180–187. doi:10.1188/13.ONE. 180–187

Rogers, E. (2003). *Diffusion of Innovations* (5th ed.). New York, NY: Free Press.

Shirey, M. R. (2007). An evidence-based solution for minimizing stress and anger in nursing students. *Journal of Nursing Education, 46*(12), 568–568.

Shirey, M. R., Ebright, P. R., & McDaniel, A. M. (2008). Sleepless in America: Nurse managers cope with stress and complexity. *The Journal of Nursing Administration, 38*(3), 125–131. doi:10.1097/01.NNA.0000310722.35666.73

Shirey, M. R., Ebright, P. R., & McDaniel, A. M. (2013). Nurse manager cognitive decision-making amidst stress and work. *Journal of Nursing Management, 21*, 17–30. Retrieved from http://dx.doi.org/10.1111/j.1365–2834.2012.01380.x

Shirey, M. R., McDaniel, A. M., Ebright, P. R., Fisher, M. L., & Doebbeling, B. N. (2010). Understanding nurse manager stress and work complexity. *The Journal of Nursing Administration, 40*(2), 82–91.

Sitzman, K., & Watson, J. (2014). *Caring science, mindful practice: Implementing Watson's Human Caring Theory.* New York, NY: Springer Publishing.

Torres, C. (2012). *Report: Health spending will climb to nearly one fifth of GNP.* Kaiser Health News. Retrieved from http://kaiserhealthnews.org/news/ report-health-spending-will-climb-to- nearly-one-fifth-of-GNP

Watson, J. (1999). *Postmodern nursing and beyond.* Edinburgh, Scotland: Churchill Livingstone.

Watson, J. (2008). *Nursing: The philosophy and science of caring* (Rev. ed.). Boulder: University Press of Colorado.

Watson, J. (2012). *Human caring science a theory of nursing* (2nd ed.). Sudbury, MA: Jones & Bartlett.

DNP Scholarly Projects: Students' Experiences

FAMILY NURSE PRACTITIONER SEEKS TO BETTER IDENTIFY AND COUNSEL VACCINE HESITANT PARENTS

JOHN T. CONNORS

The basis for my doctor of nursing practice (DNP) project was my research findings from my master's thesis (barriers and facilitators to childhood vaccination), where I identified the themes of provider characteristics (knowledge about vaccines and offering immunizations) and targeted education as affecting the immunization status of children (Connors et al., 2012). In my subsequent clinical practice as a family nurse practitioner (FNP), I noted the difficulty in speaking with vaccine hesitant (VH) parents and identifying and discussing their specific vaccination concerns in an efficient and efficacious manner. I delved into the literature in an attempt to discern how to maximize the ability of a clinical practice to identify VH in parents, increase the quality of the provider–parent interaction, and decrease the level of VH, thereby increasing the level of vaccination in the patient population. However, the research evidence did not support any definitive answers to improve my ability to identify VH and increase my technical and communication competency in dealing with VH parents.

As such, I incorporated current research evidence (screening questionnaires, identified categories of VH, and provider–parent communication practices) to develop my DNP project which sought to determine whether using a VH screening tool in conjunction with increased provider competency in addressing parental vaccination concerns during face to face provider–parent interactions would impact the parental intent to vaccinate (ITV). Additionally, I hoped to generate evidence-based data applicable to providers treating pediatric patients in support of increasing VH screening and decreasing VH among parents.

■ CHALLENGES: IDENTIFYING AND CATEGORIZING FACTORS THAT CONTRIBUTE TO VH AND WHERE TO INTERVENE TO AFFECT CHANGE IN A PARENT'S VACCINATION BEHAVIOR

Major challenges that I encountered while developing my DNP project include the difficulty categorizing the components of VH identified from the literature and identifying the point where an intervention is possible to affect parental behavior with regards to vaccination. In essence, I had difficulty finding a theoretical framework that would overall guide the study design. Discussions regarding these issues with my research advisor and several professors allowed me to refine a conceptual map that identified the different components of VH and their relationships to one another as well as the ITV. One of my professors suggested that the theory of planned behavior (TPB) as put forth by Ajzen (1991) would allow an examination of the components that affect the provider–parent interaction as well as the parent's decision not to vaccinate his or her child.

The TPB helped me refine my literature search and focus in on the factors that contribute to VH and how these factors might be affected by the provider–parent interaction. Utilizing the TPB, I found that the VH components that contributed the most to parental VH were generally able to be categorized in one of four categories. These categories were unease about vaccine efficacy, vaccine safety, prevalence of vaccine preventable disease in the community, and trust in the provider. The challenges of categorizing these findings from the literature and making a coherent argument that focused on the parental beliefs that lead to VH would not have been possible without using the TPB as a framework. The TPB also identified the point where an intervention is possible to affect the identified determinants of behavior as well as provide a framework to measure the parent level of VH and the parent ITV.

■ CHALLENGE: PERFORMING EFFECTIVE PROVIDER–PARENT EDUCATION

An additional challenge that I encountered was the lack of time that the provider has to discuss a parent's concerns regarding vaccination. This lack of time has been listed as being the most common barrier to discussing vaccination concerns with parents (Davis et al., 2001). Hence, I had to find an educational framework for providers to use with parents that was seen to be not only efficacious but efficient as well. After a discussion with several professors on patient teaching frameworks, I was able to identify the representational approach (RA) to patient education as put forth by Ward, Heidrich, and Donovan (2007) as an additional theoretical framework that could be used to guide the provider–parent discussion. The RA uses a five-step process to perform individualized patient education. The five steps as outlined in an article by Donovan and Ward (2001) are as follows: representational assessment (patient account), exploring misconceptions, creating conditions for conceptual change (link between mistaken beliefs and acting on them), introducing replacement information, and summarizing. The providers at the clinical site where my project was performed were amenable to utilizing the RA to patient education as this framework allowed a focused and participatory discussion over parental vaccination concerns and misconceptions in an efficient manner.

■ SUMMARY AND CONCLUSION

My relationships with course professors and my research chair were helpful in aiding me to identify the TPB and the RA to patient education as frameworks that informed my overall project design. These frameworks helped to guide my intervention, measure VH, guide the provider–parent interaction, and increase provider technical and communication competency during discussions about parent vaccine concerns.

CAREGIVER ASTHMA KNOWLEDGE AND CHILDREN'S ASTHMA CONTROL: CHALLENGES ENCOUNTERED

PAULETTE D. LONG

My lifework as a pediatric nurse practitioner (NP) and educator spans over three decades and has been devoted to providing care for underserved children living with asthma. Most of the children are from impoverished Black families residing in urban metropolitan communities, have limited access to optimal healthcare services, and are five times more likely to die from asthma than their counterparts (Akinbami, Moorman, & Liu, 2011). Whether providing nursing care in an inner-city school setting, emergency department, or ambulatory care clinic, asthma education was an essential component of the services offered in an effort to empower caregivers of children most adversely affected. The many years spent providing pediatric asthma care proved to be effective, resulted in favorable health outcomes, but did not generate evidence-based research that would impact clinical practice guidelines.

■ THE DECISION TO ACCEPT THE CALL

While attending a pediatric nurse practitioner conference, the participants were challenged to consider enrollment in a DNP program. The thought-provoking message spoke to the emerging role of the DNP leader, the generation and translation of evidence-based research, and "giving credit" to nurses for care previously and now rendered in multiple healthcare settings. The "call" was a challenge that I was willing to explore. The epiphanic decision to accept the challenge was a pivotal moment in my nursing career. The demands and rigor of the program, initially, were not fully realized. The enormous amount of time that would be needed, while juggling multiple roles and responsibilities, became actualized during the culminating processes of project development and program completion.

■ AN OBSERVED PHENOMENA

My retrospective observation of early asthma management includes the bronchodilator effect of home remedies such as Vicks VapoRub, Coca Cola, and make-shift mist tents. The emergence of evidence-based recommendations and an intradisciplinary approach would later progress asthma management to the use of rescue inhalers, nebulization, corticosteroids, leukotriene inhibitors, peak flow meters, and individualized asthma action plans. Further medical advancement led to focusing on environmental control and genomic considerations (Szefler, 2010). Despite the noteworthy medical strides achieved and development of the national asthma prevention and management guidelines, emphasis on caregiver education remains one of multiple gaps observed in pediatric asthma care (National Heart, Lung, and Blood Institute, 2015). Thus, the aim of my DNP scholarly project would examine the impact of caregiver education on asthma control in children.

■ MEETING THE DEMANDS

Numerous challenges were faced throughout the process of completing the DNP program. The greatest challenge was establishing a timeline instituting effective time-management strategies. Once the program requirements were realized, the initial step was to enlist the support of my spouse, family and friends, and colleagues. All were informed about the vast amount of time that would be relegated to the project and program of study. The course work, development of research papers, extensive practicum hours, obtaining institutional review board (IRB) approval, collecting and analyzing data, and preparing for presentations and the final defense would be arduous and time-consuming. Having significant support from all stakeholders was an invaluable resource and necessity.

Each program course required extensive data gathering, research synthesis, and analytics. Scheduled and ad hoc committee and group meetings became the new norm. Virtual and on-campus presentations were a given in the hybrid program of study. While there were other challenges, the greatest challenge throughout the completion process was the immeasurable amount of time that was required during each phase of the program.

The recruitment of project participants was most time-consuming. Although the participants were selected from a convenience sample, many did not maintain scheduled appointments, meet the inclusion criteria, or opted not to participate in the project. Data collection was conducted twice a week for 8 hours each day. The entire process spanned a 6-month period instead of the expected 3 months. Albeit the selection survey tools were appropriate for the reading level of the study participants, the extended amount of time actually spent completing the surveys was not anticipated. Once the data were collected and entered for statistical analysis, progress was interrupted with an unexpected occurrence involving a computer glitch and faulty software package. Reentry of the data and analyses required additional trips to the university's computer lab to complete the final statistical analysis. Unforeseen occurrences and delays required determination, perseverance, and flexibility.

Administrative support is essential as is a "good fit" work environment that encourages and promotes nursing faculty to pursue doctoral education. Additional work-release hours were required and approved by nursing administration in order to meet the program's requirement. Countless hours were spent researching the literature, developing and revising course work and presentations. Unexpected interruptions in the pre-established timeline mandated considerable flexibility, determination, and perseverance. The effective use of time management and prioritization, within a realistic timeline, were key strategies in order to avoid burnout and exhaustion.

■ THE FINAL ANALYSIS

Feedback from colleagues, the committee chair, and committee members resulted in constructive dialogue that was fundamental to the development and defense of the final DNP project. The original title of the preliminary descriptive correlational study was dubbed *Asthma Knowledge Among Caregivers of Urban Black School-Age Children and the Children's Asthma Control in a Pediatric Ambulatory Care Setting*. The final title was later changed to *Caregiver Asthma Knowledge and Children's Asthma Control*. The project findings were well supported in the current literature, promoted further inquiry, and resulted in translational research that would influence current clinical practice guidelines in pediatric asthma care. In the end, the long hours and tedious work proved to be well worth the undertaking and inestimable journey.

ADULT GERONTOLOGY ACUTE CARE NP SEEKS TO IMPROVE PERFORMANCE WITH ANTICOAGULATION MANAGEMENT

PAMELA A. BESSMER

■ NARROWING DOWN A TOPIC

As nurses, we are constantly observing the world around us. We work to improve the experience and outcomes for our patients and for our profession. Throughout my doctoral coursework and while working in cardiac surgery as an acute care NP, I had developed several areas of interest I wanted to further investigate for my DNP scholarly project.

The first topic I chose was preoperative skin preparation, specifically around intranasal mupirocin (MPN). In my clinical practice, we had been utilizing intranasal MPN for all patients preoperatively, as a part of the prophylactic antibiotic initiative of the surgical care improvement project (SCIP) created by the Centers for Medicare and Medicaid Services (CMS) and The Joint Commission (2010). I had observed in my practice that not every patient completed the MPN and chlorhexidine (CHG) baths preoperatively, not every patient was a carrier of methicillin-resistant *Staphylococcus aureus* (MRSA), and a few patients were still developing sternal wounds postoperatively. My initial thought for my scholarly project was to develop or refine an existing guideline for preoperative skin preparation. Once I really delved into the subject area, I found that I was getting deeper and deeper into a subject that would be hard to engage all the different elements (inpatients, outpatients, scheduled, and emergent surgeries) and engage all the stakeholders (outpatient and inpatient providers, pharmacists, physicians, perioperative providers, nurses, just to name a few) in order to complete and institute a new guideline effectively. The project was much larger than what would be practical for a scholarly project. My professors and advisor were invaluable in helping me come to this realization early in the process, which allowed me to transition to a new topic.

The second topic of interest for my scholarly project was postdischarge follow-up phone calls to improve satisfaction and outcomes in our patient population. I had completed the literature review, made contacts with and obtained permissions from authors of previous studies whose material I wanted to incorporate in my study, and I had began to put together a list of questions that had been well validated when I approached key stakeholders at the institution where I would be implementing my performance improvement (PI) project. It was at this stage that I discovered that the institution was already planning on initiating postdischarge phone calls and were going to be utilizing questions that another surgical department had already put into use. As a result, I abandoned my second potential project topic.

The third and final topic that I chose for my scholarly project was a PI project around a novel method to improve tracking for warfarin anticoagulation management. My target population would be patients discharged home with no plans for long-term management at time of discharge. In my practice setting, we had recently implemented an electronic medical record (EMR), which had been used at other institutions to aid in tracking anticoagulation management. As our provider team had grown and had become less centralized in one workspace, former methods of tracking these patients discharged on warfarin anticoagulation, on a white board or via email, had become more challenging to utilize effectively. Therefore, the goal was that through the implementation of a tracking system within the EMR we would improve our ability to track these patients.

As a result of my previous experiences with my first two topic choices and as a result of all the feedback I received from my professors, advisor, and committee members, I knew that I had to keep my topic very narrowed and involve key stakeholders very early on in the process in order to be successful. As soon as I had identified my third topic area, I developed a list of key stakeholders from all disciplines that could be involved in the successful implementation of my PI project and approached these key stakeholders to engage them. My goals were simple: to seek their buy-in, obtain suggestions for ways I might improve and better focus my project, and obtain their approval. Given that my scholarly project involved medication, I involved pharmacy; the EMR, I involved information systems and technology because of the EMR component;

and in order to be successful with implementation, I involved subject matter experts: clinical leaders, attending physicians, and practitioners on the inpatient team.

■ SUMMARIZING LESSONS LEARNED

From the varied experiences I had in an effort to decide on a topic, I learned one of the most important lessons along the journey to complete my scholarly project: involve key stakeholders as early as possible and keep them involved throughout the course of your project and during your implementation. These stakeholders can make or break your efforts and be your best ally.

Once you have decided on an area of interest or a topic, remember to keep your project focused. Have a solid idea of what you want to accomplish and then get even more focused from there. Unfortunately, the DNP scholarly project isn't meant to be a discipline-changing contribution; you are just demonstrating what you have learned throughout your coursework and are putting it to task—working through the process. Do not be disappointed! You are demonstrating through your scholarly project all that you have learned throughout your doctoral coursework. Save the discipline-changing work for your next project after you graduate!

Timelines are very helpful in keeping you focused. Make a general timeline and be prepared to revise it as you go. Some tasks will be faster than others to accomplish and others will take longer. Have patience with yourself and with the process. Speaking of patience, be prepared to revise your paper. Your committee members, peers, and advisors are offering you excellent advice—take it! Revise, revise, and revise again. Heed their suggestions. They have been where you are!

Congratulations! You are on your way to creating the seminal contribution toward your doctoral degree. Now is the time for you to synthesize all of your experience and education and show off all that you have learned.

PSYCHIATRIC MENTAL HEALTH NP TACKLES POLICY REDESIGN TO IMPROVE OUTCOMES FOR PATIENTS DUALLY DIAGNOSED

CENEAN WALLS RAPHEMOT

In clinical practice as a board-certified psychiatric mental health NP, I bear intimate witness to great pain, suffering, and hopelessness. For those lives dually diagnosed with the cooccurring presence of at least one psychiatric disorder as well as an alcohol or drug use disorder, the pain swells in neglect by a health system largely lacking the capability to provide best care—an integrated, concurrent delivery of mental health and substance use treatment (Barrowclough et al., 2001; Carmichael, Tackett-Gibson, & Dell, 1998; Drake et al., 2001; Mangrum, Spence, & Lopez, 2006; Tiet & Schutte, 2012; Torrey et al., 2002). According to McGovern, Lambert-Harris, Gotham, Claus, and Xie (2014), scarcely 18% of addiction treatment centers and 9%

of mental health programs met criteria for dual diagnosis-capable services. The lack of behavioral health treatment programs with the capability to serve patients with dual diagnosis has negatively impacted treatment in this population—a population already primed for poorer outcomes, including higher rates of relapse, chronic medical conditions, suicide, homelessness, violence, incarceration, inpatient hospitalization, and a lower quality of life (Baillargeon, Binswanger, Penn, Williams, & Murray, 2009; Hunt, Bergen, & Bashir, 2002; Rosenberg et al., 2001).

Attempting to cure the ailment without attending to known inadequacies in treatment delivery (i.e., behavioral health settings without dual diagnosis capability) overlooks the essence of healthcare and allows for the sustainment of poor outcomes among individuals suffering with dual diagnosis. Patient after patient, I met the moment of having little more to extend other than fragmented care—more referrals to intensive outpatient programs, more appointments, and more prescriptions from health practitioners all separate and noncollaborative in care. The concern was sobering: if nothing changed I could likely find myself a part of the pain in a patient's life, and not a part of the healing. The question weighed heavy: Could using programmatic guidance and evaluation instruments—such as the Dual Diagnosis Capability in Addiction Treatment (DDCAT) and COMPASS-EZ— successfully facilitate the development of an integrated, concurrent delivery of mental heath and substance use treatment in community-based behavioral health agencies? I knew something had to change, and after years of studying human behavior I knew that change was never easy.

■ THE CHALLENGES OF ORGANIZATIONAL CHANGE AND INNOVATION

And so, if we were sharing a cup of tea like old friends in a quaint tucked away café, I would tell you that my DNP project experience was not the picture of smooth sails riding graceful winds; it will always be my constant reminder that navigating quality improvement (QI) in clinical practice requires grit, committed champion-stakeholder collaboration, and a dogged prioritization toward best practice, best outcomes. Systematic program evaluation and analysis using the DDCAT and COMPASS-EZ unearthed 15 service gaps barring agency capability to serve clients with dual diagnosis. Fifteen! I took a deep breath—the "weight of the world on your shoulders" kind of breath, inhaling and exhaling one thought: How are we ever going to do it all? The challenges of QI include the reality that there are often many things to improve.

Collecting each voice in roundtable discussion, I listened closely; all stakeholders (i.e., patient, provider, administration, state funding entities, etc.) upheld their chief concerns for QI action with benevolently competing priorities. Every service gap *was* important to address, however the very real limitations of community behavioral health resources and time would also mean I would need to exercise the very real opportunity of acute decision making. Some organizational changes would lead first while others would inevitably be tackled in a different season. A DNP progression in scholarship (research), theory, finance, and healthcare leadership would offer me the knowledge base to elect these lead changes with strategic confidence. I would come to learn that at the core of any successful organizational change is *in actuality* successful change in organizational members' behavior; that changes at the system level within a healthcare organization have the upstream concentration of stimulus and sustainability to alter the infrastructure for all acts (behaviors) of clinical service and administration; and that, accordingly, system-level changes such as policy development and/or protocol redesign would yield the greatest return (i.e., improving patient outcomes, quality of the patient care experience, healthcare costs, and welfare of clinician and staff) for that which was invested.

■ "LOCATING THE LIGHTHOUSE" — SUCCESSFUL QI NAVIGATION

As the operational lighthouse navigates maritime pilots to increasing safety, likewise the collective application of two independent instruments proved increasingly useful to guide and measure the efficacy of QI efforts across "unchartered waters." The decision to use two instruments for program evaluation rather than a single tool was the turning point of this DNP project. First, all evidence-based instruments in the evaluation of dual diagnosis capability were collected and examined for application to the project. Appropriate in validity and reliability and suited to the project's population and clinical milieu, two independent instruments—DDCAT and COMPASS-EZ—emerged for judicious discussion with the doctoral chair and the DNP project committee (Substance Abuse and Mental Health Services Administration [SAMHSA], 2011; ZiaPartners, Inc., 2016). I entered the conference of mentors convinced that the significant question of decision was "Which instrument should I determine to use?" and left actively searching the significance of a different question, "Why not use both?"

And so, the DDCAT and COMPASS-EZ were both employed—not for means of comparison, rather dually operated for a concerted effect adding breadth (scale) and depth (penetration) of evaluation and QI action. Utilization of the two tools side-by-side granted distinctive value in the detection of programmatic service gaps not fundamentally apparent with either tool in use separately. I labored successfully in increasing dual diagnosis capabilities within the partnered community behavioral health agency, returning best care and best outcomes through an integrated, concurrent delivery of mental health and substance abuse (MH/SA) treatment. And I learned a fortifiable lesson: Do not hesitate to use every tool available to make a difference. The DNP-prepared APRN is impeccably equipped to make a resounding difference in our world. Let us use *every* tool we find available to do so; for that beacon of light alone, like a lone lighthouse, may usher many to safety and welfare.

THE DEVELOPMENT OF AN NP POST–STROKE DEPRESSION SCREENING AT 2 AND 4 WEEKS POSTDISCHARGE

KAREN L. YARBROUGH

■ ESTABLISHING THE DNP STUDENT QUESTION: BACKGROUND AND LITERATURE REVIEW

An ischemic stroke is an episode of neurological dysfunction caused by focal cerebral, spinal, or retinal infarction (Sacco et al., 2013). In the United States, the incidence of new or recurrent stroke is approximately 795,000 people per year and is the fifth leading cause of disability in the United States (Mozaffarian et al., 2015). Medical management focuses on targeted goals for both physical and psychological sequela of stroke. However, post-stroke depression (PSD) screening is not routinely performed in the acute recovery period. PSD is described as a depressed mood which develops after experiencing a stroke (American Psychiatric Association, 1994).

The prevalence of PSD is estimated to be 30% and can be diagnosed within 2 weeks after stroke (Ayerbe, Ayis, Rudd, Heuschmann, & Wolf, 2011). Correlations have been made between PSD and increased stroke mortality (Bartoli et al., 2013), recurrent stroke, and decreased quality of life (Pan, Sun, Okereke, Rexrode, & Hu, 2011). Meader, Moe-Byrne, Llewellyn, and Mitchell (2014) performed a meta-analysis which validates the reliability of using the Patient Health Questionanire-9 instrument (PHQ-9) to assess for PSD. The literature provided evidence a practice gap existed for performing a PSD screening in the acute stroke recovery phase. To address this gap, I identified an opportunity to improve clinical practice by implementing a PSD screening guideline for my DNP project.

■ STRATEGIES FOR A DIRECTED PI TEAM

With a practice issue firmly established, I developed a PI project to address the practice gap. I formed a PI team to facilitate engagement of organizational stakeholders. The first challenge was to identify stakeholders who agreed the project had scientific merit and clinical utility. Stakeholders were chosen for their clinical expertise and represented an interdisciplinary team. This team represented experts who could assist me in identifying barriers to accomplishing the project goals.

An effective strategy to engage stakeholders was to use the organization's model of process improvement. In this instance, the Plan, Do, Study, Act Cycle was used for this PI project (Institute of Healthcare Improvement, 2015). The DNP student team leader provided a PowerPoint lecture including a review of the literature, specific aims, and methods. The team was encouraged to provide constructive criticism of the proposed project. This proved to be an invaluable strategy to convey the project had clinical utility to the organization. In addition, team members were convinced the project could be completed within my required 3-month time frame. Team members were sent biweekly updates to facilitate engagement.

A critical step in the PI process was to develop a project which has clearly defined aims. Aims need to be measurable and support the transformation of data into clinical practice. The primary aim of this PI project was to measure resource utilization created when a NP administered a PSD screening in the acute ischemic stroke patient discharged home using the PHQ-9 in a clinic setting at 2 and 4 weeks post-stroke via telehealth. NP resource utilization was determined by calculating the time in minutes required to administer the PSD screening and complete all tasks associated with the PSD screening. Data analysis included the proportion of completed NP PSD screenings in the clinic and by telephone, as well as the number of patients who had PHQ-9 scores greater than 5 that resulted in prescribing antidepressants and referral to a behavioral health clinician.

■ SUMMARY OF PROJECT: METHODS, SETTING, AND RESULTS

This PI project was implemented at the clinical site where I was employed. This ensured that I had access to patients who were included in the targeted population. Two weeks postdischarge, patients were assessed in our stroke transitional discharge practice. Patients were asked to complete the PHQ-9 or I completed it with the patients. Four weeks after discharge, I administered a PSD screening using the PHQ-9 via telephone. The scores of the PHQ-9 for both visits were entered into EPIC, the organization's EMR. The office visit consultation was faxed to the patient's primary and neurology clinicians. For any patient with a PHQ-9 score more than 5, the patient's primary clinician was notified immediately. A score more than 5 was not the only criteria which was used to make a diagnosis of PSD. The patient had an in-depth clinical evaluation to confirm a diagnosis of PSD. A procedure was in place if the patient verbalized suicidal ideations. This included notifying the behavioral crisis team immediately to evaluate the patient. If the patient verbalized suicidal ideations during the telephone call, the patient and caregiver were going be counseled to seek evaluation in the organization's behavioral health emergency department. Feasibility for measuring a NP PSD screening included reporting the proportion of completed NP PSD screenings in the clinic and by telephone and the number of patients who had PHQ-9 scores greater than 5 that resulted in prescribing antidepressants and referrals to a behavioral health clinician. In summary, team members approved the project's aims because they reflected the safeguards required for patients with behavioral health issues.

Fifty-two patients were screened during a 3-month data collection period. Twenty-two patients were excluded due to premorbid depression ($n = 15$) or aphasia ($n = 8$). The resulting sample included 30 patients. The mean age was 57 years (SD ± 14) and 65% were female (19/29) and 35% were male (10/29). Racial distribution was 62% African American ($n = 18/29$) and 38% were White ($n = 38\%$). All patients had a diagnosis of mild ischemic stroke with a National Institutes of Health Stroke Scale (NIHSS) less than 4. The mean time in minutes to complete the PHQ-9 in the clinic was 7 minutes (SD ± 2.5 minutes). The mean time to complete the PHQ-9 via telephone was 8 minutes (SD ± 3.5 minutes). In the clinic, 28% of the patients ($n = 8/29$) had a PHQ-9 score greater than 4, classified as mild depression. Sixty percent ($n = 5/8$) of these patients were started on an antidepressant by their primary medical provider. The proportion of patients who had a PHQ-9 assessment completed in the clinic was 100% (29/29) and 90% (26/29) via telephone at 4 weeks. The PSD screening guideline is now part of daily practice in the outpatient stroke practice.

■ LESSONS LEARNED: PRACTICAL STRATEGIES TO ENHANCE PROJECT IMPLEMENTATION

This PI project was completed successfully because several strategies were applied to avoid unexpected barriers to success. Tactics to avoid making mistakes and facilitate effective implementation were to (a) identify a practice gap using evidence to support the desired clinical change, (b) develop a PI team with varied expertise which can identify barriers to implementation, (c) disseminate findings with stakeholders frequently during implementation, (d) develop aims which are measureable, and (e) develop a timeline with specific targeted goals with a date in which they need to be completed. By adopting these simple strategies, stakeholders will value the DNP student's role in successfully completing a project which improves the practice and safety of patients.

■ REFERENCES

Ajzen, I. (1991). The theory of planned behavior. *Organizational Behavior and Human Decision Processes, 50*(2), 179–211. doi:10.1016/0749-5978(91)90020-T

Akinbami, L., Moorman, J., & Liu, X. (2011). Asthma prevalence, health care use, and mortality: United States, 2005–2009. *National Health Statistics Report, 32*, 1–16.

American Psychiatric Association. (1994). *Diagnostic and statistical manual of mental disorders* (4th ed.). Washington, DC: Author.

Ayerbe, L., Ayis, S., Rudd, A., Heuschmann, P., & Wolfe, C. (2011). Natural history, predictors, and association of depression 5 years after stroke: The South London Register. *Stroke, 42*, 1901–1907. doi:10.1161/STROKEAHA.110.605808

Baillargeon, J., Binswanger, I. A., Penn, J. V., Williams, B. A., & Murray, O. J. (2009). Psychiatric disorders and repeat incarcerations: The revolving prison door. *American Journal of Psychiatry, 166*(1), 103–109. Retrieved from http://www.antoniocasella.eu/archipsy/Baillargeon_revolving_2009.PDF

Barrowclough, C., Haddock, G., Tarrier, N., Lewis, S. W., Moring, J., O'Brien, R., . . . McGovern, J. (2001). Randomized controlled trial of motivational interviewing, cognitive behavior therapy, and family intervention for patients with comorbid schizophrenia and substance use disorders. *American Journal of Psychiatry, 158*(10), 1706–1713. doi:10.1176/appi.ajp.158.10.1706

Bartoli, F., Lillia, N., Lax, A., Crocamo, C., Mantero, V., Carrà, G., . . . Clerici, M. (2013). Depression after stroke and risk of mortality: A systematic review and meta-analysis. *Stroke Research and Treatment, 2013*, 1–10. doi:10.1155/2013/862978

Carmichael, D., Tackett-Gibson, M., & Dell, O. (1998). *Texas dual diagnosis project evaluation report, 1997–1998.* College Station: Texas A&M University Public Policy Research Institute.

Connors, J., Arushanyan, E., Bellanca, G., Delgado, A., Hoeffler, A., Racine, R., & Gibbons, S. (2012). A description of barriers and facilitators to childhood vaccinations in the military health system. *Journal of the American Academy of Nurse Practitioners, 24*(12), 716–725. doi:10.1111/j.1745-7599.2012.00780.x

Davis, T. C., Fredrickson, D. D., Arnold, C. L., Cross, J. T., Humiston, S. G., Green, K. W., & Bocchini, J. A. (2001). Childhood vaccine risk/benefit communication in private practice office setting: A national survey. *Pediatrics, 107*(2), E17. Retrieved from http://www.pediatrics.org/cgi/content/full/107/2/e17

Donovan, H., & Ward, S. (2001). A representational approach to patient education. *Journal of Nursing Scholarship, 33*(3), 55–69.

Drake, R. E., Essock, S. M., Shaner, A., Carey, K. B., Minkoff, K., Kola, L., . . . Rickards, L. (2001). Implementing dual diagnosis services for clients with severe mental illness. *Psychiatric Services, 52*(4), 469–476. doi:10.1176/appi.ps.52.4.469

Hunt, G. E., Bergen, J., & Bashir, M. (2002). Medication compliance and comorbid substance abuse in schizophrenia: Impact on community survival 4 years after a relapse. *Schizophrenia Research, 54*(3), 253–264.

Institute of Healthcare Improvement. (2015). *How to improve.* Retrieved from http://www.ihi.org/resources/Pages/HowtoImprove/default.aspx

Mangrum, L. F., Spence, R. T., & Lopez, M. (2006). Integrated versus parallel treatment of co-occurring psychiatric and substance use disorders. *Journal of Substance Abuse Treatment, 30*(1), 79–84. doi:10.1016/j.jsat.2005.10.004

McGovern, M. P., Lambert-Harris, C., Gotham, H. J., Claus, R. E., & Xie, H. (2014). Dual diagnosis capability in mental health and addiction treatment services: An assessment of programs across multiple state systems. *Administration and Policy in Mental Health and Mental Health Services Research, 41*(2), 205–214. doi:10.1007/s10488-012-0449-1

Meader, N., Moe-Byrne, T., Llewellyn, A., & Mitchell, A. (2014). Screening for post stroke major depression: A meta-analysis of diagnostic validity studies. *Journal of Neurological Neurosurgery Psychiatry, 85*, 198–206. doi:10.1136/jnnp-2012-304194

Mozaffarian, D., Benjamin, E., Go, A., Arnett, D., Blaha, M., Cushman, M., . . . Turner, M. (2015). Heart disease and stroke statistics—2015 update: A report from the American Heart Association. *Circulation, 131*, e29–e322. doi:10.1161/CIR.0000000000000152

National Heart, Lung, and Blood Institute. (2015). *National asthma education and prevention program: Program description.* Retrieved from https://www.nhlbi.nih.gov/about/org/naepp

Pan, A., Sun, Q., Okereke, O., Rexrode, K., & Hu, F. (2011). Depression and the risk of stroke morbidity and mortality: A meta-analysis and systematic review. *Journal of the American Medical Association, 306*(11), 1241–1249. doi:10.1001/jama.2011.1282

Rosenberg, S. D., Goodman, L. A., Osher, F. C., Swartz, M. S., Essock, S. M., Butterfield, M. I., . . . Salyers, M. P. (2001). Prevalence of HIV, hepatitis B., and hepatitis C in people with severe mental illness. *American Journal of Public Health, 91*(1), 31–37.

Sacco, R., Kasner, S., Broderick, J., Caplan, L., Connors, J., Culebras, A., & Vinters H. (2013). An updated definition of stroke for the 21st century: A statement for health care professionals from the American Heart Association/American Stroke Association. *Stroke, 44*, 2064–2089. doi:10.1161/STR.0b013e318296aeca

Substance Abuse and Mental Health Services Administration. (2011). *Dual diagnosis capability in addiction treatment (DDCAT) toolkit, version 4.0.* Rockville, MD: U.S.

Department of Health and Human Services. Retrieved from http://ahsr.dartmouth.edu/docs/DDCAT_Toolkit.pdf

Szefler, S. (2010). Defining asthma phenotypes: Focusing the picture. *Journal of Allergy and Clinical Immunology, 126*(5), 939–940.

The Joint Commission. (2010). *Specifications Manual for Joint Commission National Quality Core Measures* (2010A1). Retrieved from https://manual.jointcommission.org/releases/archive/TJC2010B/SurgicalCareImprovementProject.html

Tiet, Q. Q., & Schutte, K. K. (2012). Treatment setting and outcomes of patients with co-occurring disorders. *Journal of Groups in Addiction & Recovery, 7*(1), 53–76. doi:10.1080/1556035X.2012.632330

Torrey, W. C., Drake, R. E., Cohen, M., Fox, L. B., Lynde, D., Gorman, P., & Wyzik, P. (2002). The challenge of implementing and sustaining integrated dual disorders treatment programs. *Community Mental Health Journal, 38*(6), 507–521.

Ward S. E., Heidrich S. M., & Donovan, H. S. (2007). An update on the representational approach to patient education. *Journal of Nursing Scholarship, 39*(3), 259–265.

ZiaPartners, Inc. (2016). *Compass-EZ™: A self-assessment tool for behavioral health programs.* Retrieved from http://www.ziapartners.com/tools/compass-ez

SECTION THREE

Application of the Essentials to Advanced Nursing Practice

SHEILA M. DAVIS

The curricular elements and competencies that must be present in programs conferring The doctor of nursing practice (DNP) degree are articulated by the American Association of Colleges of Nursing (AACN) in *The Essentials of Doctoral Education for Advanced Practice*. The successful application of the essentials to advanced nursing practice is the essence of successful DNP practice. How a graduate successfully translates knowledge obtained in school to everyday practice is often elusive, and lessons learned from experienced DNPs can be informative, guiding, and most importantly inspiring. This section explores the application of the DNP Essentials to advanced nursing practice (AACN, 2006). This section begins with Chapter 8 and the reflections of seven experienced DNPs currently working in very different settings with a wide span of level of organizational responsibility, scope of practice, and health system influence sharing their thoughts when asked to reflect on the DNP and their professional journey.

Leadership at all levels is an integral part of DNP practice. Doyle-Lindrud and Kwong in Chapter 9 explore leadership skills needed for all advanced practice nurses. They identify key common themes that relate to leadership including collaboration, communication, evaluation, and leading others. Pragmatic strategies to develop key leadership skills that will advance practice and professional growth are outlined along with guidance on incremental steps that can be taken to become a strong leader.

Executive nurse leaders carry an ever-expanding level of responsibility for leading in all aspects of healthcare, requiring an expansive range of leadership skills. In Chapter 10, Ives Erickson, Ditomassi, and Adams discuss the critical need for knowledge-based practice (KBP) within the context of nursing administration and executive nurse leadership roles. They share their experiences developing a knowledge-based nursing leadership practice inclusive of research and theory that has long been a part of efforts at the Massachusetts General Hospital (MGH).

Webb and McKinnon-Howe discuss how DNP-prepared nurses define themselves in education, policy, and practice in Chapter 11. Exploration of pivotal moments in DNP education are illustrative of the challenges that emerged in the evolution of the degree and highlight where additional advocacy is needed to further understanding and development. The implications that barriers to advance nursing practice affect access to quality healthcare is explored, and the call to action for DNP-prepared nurses to take their rightful place in driving policy is highlighted.

Hearing from the DNP community is important and a necessary part of our evolution. In Chapter 12, O'Dell shares highlights from the survey that was administered to DNP graduates by doctors of nursing practice, Inc. (DNP, Inc.) The first survey was completed in 2011 and subsequent surveys were administered in 2012, 2013, 2015, and 2017. As a DNP professional community, we need to continually challenge ourselves to respond to the ever-changing healthcare environment.

■ REFERENCE

American Association of Colleges of Nursing. (2006). *The essentials of doctoral education for advanced practice nursing.* Retrieved from http://www.aacnnursing.org/Portals/42/Publications/DNPEssentials.pdf

CHAPTER EIGHT

Personal Perspectives on Role Integration

As the number of doctor of nursing practice (DNP) graduates has continued to grow, we are able to learn from experienced DNPs about their professional paths, current positions, and personal guiding principles. Although the DNP degree does not expand the legal scope of practice or clinical preparation leading to credentialing and licensure, the education exposes graduates to a broad area of knowledge and skills. In this chapter, experienced doctors of nursing practice were asked to reflect on their professional journeys. Their interpretations of the question asked were as diverse as the reflections they share.

ANTICIPATED AND UNANTICIPATED CONSEQUENCES

JOANNE HOGAN

Nursing knowledge is forever expanding. After 25 years of practicing nursing, I felt compelled to advance my own knowledge through attainment of the DNP. Fueled by my passion for the profession, personal experiences, and support from colleagues who knew the difference that would come from obtaining a terminal degree, I embarked on the academic journey. My DNP resulted in intended and unanticipated consequences.

I began my nursing career as a primary nurse in an academic medical center. This is where I learned my commitment to nursing and patient- and family-centered care. It was very important to me to continuously improve practice by supporting development of self and others while collaborating with nurse scholars in expanding nursing knowledge. An environment of continuous learning and support for advancing practice helped me realize that at least one advanced degree was in my future.

I decided to pursue a master's degree in nursing administration as a means of developing leadership and management competencies. Subsequently, I assumed administrative nursing roles in another academic medical center as my career advanced. I accomplished all this while maintaining a happy marriage, raising two wonderful children, and supporting aging parents. It can be done.

My good fortune came from the learning and support of many expert nurse leaders with terminal degrees. I was struck by their depth and breadth of knowledge and willingness to encourage and support other nurses toward continued education. These leaders had the underpinnings of the DNP Essentials (American Association of Colleges of Nursing [AACN], 2006). They were well versed in theory and science as foundations for practice; they were system-thinkers who wielded large bodies of work across organizations, systems, and communities; evidence and outcomes drove their practice; they practiced externally in policy and academic arenas and collaborated interprofessionally to improve patient outcomes and population health; and they supported continued education and development of nurses. In short, they were committed to expanding nursing knowledge. I longed to be more like them.

The intended consequences of my DNP came with each component of the curriculum. Theory, practice, and outcomes were interwoven and built upon each other. I had the opportunity to delve into nursing, leadership, and systems theories while also applying and testing them in my everyday practice. My DNP project (Hogan, 2016) centered on Jean Watson's Caring Science Theory (Watson, 2012) as the foundation to nursing practice. With caring theory as the scientific underpinning, I analyzed caring practices of nurses with patients enrolled in a successful high-risk care management program. This required gaining knowledge in health policy, population health, outcomes measures, information systems, and engaging nursing and interprofessional colleagues.

Self-discovery serves as the foundation of the unanticipated consequences of my DNP. A backdrop of authentic leadership theory (Walumbwa et al., 2008) brought clarity and focus to a quest for continued self-development and awareness. Discovering my purpose and values led to an uncompromising stance as a nurse leader. Congruency of my leadership style and behaviors with stated values became of utmost importance to me, and this continues to drive my practice. I find myself making decisions and taking actions unlike those made in the past. Clarity enables the confidence, courage, and risk-taking required to lead. Rooted in purpose, values, and knowledge of the contributions of nurses to the health of individuals and societies, the DNP has provided me the courage to lead, collaborate, study, and convey the contributions of nurses to patients and health systems.

Healthcare reform is driving significant changes in the delivery of care. Our contemporary healthcare environment requires nurse leaders well versed in nursing science, systems-thinking, outcomes measurement, technology, policy, inter- and intraprofessional collaboration, and an unwavering focus on the contributions of nurses to the health and well-being of individuals and societies. The knowledge and skill obtained through the DNP are essential for nurse leaders now and in the future.

THE DNP EXECUTIVE

LAURA J. WOOD

I was employed as a registered nurse for over three decades when I decided to pursue DNP studies in 2010. I suspect I was viewed as an improbable DNP program applicant given both my age and career stage. Prior to pursuing a DNP degree, I gained significant clinical and leadership experience within leading children's hospitals, academic health centers, and a global healthcare information technology organization. Yet, despite my considerable professional practice experience, I had long felt there was more I might contribute upon the completion of doctoral-level education.

My appreciation for the impact of nurses and the profession of nursing has been a lifelong focus. The experience I had as a 5-year-old patient with my own nurse mother as advocate at my side throughout an extended hospitalization in a pediatric specialty hospital created a lasting impression. With a deeply held commitment to education, I enrolled in a doctor of philosophy (PhD) degree program after a decade in clinical practice. The PhD degree was widely considered the terminal degree in nursing prior to the conceptualization of the DNP degree. I completed PhD coursework while employed in nursing full time, but found dissertation completion mistimed when the confluence of parenting, family caregiving, and work demands all coalesced. Continued life demands, coupled with the additional complexity of significant travel in a nationally focused industry role, led me to imagine that my successful completion of a doctoral degree in nursing might well remain out of reach.

Over time, I came to appreciate my strongest professional commitments were no longer related to the mastery of nursing research science. Rather, my investment as a practice-focused nurse leader guided my strong desire to strengthen healthcare leadership methods, improve health system quality and safety, enhance the well-being of nurses and team members, and contribute to care delivery transformation. The opportunity to challenge myself through enrollment in an academically rigorous DNP program, collaborate with nationally recognized faculty and practice-focused leaders in quality and safety, and pursue elective studies with national nurse leaders proved to be extremely gratifying. I am tremendously grateful for this new opportunity, as the flexibility of an asynchronous learning program with a deep practice focus simply did not exist earlier in my career.

As I progressed through my DNP program, I worked closely with several generous faculty mentors and began to set more ambitious goals for my professional future. I was extremely humbled to be one of two students in my DNP cohort selected to participate in a yearlong Nurse Leader Mentorship Program that provided mentorship and educational opportunities to build leadership capacity. Through this award, I received funding to complete a course of online study through a leading user-centered design and traveled nationally to complete a program of study and site visits to leading healthcare delivery transformation design programs. Also invited to join in authorship with four preeminent nurse leaders, I contributed to a multiyear qualitative analysis of nurse-led innovators with the CEO and president of the American Academy of Nursing. In the course of this collaboration, I was encouraged to apply for a postdoctoral fellowship to continue to build my nursing leadership capacity.

As I look back, the new academic tools and leadership skills I gained while a DNP student led me to challenge myself in new ways. The month following my DNP graduation, I was notified of my selection as a Robert Wood Johnson Foundation Executive Nurse Fellow; I became one of 20 nurse leaders selected nationally for this 3-year fellowship. Approximately 1 year after graduation, I was appointed senior vice president, patient care operations and chief nursing officer (CNO) within a leading children's hospital. It is a distinct privilege to lead the discipline of nursing, to support approximately 5,000 patient care team members, and to contribute to the mission of a remarkable organization that is at the forefront of shaping children's health policy regionally, nationally, and beyond. I serve on the organization's Board of Trustees, several board subcommittees, and am an appointed member of national CNO advisory groups for a leading safety and regulatory organization, a leading patient/family experience advisory organization, and as part of several academic health system advisory groups spanning both healthcare ethics and nursing education.

As a tenured nurse leader joining a remarkable organization and exceptional group of front-line leaders, my focus 5 years post-DNP degree completion has now turned toward a wide range of initiatives to strengthen our professional practice environment and to translate similar improvements more broadly within nursing and healthcare. Examples include

- Fostering original clinical scholarship, nursing science, and evidence-based practice initiatives with a focus on risk reduction, illness prevention, and health maintenance to improve the care of children, families, and populations
- Creating clinical/promotional ladders, peer review processes, and shaping policy to meet the practice requirements of a rapidly expanding advanced practice registered nurse (APRN) and specialty workforce
- Shaping healthcare policy and leadership including the translation of mandatory nurse staffing models and contributions to national policies related to care delivery innovation during my 5-year tenure as national co-chair, Nursing Informatics Working Group Policy Committee, American Medical Informatics Association (AMIA)
- Refining the business and clinical use of the organization's enterprise data warehouse to promote continuous improvement and build the business case for data-driven healthcare from both a finance and quality/safety perspective
- Strengthening organization and systems leadership through the application of reliability science within healthcare to advance the health and well-being of both employees and patients

- Designing and implementing new care delivery models that effectively align health system and community population health resources to strengthen the cost-quality value equation

DNP preparation contributed greatly to my readiness to lead at new levels. I look forward to noting the impact of current and future DNP-prepared nurse leaders who have similar opportunities to contribute to the profession of nursing and to the improvement of health and healthcare delivery.

MOVING OUT OF THE NURSE LEADER COMFORT ZONE TO EFFECT CHANGE

ELAINE BRIDGE

As a professional nurse for many years, I have had several opportunities to contribute to the care of patients, often in traditional roles and settings. As a critical care bedside nurse, I delivered direct care to patients in intensive care units and in emergency department settings and saw immediate and tangible results of my efforts.

As I moved into management and then into hospital administrative roles as a chief nurse and interim COO, I influenced the care and the environment in which it was delivered, within a given organization. It was not always immediately evident what impacts I had as a healthcare leader, but over time these efforts typically translated into measurable outcomes with which to gauge my leadership effectiveness. Many of my efforts as a member of various leadership teams resulted in evidence that highlighted that the care delivered resulted in positive patient outcomes and the longer term success of the institution because of those outcomes. This was measured by positive patient experiences and staff engagement, as well as financial health and community commitment to the organizations.

When presented with the opportunity to move into a corporate position joining a team responsible for implementing an enterprise electronic health record (EHR), I considered my professional goals and my desire to thoughtfully choose my next career move. This evaluation included consideration for the specific role and the sphere of influence such a position might afford me as a nurse leader, clinician, and one committed to improving the care of patients across a complex system.

I also considered the fact that this role would move me further from direct care and that the impacts of this role would be much more difficult to evaluate. Having completed my doctorate in nursing practice 3 years prior, I reflected on my DNP learnings during my evaluation of this opportunity. As I progressed through the DNP curricula, it became very clear to me that, as a nurse leader, it was important to seek opportunities in unconventional roles to broaden the nurse leader sphere of influence. I recalled that it was incumbent upon all nurse leaders to ensure that nursing had a voice when decisions were being made that would impact care and the care environment. And it was, therefore, more imperative than ever that nurse leaders think more broadly and more boldly about opportunities to influence decisions impacting the care environment.

It was in this context that I evaluated this opportunity to participate in a less conventional nursing leadership position as my system embarked on this enterprise transformation. The project had already formed with the inclusion of substantial physician representation, which was necessary. However, the lens and voice of nursing and other care providers was lacking at the decision-making level of the project. As a DNP, I knew it was essential that a nurse leader serve in an influential role on a project that was so foundational to the future success of the enterprise. If the enterprise was going to move beyond its current structure, maintain the focus on patient care, and improve the coordination and efficiency of that care, this project was an essential next step and nursing had to be represented at the executive level of the project.

The opportunity to collaborate with many disciplines across the enterprise, to appreciate the multiple cultures, priorities, and challenges, and to gain even broader knowledge of how complex systems function and how to effectively manage change all contributed to my interest in this next professional challenge and role. As I embarked on this new role, it became apparent that this was not going to be an easy role to fulfill—not a completely surprising realization given the disruptive nature of this project and what we know about change and change management. Asking clinicians and others to completely rethink their approach to the care they provided and the way in which they delivered that care was not insignificant.

As such, I feel it would have been much more difficult to be successful in this role had I not had the education as a DNP to reflect upon. I relied on evidence-based research when challenged about certain project decisions and learned more about leadership accountability. Standing up to the difficulties associated with high-level change, which occasionally manifested in anger, blame, and dissatisfaction, allowed me to grow as an empathic, authentic leader.

Further, as I recalled from my DNP learnings, the principle of developing strong relationships, essential to success as a leader, was apparent throughout my time in this challenging role and it was clear how much more difficult the challenge would have been and how outcomes might well have suffered without strong relationships. It was also important to acknowledge that technology is never a substitute for human competency and caring, something nurses and other care providers know intrinsically. Implementing a technology solution was not intended to supplant the caregiver, but rather was intended to enhance coordinated, efficient care. My ability to relate to this sentiment allowed me to be seen as an advocate for both the project and the people impacted by this transformation.

For all that I may have contributed to this project, I learned as much or more. It became obvious that change is seldom easily accomplished. It also became clear that different groups respond differently when confronted with change. Perhaps the biggest take away for me is that the culture of an organization directly impacts the ease or difficulty with which an organization will adopt and adapt to change.

Finally, had I not studied for my DNP, I firmly believe that I would not have had the ability to succeed in moving the most resistant individuals and groups forward, however grudgingly, as I believe they would not have taken me as seriously. Having a DNP has opened doors for me by opening the minds of others, in ways I would never have anticipated. I am proud to have earned this degree and to use the DNP designation with as much pride as I have used my RN designation for so many years.

WHO BETTER TO LEAD?

LISA SGARLATA

In 1931, Robert Wood Johnson, in his booklet *Service to the Patient*, addresses the need to empower nurses to make care decisions to ensure high-quality patient care. His words now echo in the Institute of Medicine's (IOM) *Future of Nursing* report (IOM, 2011). The IOM recommended the development of a nurse workforce whose members are diverse, well-educated, and prepared to practice to the full extent of their education and training. The report speaks to the need for nurses to meet the emerging needs of patients but also act as a full partner in reforming the nation's healthcare system (IOM, 2011). Personal and professional growth, leadership development, mentoring programs, and opportunities to assume leadership positions across all levels are addressed in this influential report; but how do we, as nurses, get there?

While my path was not clearly defined in my early years, an innate passion for education and personal growth has become a foundation for my belief in quality and compassionate leadership. The most influential opportunity for me lies within the quality of uniqueness. As a female chief officer in a male-dominated environment, I needed to capitalize on what makes me "unique" and not conform to the culture that currently existed. I was unique because I was a nurse.

Earning my DNP provided me with a key leadership opportunity to take my current position and educational background to a higher level and influence those closest to me as well as those within the larger organization. The changes needed impacted the development of expanded organizational behaviors, strategic insight, and the need to drive a consistent vision with the health system. Obtaining my DNP was a key growth opportunity in developing nursing leaders to come up with creative solutions to real problems while constantly questioning and challenging the traditional behaviors, ideas, and processes that exist in healthcare today.

As today's advanced practitioners, we are challenged to ensure that both financial and quality goals are met in an uncertain environment. The healthcare system is in a state of constant chaos, and although many changes can be perceived as barriers to good quality healthcare delivery, I truly believe that they are not insurmountable. The healthcare system is continually evolving and there has to be an unwavering commitment to ensuring that the voices of nurses are heard and that nursing is positioned to contribute as full partners in a transformed system.

The DNP education provided the skills and knowledge I needed to successfully communicate a consistent vision and the ability to successfully implement change without losing sight of our current mission of improving patient care and outcomes. Having the ability to expand my knowledge beyond the healthcare realm gave me the opportunity to combine the autonomy of my nursing background with a solid strategic understanding needed within the executive team structure and broader healthcare environment. François de la Rochefoucauld said: "The only thing constant in life is change" (1613–1680). Who better to lead that change than a doctoral-prepared nurse?

GROWTH OPPORTUNITIES

CLAIRE SIMONE

Not long after completing my training as a nurse practitioner in 1995, I knew I wanted to take my education to the next level. Despite the value inherent in the breadth of knowledge and skills a family nurse practitioner (FNP) must employ in their daily clinical practice, I wanted to give myself the gift of focusing intently on a specific area of study. I entertained applying to PhD programs more than a few times, but always pulled back, feeling the fit was not quite right.

I am a practical person always searching for the next thing to improve clinical practice. After two decades of clinical practice in HIV care and substance use treatment, all the while nurturing a growing passion for continuous quality improvement, I discovered the DNP degree and found a program that was the right match for my goals and interests. At a relatively late stage in my career, why invest the time, money, and sleepless nights in a new degree? I hoped my investment in a DNP education would complement my clinical practice by accelerating my learning and expertise in the quality and systems of healthcare. My career goals also included increasing my value and capacity for teaching and consultancy. The DNP degree did just that.

Contrary to my original plans, I chose to keep my current job after graduation. Almost seamlessly during my course of study, as I grew in my ability to understand, analyze, and improve evidence-based practice, my clinical job became enriched with opportunities to employ the skills I was developing in my DNP program. This trajectory continued after graduating. I am now seen as a colleague with expertise and leadership in data, systems, and practice improvement, and I am invited to sit at the table with upper management as we develop specific projects to meet current and future program goals. I have been given additional resources to support this work while it complements my ongoing clinical practice.

My DNP education matured my perspective and understanding about the relationship of my clinical work in substance use treatment and public health. I grew in confidence to reach beyond our day-to-day work and collaborate with community leaders to improve both patient and public health outcomes, partnering on grant opportunities, citywide initiatives, consultancy, and research.

A further benefit of my DNP program was gaining confidence and skills as an educator. Though becoming tenured faculty is not a goal of mine, I have always loved learning and sharing that passion as a teacher and mentor. I witnessed a marked improvement in my skills mentoring master's students in an evidence-based practice course. My comfort developing and presenting talks or workshops grew stronger, and I have subsequently been invited to present locally and nationally in the areas of HIV, substance use, and integrated services. I have always loved to write, but lacked the confidence that my professional interests would be applicable or of interest to others. My DNP program had a heavy emphasis on professional writing, which allowed me to hone the skills of researching and analyzing literature, precise writing and editing, and, above all, a confidence to submit my work for presentation or publication. It has been a wonderful journey for sharing the work that inspires me with the broader community, continually expanding and deepening my professional circle.

As time passes, I am continually presented with new opportunities to further grow the skills and expertise that were fostered by my DNP program. In the not-too-distant future, I plan to transition out of my current clinical practice and focus on growing opportunities for teaching and consulting domestically and internationally. This was an original career goal when I considered the DNP degree, and I believe I was well served by my program of education.

CLINICIAN AND EDUCATOR

MICHAEL SANCHEZ

The DNP degree has prepared me to meet the demands of the continually evolving and complex healthcare system. While not only broadening my perspective of healthcare, the DNP degree provided the ability to implement evidence-based changes and lead practice change initiatives which will ultimately improve the care patients receive.

The way in which one can fully drive healthcare initiatives, innovation, and overall care as a DNP may vary depending on your employment setting and organization. Upon finishing my DNP program, I was working for a private practice. Due to the specific job duties and expectations as a nurse practitioner and limitations by organizational leadership, opportunities to implement practice changes aimed at the complex healthcare environment were not fully supported. Larger clinical settings may offer broader support of DNP-prepared nurses.

As a clinician and educator, I continually aim to impact nursing practice at all levels. I was recently given a clinical appointment as a nurse practitioner at the John G. Bartlett Specialty Clinic in Baltimore with a joint appointment with the Johns Hopkins School of Medicine, Division of Infectious Diseases. As a clinician in this setting, I provide HIV and primary care services to patients living with HIV and offer clinical services directed at HIV prevention. Through interprofessional collaborations with other clinicians and researchers, I also offer implementation strategies of practice guidelines for HIV prevention and incorporate screening, brief intervention, and referral to treatment of alcohol and substances use disorders. In this role, I provide expertise to students on the topic of HIV prevention and present chronic management in HIV theory courses and clinical experiences.

As an educator, I have taught and coordinated courses across both prelicensure and nurse practitioner programs. Since stepping into the role of a teacher, my intent is to successfully deliver courses incorporating the use of technology, case studies, and adult-learning techniques to promote critical thinking and retention. Further, as co-investigator on a Substance Abuse Mental Health Services Administration (SAMSA)-funded grant, I have taken a leadership role in ensuring the core content of substance use screening, brief intervention, and referral to treatment education are successfully integrated into the Entry to Nursing curriculum.

In summary, this terminal degree of nursing practice has been an essential part of my career. It has prepared me to care for my patients beyond the clinical groundwork of my FNP program. This degree has enabled me to work in administrative and leadership roles, which broadened my views on the complexities of the healthcare system and equipped me to implement practice changes.

NURSE INFORMATICIST

JOHN ROBERTS

My introduction to health information technology (HIT) came during my master's preparation as a cardiovascular nurse specialist. I was drawn to the monitoring and assistive devices required to nurse critically ill persons back to health after devastating trauma or dramatic, life-saving surgeries. It is a challenge to maintain human connections and nurturance, so very important to recovery, in the midst of technology. I practiced critical care and emergency nursing for a decade before seeking a certificate of advanced graduate study to become an adult nurse practitioner. This was a decidedly low-tech lifestyle in comparison to my prior practice that began the lugubrious process of transition into the information age, kicking and screaming.

I had become interested in information technology as a personal quest, acquiring a Commodore 64 computer using 8-inch floppy discs, making connection to the new development, the Internet. In my clinical practice, I used every iteration of the Palm® devices for information storage and some reference applications. When my practice began to install personal computers on desktops, I became the go-to person for help with these devices and their software. When a grant opportunity became available to trial an Internet-based application to dictate and deliver documentation of clinical care, I was front and center to take that opportunity. Shortly after that, our health center began to investigate moving to an EHR. As a member of a workplace group that was charged with assessing software options, I helped to make a selection from the few, rudimentary options available to us. Thus began a journey through implementation, development, and support challenges that continues today.

I hold the position of clinical information specialist in my organization that operates four federally qualified community health centers in Massachusetts. I participate in the implementation of our chosen EHR and continue to be involved in day-to-day operations. My principle focus is end-user support, training new users, updating current users, and problem-solving issues that arise. I also advise on EHR configuration and development and the planning necessary to stay current with our software product and its supporting hardware. I maintain a clinical practice because I enjoy direct patient care as well as staying current with the experience of the users I support, their joys and pains.

After several years in my position, I felt the need to seek additional understanding of the underpinnings of the technology I support. I returned to graduate school to a DNP program with a specialty in informatics. There I learned about the thought processes that underlie HIT. We examined the coding structures that ensure data are retrievable, aggregable, and analyzable. We considered health policy initiatives such as the Health Information Technology for Economic and Clinical Health (HITECH) Act of 2009 that created a federal program and funding to support healthcare's transition to HIT, including the certification of EHRs and the meaningful use (MU) initiative, which incentivized the adoption of EHRs in hospital and ambulatory practices. My course work involved not only courses specific to HIT, but also about healthcare finance, population health, project management, leadership, and quality measurement. Although I remain in the same position, achievement of my DNP allows me to bring other skills that I previously had not acquired.

One key area of focus for my informatics practice is to examine strategies to optimize our EHR and improve usability. As Staggers (2003) asserts, usability considers how well we are able to meld the observations and efforts of our thought processes with the computer tool that we use to reflect those observations and efforts in the patient care record. I am able to analyze human factors that can interfere with successful use of technology as well as the limitations of technology design. For example, a key argument for EHR adoption is to make data about clinical care available for research as well as sharing across the continuum of care. At this stage of development, entry of this information sharing requires much of the data to be analyzed in a structured manner. Structured data entry is often at odds with usability, as it calls on users to focus energy on recording of data instead of capturing the patient's clinical story. I continue to seek ways to help users to see the value in these data, but also to discover strategies to ease the data entry burden, such as making sure that data need not be entered more than once, yet are available for review in multiple locations where it is clinically appropriate. Structured data entry is also key when considering the sharing of clinical data across systems by health information exchange so that data from different software platforms represent the same clinical findings and reflect the same care in each system.

A significant portion of my role is implementing novel applications of technology in healthcare. Electronic prescribing allows the transmission of legible prescriptions directly to the pharmacy. Direct integration of prescriptions into the pharmacy software improves accuracy and speeds the filling process, increases security when prescribing medications, reduces opportunities for drug diversion, and allows clinical decision support in the form of drug–drug, drug–condition, and drug–allergy interaction checking thereby improving patient safety. In addition, electronic prescribing ensures entry of information into a state's prescription monitoring program to allow assessment of a patient's prescribing history for potential drug abuse. Additionally, we have begun the use of dermatologic imaging equipment that allows high definition image capture of skin lesions with transmission to consulting dermatologists at remote locations. This greatly speeds assessment of skin disorders, providing a clinical diagnosis and treatment advice within 3 business days. The next step in this project will be full integration with our EHR.

A different role that my DNP has supported for me is as informatics educator. I teach in on-line master's programs for FNPs. I am passionate about this subject, as I believe that healthcare cannot continue to advance, nor practice safely happen, without the tools and opportunities to collect and analyze data that informatics, and specifically EHRs, bring. Population data is a key to effective, evidence-based practice and cannot be gathered, let alone compared across settings, without a robust solution for data collection.

Nurse informaticists are involved in projects to advance patient engagement, as well as meeting reporting requirements for grant funding and management, performance monitoring, and project management. We provide leadership for organizational development. We craft policy to improve institutional and governmental support of healthcare. We pursue data to better describe and quantitate nursing care, improving the visibility of nurses' role in the healthcare system. Training and workflow analysis and redesign are fundamental job expectations. I am better able to meet these challenges and advance transformation of the healthcare system because I am prepared as a DNP.

■ SUMMARY

The reflections by the seven DNP-prepared nurses in this chapter illuminate the vast depth and breadth of experience. From the bedside to the boardroom, a commitment to quality care for their patients is evident. Many used the DNP to catapult their careers into areas previously seen as purely administrative or physician-led areas. All champion the advancement of healthcare delivery, and their proximity to patients gives them a unique advantage to do so. These perspectives of executive nurse leaders—their challenges and the successes—provide insights into the complexities in leadership at the highest level. Although all of the contributors shared different parts of their professional journeys, the commitment to improving the lives of those who care, whether at the bedside or in the boardroom, is inspiring.

■ REFERENCES

American Association of Colleges of Nursing. (2006, October). *Essentials of doctoral education for advanced nursing practice.* Retrieved from http://www.aacnnursing.org/Portals/42/Publications/DNPEssentials.pdf

Hogan, J. (2016). *Examining caring behaviors of RN care coordinators in complex care management.* Unpublished manuscript, MGH Institute of Health Professions, Charlestown, MA.

Institute of Medicine. (2011). *The future of nursing: Leading change, advancing health.* Retrieved from http://nationalacademies.org/hmd/reports/2010/the-future-of-nursing-leading-change-advancing-health.aspx

Staggers, N. (2003). Human factors: Imperative concepts for information systems in critical care. *AACN Clinical Issues, 14*(3), 310–319.

CHAPTER NINE

Leadership Skill Set for the Advanced Practice Registered Nurse

SUSAN DOYLE-LINDRUD AND JEFFREY KWONG

The doctor of nursing practice (DNP) graduate has many opportunities available upon graduation. For most registered nurses electing to pursue advanced practice roles, the DNP represents the first step in gaining a combination of both new clinical skills and a new identity as an advanced practitioner. The DNP degree prepares individuals to work in a variety of different settings and roles, ranging from direct patient care, to administrative, to education, to policy, to entrepreneurial, and much more. For master's-prepared nurses who elect to complete a DNP program, this new degree serves as a means of broadening their existing scope of practice by focusing on a larger systems perspective. For baccalaureate-prepared nurses entering DNP programs, the degree may prepare them to work as an advanced practice nurse in the role of a nurse practitioner, administrator, or other advanced practice clinician.

Although DNP programs may vary with regard to their emphasis on administrative or clinical tracks, all DNP programs will have curricular content that includes the same core competencies. These core competencies are articulated in *The Essentials of Doctoral Education for Advanced Practice Nursing*, the curricular content present in DNP programs developed by the American Association of Colleges of Nursing (AACN), the voice for graduate nursing education (AACN, 2006). The DNP position statement identifies the importance of the development of advanced competencies for complex practice and leadership roles (AACN, 2006).

In 2011, the Institute of Medicine (IOM) published a report, *The Future of Nursing: Leading Change, Advancing Health*, which emphasized the key role nurses play in the delivery, creation, and advancement of healthcare. The report places an emphasis on leadership roles and responsibilities that nurses across the practice continuum must possess to actively participate as a change agent in the healthcare system. Two key messages of this report are that "Nurses should be full partners, with physicians and other health professionals, in redesigning healthcare in the United States" and "Leadership from nurses is needed at every level and across all settings."

Also stated in the report, it is critical that leadership competencies be included in nursing education (IOM, 2011, p. 221, 225). This overlaps well with *The Essentials of Doctoral Education for Advanced Practice Nursing*. A curricular element of the DNP Essentials asserts "Organizational and systems leadership are critical for DNP graduates to improve patient and healthcare outcomes." This competency describes the need for the DNP graduate to develop quality improvement initiatives within their practice setting or organization and develop new care delivery models (AACN, 2006, p. 10).

Dwight D. Eisenhower defined leadership as "the art of getting someone else to do something that you want done because he wants to do it, not because your position of power can compel him to do it" (NARA, 2017). This definition applies well to the role of the advanced practice nurse in that they educate and counsel patients about their medications, dietary modification, and/or exercise to improve health outcomes. The AACN emphasizes that the DNP-prepared nurse is a practice expert who possesses an array of knowledge as it applies to evidence-based practice, quality improvement, and systems-level thinking (AACN, 2006).

Exactly what are "leadership skills" and how does one develop these skills? The AACN has included leadership within several of the major core competencies in the DNP Essentials. The competencies associated with leadership are listed in Exhibit 9.1. It is clear, based on the competencies, that the DNP graduate is expected to be proficient in several areas often found in leadership roles, ranging from policy to financial and cost analysis, quality improvement, and clinical leadership. However, as the saying goes, "Rome wasn't built in a day." Likewise, the skills of becoming a leader often take time to develop. So, the question remains, how can one develop these skills?

Most academic programs offer theory and education related to the foundational components of leadership. The study of leadership has roots in psychology and business and there are numerous theories on leadership, organizational strategy, and leadership style, and the review of these theories and principles of leadership are beyond the scope of this chapter. DNP programs include leadership content in the curriculum through various methods, which include stand-alone nursing leadership courses, integration of leadership content into the coursework, or by integrating leadership courses offered through other programs such as schools of business or public administration. Regardless of how leadership theory is taught, there still lies the challenge of gaining practical "hands-on" experience. Just as a nurse may be well versed in the pathophysiology of congestive heart failure (CHF), it is not until the nurse has to care for a patient in acute CHF that the nurse learns to combine the theoretical knowledge with the practical aspects of caring for someone presenting with signs and symptoms of the disease. The focus of this chapter, therefore, is to provide a brief guide on how to gain practical experience that will benefit the new DNP graduate in developing and applying the skills necessary to fulfill the role of DNP.

If one reviews the competencies required of the DNP degree as established by the AACN, it would seem as if the DNP graduate is prepared to solely take on an overwhelming responsibility. One person having all of the characteristics and skills needed to be the complete leader is not required. It is better to understand one's own strengths and weaknesses and motivate others to utilize their strengths to accomplish team objectives (Marshall, 2010). However, if one looks for broad themes within the DNP competencies, which can then be broken down to a few commonalities, the leadership role is achievable. The common themes that arise as they relate to leadership include collaboration, communication, evaluation, and leading others. These domains seem self-explanatory, but learning or gaining experience in these areas can be challenging. This holds true especially for those with limited clinical experience or for those who may not view themselves as being in a leadership position in their current setting.

EXHIBIT 9.1 Leadership-Themed Competencies of the DNP

Essential I: Scientific underpinnings for practice

The DNP program prepares the graduate to:

- Use science-based theories and concepts to evaluate outcomes.
- Develop and evaluate new practice approaches based on nursing theories from other disciplines.

Essential II: Organizational and systems leadership for quality improvement and systems thinking

The DNP program prepares the graduate to:

- Develop and evaluate care delivery approaches that meet current and future needs of patient populations based on scientific findings in nursing and other clinical sciences as well as organizational, political, and economic sciences.
- Ensure accountability for quality of healthcare and patient safety for populations with whom they work.
- Use advanced communication skills/processes to lead quality improvement and patient safety initiatives in health systems.
- Employ principles of business, finance, economics, and health policy to practice initiatives that will improve the quality of care delivery.
- Develop and/or monitor budgets for practice initiatives.
- Demonstrate sensitivity to diverse organizational cultures and populations, including patients and providers.
- Develop and or evaluate effective strategies for managing the ethical dilemmas inherent in patient care, the healthcare organization, and research.

Essential III: Clinical scholarship and analytical methods for evidence-based practice

The DNP program prepares the graduate to:

- Design and implement processes to evaluate outcomes of practice, practice patterns, and systems of care within a practice setting, healthcare organization, or community against national benchmarks to determine variances in practice outcomes and population trends.
- Design, direct, and evaluate quality improvement methodologies to promote safe, timely, effective, efficient, equitable, and patient-centered care.
- Function as a practice specialist/consultant in collaborative knowledge-generating research.
- Disseminate findings from evidence-based practice and research to improve healthcare outcomes.

Essential IV: Information systems/technology and patient care technology for the improvement and transformation of healthcare

The DNP program prepares the graduate to:

- Design, select, use, and evaluate programs that evaluate and monitor outcomes of care, care systems, and quality improvement, including consumer use of healthcare information systems.
- Analyze and communicate critical elements necessary to the selection, use, and evaluation of healthcare information systems and patient care technology.
- Provide leadership in the evaluation and resolution of ethical and legal issues within healthcare systems relating to the use of information, information technology, communication networks, and patient care technology.
- Evaluate consumer health information sources for accuracy, timeliness, and appropriateness.

Essential V: Healthcare policy for advocacy in healthcare

The DNP program prepares graduates to:

- Critically analyze health policy proposals, health policies, and related issues from the perspective of consumers, nurses, other health professionals, and other stakeholders in policy and public forums.
- Demonstrate leadership in the development and implementation of institutional, local, state, federal, and/or international health policy.
- Influence policy makers through active participation on committees, boards, or task forces at the institutional, local, state, regional, national, and/or international levels to improve healthcare delivery and outcomes.

- Educate others, including policy makers at all levels, regarding nursing, health policy, and patient care outcomes.
- Advocate for the nursing profession within the policy and healthcare communities.
- Develop, evaluate, and provide leadership for healthcare policy that shapes healthcare finance regulation and delivery.
- Advocate for social justice, equity, and ethical policies within all healthcare arenas.

Essential VI: Interprofessional collaboration for improving patient and population health outcomes

The DNP program prepares the graduate to:

- Employ effective communication and collaboration skills in the development and implementation of practice models, peer review, practice guidelines, health policy, standards of care, and/or other scholarly products.
- Lead interprofessional teams in the analysis of complex practice and organizational issues.
- Employ consultative and leadership skills with professional and interprofessional teams to create change in healthcare and complex healthcare delivery systems.

Essential VII: Clinical prevention and population health for improving the nation's health

The DNP program prepares the graduate to:

- Evaluate care delivery models and/or strategies using concepts related to community, environmental and occupational health, and cultural and socioeconomic dimensions of health.

Essential VIII: Advanced nursing practice

The DNP program prepares the graduate to:

- Design, implement, and evaluate therapeutic interventions based on nursing science and other sciences.
- Develop and sustain therapeutic relationships and partnerships with patients and other professionals to facilitate optimal care and patient outcomes.
- Demonstrate advanced levels of clinical judgment, systems thinking, and accountability in designing, delivering, and evaluating evidence-based care to improve patient outcomes.

- Guide, mentor, and support other nurses to achieve excellence in nursing practice.
- Educate and guide individuals and others through complex health and situational transitions.
- Use conceptual and analytical skills in evaluating the links among practice, organizational, population, fiscal, and policy issues.

Source: Adapted with permission from the American Association of Colleges of Nursing (AACN). (2006). *The essentials of doctoral education for advanced nursing practice.* Retrieved from http://www.aacn.nche.edu/dnp/pdf/essentials.pdf

■ THE SKILLS

COLLABORATION

Collaborative leadership describes a leadership style that involves seeking out and using the input from individuals from different backgrounds, generations, and cultures within a group or team, while respecting all different perspectives. According to Archer and Cameron (2009), one of the key goals of the collaborative leader is being able to achieve value from inherent differences. This is especially true for the DNP graduate who is prepared to work with various leaders within an institution as well as those from partnering organizations who may not necessarily have all of the same objectives or goals. The DNP must be able to lead the team effectively, by gathering ideas and resources in an environment of open communication that ultimately leads to action. Collaboration is more than being able to get along well or build consensus. Collaboration involves specific skills that require a big picture perspective of a situation, the ability to recognize the obstacles to achieving an objective, the ability to resolve conflict, and, ultimately, facilitating the steps to attain a successful outcome (Fitzpatrick, 2013). In today's workforce, interprofessional collaboration is critical for the sustainability of healthcare systems. Interprofessional approaches can solve problems within healthcare systems by drawing from the expertise of all disciplines. This type of collaboration can be fostered through interprofessional education, which is now incorporated into the curriculum of many academic programs for healthcare professions. Nurse leaders in practice settings have demonstrated the ability to collaborate with other healthcare professionals and this has led to a cultural shift in healthcare organizations with more nurses having a seat at the table (Fitzpatrick, 2013).

COMMUNICATION

Another theme that is evident in the AACN *Essentials of Doctoral Education for Advanced Practice Nursing* is communication (AACN, 2006). Effective communication is at the heart of leadership and can come in many forms, such as talking, writing, body language, and actions. As nurses, we have the advantage of having experience in communicating with others, and the art of communication is inherent in the work we do with patients. Nurses must be able to provide empathic care to the infirmed, provide education to someone who was recently diagnosed with a life-threatening diagnosis, or communicate the importance of preventive health screening to populations at risk for disease.

James Clawson is an author and professor of business administration at the University of Virginia. In his book titled *Level Three Leadership: Getting Below the Surface*, Clawson describes leadership as "managing energy . . . first in yourself and then in others" (2006, p. 3). He categorizes leadership on three different levels based on how the leader is able to view, understand, and communicate with others. *Level one* leadership is more of a superficial level of leading others. Leaders who practice at this level tend to make assessments based on others' visible behaviors. *Level two* leaders require a deeper level understanding based on individuals' conscious thoughts. *Level three* leaders lead and influence others by understanding the deep-rooted values, attitudes, behaviors, and expectations (or as Clawson terms them, VABEs) of others and knowing how to influence individuals on this much deeper level. He goes on to state that effective level three leaders are able to "understand the basic assumptions and values of employees and to match them or educate them toward harmony with the goals and strategic directions of the firm." He believes that new or potential level three leaders "must develop new skills, including the ability to view what people are thinking and feeling" (Clawson, 2006, p. 60). The first step in being able to lead at level three begins with understanding and clarifying one's own VABEs.

Effective leaders communicate a vision to a team and the team develops a plan to make the vision a reality. Nurses, during their graduate education, learn about the importance of communication and self-reflection. One of the most important tools we have for good communication is listening. Nurses can develop strong listening skills, empathy, ways to recognize and manage personal emotions, and the ability to pay attention to others over time through patient interactions. Daniel Goleman, a psychologist, refers to these skills as *emotional intelligence* (1998). Emotional intelligence is the ability to understand and manage your own emotions and those of the people around you. Goleman describes five main elements of emotional intelligence: self-awareness, self-regulation, motivation, empathy, and social skills. As a leader, the more you are able to manage these elements, the higher your emotional intelligence. Goleman notes that, while the core elements of emotional intelligence are developed in childhood, these same elements can be developed in adulthood with training (Goleman, 1998). Nurses use emotional intelligence, or at least most components of emotional intelligence, as part of their everyday work, and for many it becomes second nature. The DNP is able to harness these skills and apply them not only to patient encounters but can utilize these same skills to lead clinics or healthcare organizations.

By being able to communicate effectively and by using both emotional intelligence and Clawson's level three leadership techniques, the DNP-prepared nurse is able to work productively with other key personnel within organizations. The DNP is able to translate and share critical information regarding evidence-based practice with front-line clinical staff and is able to advocate for the needs of patients in the ever-changing and complex health systems.

EVALUATION

The *AACN DNP Essential III, Clinical Scholarship and Analytical Methods for Evidence Based Practice* identifies the importance of the DNP-prepared nurse designing and implementing processes that evaluate outcomes of practice, practice patterns, and systems of care within a clinic, community, or healthcare organization against national benchmarks to determine variances in practice outcomes and population trends (AACN, 2006). DNP programs prepare graduates to be able to critically review and interpret data and to understand the implications of the findings both clinically as well as from a fiscal and quality improvement perspective. By identifying new and innovative interventions, translating quality evidence into practice, and evaluating the outcomes of these interventions, DNPs are able to lead organizational change and provide patients with the best possible care. Evaluation is a skill that confers upon the DNP *expert power*. This is a concept that has been described in the theories of leadership by French and Raven (1959). Expert power has been associated with a form of leadership where others defer to a person based on their superior knowledge base or understanding of a subject matter. In essence, by having the skills and knowledge of a doctoral-prepared nurse, one is viewed by others in the field, and in the organization, as being the expert. Having the ability to provide critical evaluation of practice recommendations or evaluating the overall cost-effectiveness of an intervention is highly valued by other health professionals and administrators. It is through utilization of these skills that the DNP can find his or her niche and value to an organization.

■ LEADING OTHERS

Nursing leadership in this rapidly changing healthcare environment requires the skills previously reviewed, such as knowledge in their area of expertise, works well with others, and excellent communication and listening skills along with the ability to evaluate interventions. There are many different approaches to leadership but one that resonates with what is required to be a successful health system leader is *transformational leadership*. Transformational leadership is an approach that creates positive change in team members with the end goal of developing followers into leaders (Goleman, 2006). It can enhance the motivation, morale, and performance of the team through a variety of mechanisms, including role modeling, challenging team members to take greater responsibility for their work, and understanding strengths and weaknesses of the team members so that appropriate tasks are assigned to optimize performance (Bass, 1997). This type of leader has vision, self-confidence, self-direction, energy, honesty, commitment, and the ability to develop and implement a vision while empowering others (Barker, Sullivan, & Emery, 2006). The DNP graduate with transformational leadership skills will be able to lead healthcare teams to improve quality of care and patient safety. By utilizing knowledge, training, and skills attained through education and clinical practice, the DNP serves a pivotal leadership role by translating evidence into practice, assessing systems to improve quality, utilizing technology to improve patient care, and measuring outcomes.

■ DEVELOPING THE SKILLS

What are the steps one must take in order to develop and become competent in these skills? Several ways in which one can begin the journey to a leadership role are outlined here.

1. **Identify Leaders You Admire**

   One of the first steps in becoming a leader is to identify someone or a group of people who you feel embodies or possesses the qualities that you would like to develop. There is nothing better than seeing leadership in action. You can pick one person, but since it is difficult for one individual to possess all of the qualities that you see as ideal, you will probably need to find more than one person. The individuals you select could include a faculty member, a colleague, a boss, or someone that you know through your social network. Ideally, one or more of these individuals could mentor you in becoming a leader. The person or group of individuals you choose do not necessarily need to be a formal mentor in the classic sense of the term. A formal mentor–mentee relationship involves a mutually agreed-upon recognition of a relationship, a set of goals, and a long-term commitment of training and apprenticeship (David, Clutterbuck, & Megginson, 2013). This is not necessary for this experience.

   Once you have identified this person or set of individuals, it is important to observe and take note of exactly what it is they do in certain situations, particularly ones that involve collaboration, evaluation, conflict negotiation, communication, and leading or inspiring others. These situations do not have to be nursing or healthcare focused because the skills and the techniques that these individuals use can be adapted and applied to your work site. You may find that you like how some leaders are able to take a visionary approach to motivating others, or how certain leaders approach a situation when they have made an error. You may learn by watching how your boss is able to achieve consensus among differing groups. By observing these real-life interactions, you will soon be able to identify the techniques that are successful and integrate them into your skill set.

2. **Assess Your Skills and Leadership Style**

   Now that you have learned and identified persons who possess the skills you would like to embody, the next step is to assess your current skill set, highlighting your strengths and weaknesses. There are various self-administered leadership inventories available and many are available online. Much like a personality test, these self-assessments are one way to identify the type of leader you are and the type of leadership style that most closely resembles your personality and inherent strengths. It is important when interpreting these test results to remember that these tests are designed to give you a general sense of your traits, but it is important not to feel locked into the results. You can modify or alter certain aspects of your leadership style if you feel that it does not mesh with your current organization or the organization you envision yourself leading. Identifying your leadership style is, however, a starting point that can help you determine what areas you need to develop and strengthen.

3. **Assess What Leadership Activities You Are Currently Doing**

Many individuals may not necessarily view themselves as being in a leadership role, but may very well be in one without recognizing it. One of the first steps is to review your activities, accomplishments, and interests. This involves taking time to reflect on the things that you have done in life and what you enjoy doing. This is the time to "think outside the box" and not just focus on your professional life as a nurse. In reality, many of us may use similar skills required of the DNP degree in other activities. For example, you may be someone who is active in your child's parent–teacher association at school, coaches the soccer team, serves on the welcoming committee for your neighborhood association, or organizes the fundraiser for the local homeless shelter. These are not only personally gratifying activities, but they also provide you with the opportunity to develop important skills that you can use in your professional career.

Once you have identified the activities that you participate in, think about what types of skills you use in these activities and see if they fit into any of the main themes of leadership found in the DNP competencies, such as collaboration, communication, evaluation, and leading others. You will likely find at least one or two activities that include these skills or at least provide an opportunity for you to practice these skills in an environment or an organization that you already belong to and feel comfortable working in. Perhaps the parent–teacher association that you belong to wants to know the most cost-effective way of increasing the budget without raising parent membership fees. This task would require you to use your skills of evaluating data, looking at the financial objectives, and determining the best options. As you can see, there is a wide variety of ways to use these skills and gain practical experience in building confidence to become a recognized leader.

4. **Start Small and Then Go Big**

If you find that you lack sufficient experience with certain skills, you can look for opportunities to practice these skills on a smaller scale project. For example, you may want to volunteer to organize the next school fundraiser. This involves communication, collaboration, evaluating, and leading other parents. Perhaps you have the opportunity to volunteer on a local political campaign. This involves working within a larger system, communicating with voters and the campaign office, negotiating with others who may have differing views, and inspiring or envisioning organizational change. Once you gain confidence and experience in these smaller venues, the next step involves applying the lessons learned to aspects of your professional career.

5. **Seize the Opportunity**

If you are working as a staff nurse while in graduate school, your practice site may have working groups or committees. These committees may be unit based or hospital wide. Take (and make) the time to volunteer for these committees. Seize the opportunity to get involved and use your leadership skills. Even by serving as a working member of a committee, you automatically assume leadership responsibilities by representing your peers. Many times, these committees may have a specific focus such as patient safety, but often unit-based or hospital-based committees focus on issues related to quality improvement. This is the ideal setting for the DNP-in-training to gain first-hand knowledge of how quality improvement opportunities are identified, how strategies for improvement are implemented, and how organizational change occurs. By getting involved in these work-based activities, you will be able to put your learned skills into practice and ultimately be recognized as a valuable member of the committee. These are the initial steps you can take on the road to becoming an advanced practice nurse leader. Within these working groups, new ideas and projects may be realized and new opportunities to create and lead can be developed.

6. **Create Your Own Opportunities**

As a DNP student, you learn to look at your practice site and identify areas for needed improvement. If you are able to identify an area of needed improvement, you can develop this into a quality improvement project. For example, perhaps you want to assess the patient discharge process on your unit to identify ways of increasing efficiency, or you want to know how many patients attending your clinic received screening for tobacco use, or how many of your CHF home health clients required multiple in-home services. Be the driving force to create change. Leaders within your healthcare setting will likely be pleased to have you look into areas where there may be gaps or areas needing improvement. In some instances, you may have the opportunity to complete these activities as part of your regular work assignment, but be prepared to volunteer your time. Remember, you may be volunteering your time now, but you are gaining experience that will benefit you in the long term.

7. **Lead in the Profession**

Other areas to seek leadership opportunities include working with or joining professional organizations. Many major professional organizations have local affiliates or chapters. If you are not already a member of a specialty nursing organization, consider joining one. If you already are a member, consider volunteering for various committees or even running for a position as an officer. Professional organizations are a wonderful way to meet and network with nurses and nurse leaders outside of your place of employment. Within these organizations, you can exercise your skills of communication, collaboration, and leading others by working side by side with other recognized nurse leaders and advanced practice clinicians.

8. **Reflect, Review, and Redirect**

One of the components of learning a new skill is being able to assess and adjust what you are doing. Although self-assessment has been discussed as a first step in gaining leadership skills, it is also important to periodically reflect on your progress throughout your learning process. The skill of self-reflection is often taught to entry-level nursing students and remains an important skill for our entire careers. It is from critically appraising clinical situations that we learn what works, what does not work, and how to anticipate and prepare for future events. It is important to be able to take the time to look at how you have incorporated your new skills into your practice. What aspects of your new leadership style do you like? What seems to be less effective? What areas would you like more practice? How well do you communicate your vision? How are you at collaborating with others? Are you able to lead others? Are you able to critically evaluate information and use it to create change? If the answers to these questions is "yes," then keep doing what you are doing. If the answer to some or all of these questions is "no," then redirect your focus, identify your assets and ways to overcome your challenges, and then try out a new strategy. From this ongoing self-reflection, you will eventually find the right mix of skills and expertise to be the leader you envision yourself being.

■ JUST THE BEGINNING

Once you have gained some practical experience in leadership and using your advanced practice skills, you will be well on your way to fulfilling the role and competencies of the DNP. It is important to remember that the process of becoming a leader takes time and is an evolutionary process that is both challenging and rewarding. Leadership is both a skill and an art form. Just like any other skill, the more you do it, the easier it becomes. As you transition into the role of DNP, you will cross many milestones, and being a leader and gaining the skills to be a successful leader are included in those milestones. Now more than ever, the field of nursing and the healthcare environment are changing at speeds that far exceed the changes we have seen historically. It is truly a time of limitless boundaries, and as clinicians, visionaries, and systems-level experts, the DNP graduate of today has the opportunity to change the landscape of healthcare for generations to come.

■ REFERENCES

American Association of Colleges of Nursing. (2006). *The essentials of doctoral education for advanced nursing practice.* Retrieved from http://www.aacnnursing.org/Portals/42/Publications/DNPEssentials.pdf

Archer, D., & Cameron, A. (2009). *Collaborative leadership, how to succeed in an interconnected world.* Burlington, MA: Elsevier.

Barker, A. M., Sullivan, D. T., & Emery, M. J. (2006). *Leadership competencies for clinical managers.* Boston, MA: Jones & Bartlett.

Bass, B. (1997). *Transformational leadership: Industrial, military, and educational impact.* East Sussex, UK: Psychology Press.

Clawson, J. G. (2006). *Level three leadership: Getting below the surface* (3rd ed.). Upper Saddle River, NJ: Pearson Prentice Hall.

David, S., Clutterbuck, D., & Megginson, D. (2013). *Beyond goals strategies for coaching and menotring.* New York, NY: Routledge.

Fitzpatrick, J., & Greer, G. (2013). *Nursing leadership from the outside in.* New York, NY: Springer Publishing.

French, J. R. P., & Raven, B. (1959). *The bases of social power.* Ann Arbor: University of Michigan Press.

Goleman, D. (1998). What makes a leader? *Harvard Business Review* (pp. 82–91). Retrieved from http://www.lesaffaires.com/uploads/references/743_what-makes-leader_Goleman.pdf

Goleman, D. (2006). *Emotional Intelligence: Why it can matter more than IQ.* New York, NY: Bantam.

Institute of Medicine. (2011). *The future of nursing: Leading change, advancing health.* Retrieved from https://www.nap.edu/read/12956/chapter/10

Marshall, E. (Eds.). (2010). *Transformational leadership in nursing.* New York, NY: Springer Publishing.

NARA. (2017). *Eisenhower presidential library, museum and boyhood home.* Retrieved from https://www.eisenhower.archives.gov/all_about_ike/quotes.html

CHAPTER TEN

Developing the Leadership Skill Set for the Executive Nurse Leader

JEANETTE IVES ERICKSON, MARIANNE DITOMASSI, AND JEFFREY M. ADAMS

Opportunities and strategies for leadership improvement in the healthcare system have been well documented. Yet, direct funding and support of nursing administration research have not traditionally been a high priority for federal or private grant-making institutions. The increasing acuity of patients, the demand for reducing cost of providing health services, and the need for establishing structures that lead to a more efficient, effective, timely, equitable, safe, and patient-centered (Institute of Medicine [IOM], 2001) delivery system require expert nurse leadership. Thus, focus and development of expert executive nurse leaders are more important than ever. This chapter explores the efforts, experiences, and framing of executive nurse leadership through an organization's commitment to development and utilization of a program of research within this population.

■ EVIDENCE- AND KNOWLEDGE-BASED MANAGEMENT PRACTICE

An important distinction in setting an organizational executive nurse leadership agenda is the commitment to evidence-based practice (EBP) and, perhaps more importantly, knowledge-based practice (KBP) within the context of nursing administration and executive nurse leadership roles. EBP can be defined as the integration of best-research evidence with clinical expertise driven by patient and family values (Sackett, Straus, Richardson, Rosenberg, & Haynes, 2000). KBP can be best described as the interactive linkage among theory, research, and practice (Roy, 2007). Although evidence and data have been widely adopted as drivers of clinical practice decisions, they have not been completely integrated in administrative or leadership practice. KBP provides a framework for both basis and justification of executive nurse leadership practice. It places value on critical thinking and decision making, providing some latitude for managing social and political structures that are a daily part of executive leadership practice.

Parallel to the need for the adoption of EBP/KBP strategies, Magnet® recognition validates executive nurse leadership and highlights the presence of a strong and collaborative professional practice environment (PPE). Grounded in research, Magnet recognition is the highest honor awarded to healthcare institutions by the American Nurses Credentialing Center (ANCC) for excellence in nursing services. The current Magnet recognition model heightens the importance of demonstrating the outcomes and effects of nurses' work (ANCC, 2008). This framework challenges executive nurse leaders to utilize EBP/KBP as part of a continuous critical review toward improving the structures and processes that support care delivery.

■ ADVANCING KNOWLEDGE/FRAMING THE EFFORTS

An important part of KBP is not only the utilization of evidence, but also the participation and development of new knowledge to inform and advance the discipline and improve patient care outcomes, the PPE, and patient and staff satisfaction. Because of the impact, advancing knowledge is a high priority. The Agency for Healthcare Research and Quality (AHRQ), American Nurses Association (ANA), American Organization for Nurse Executives (AONE), and the National Institute for Nursing Research (NINR) have all identified nursing work environments, organizational structure, and patient outcomes research as funding priorities. Additionally, it can be surmised that these research initiatives will also lead to the refinement of nursing administration educational curricula and continuing education strategies for the executive nurse leader.

Shortell, Gillies, and Devers (1995) first introduced a need to understand and manage the complexities of healthcare institutions, with the recognition that new management and leadership skills are required. They proposed that healthcare leaders must generate the development of a new culture with an emphasis on managing horizontally, which calls for greater negotiation and conflict management skills, systems thinking, and team building. While this call, over two decades old, has not gone unheeded, adapting to manage the complexities of healthcare is a forever project, and success is closely tied to those with vision and focus. Within this context, tying or framing executive nurse leadership research to PPEs and/or patient outcomes serves as both a visionary approach and a focus that can be shared and supported by funding organizations; it also further defines and improves success for those in nursing executive leadership practice.

■ LEADERSHIP DEVELOPMENT TRAJECTORY—THE PROFESSIONAL PRACTICE MODEL

While a knowledge-based nursing leadership practice inclusive of research and theory has long been a part of efforts at the Massachusetts General Hospital (MGH), the coordinated efforts toward a focused executive nurse leadership strategy integrating and emphasizing the PPE began in 1996. At this time, the MGH nursing and patient care leadership first developed the MGH Professional Practice Model (PPM) as represented in Figure 10.1 (Ives Erickson, 1996). A PPM is a conceptual, theoretical,

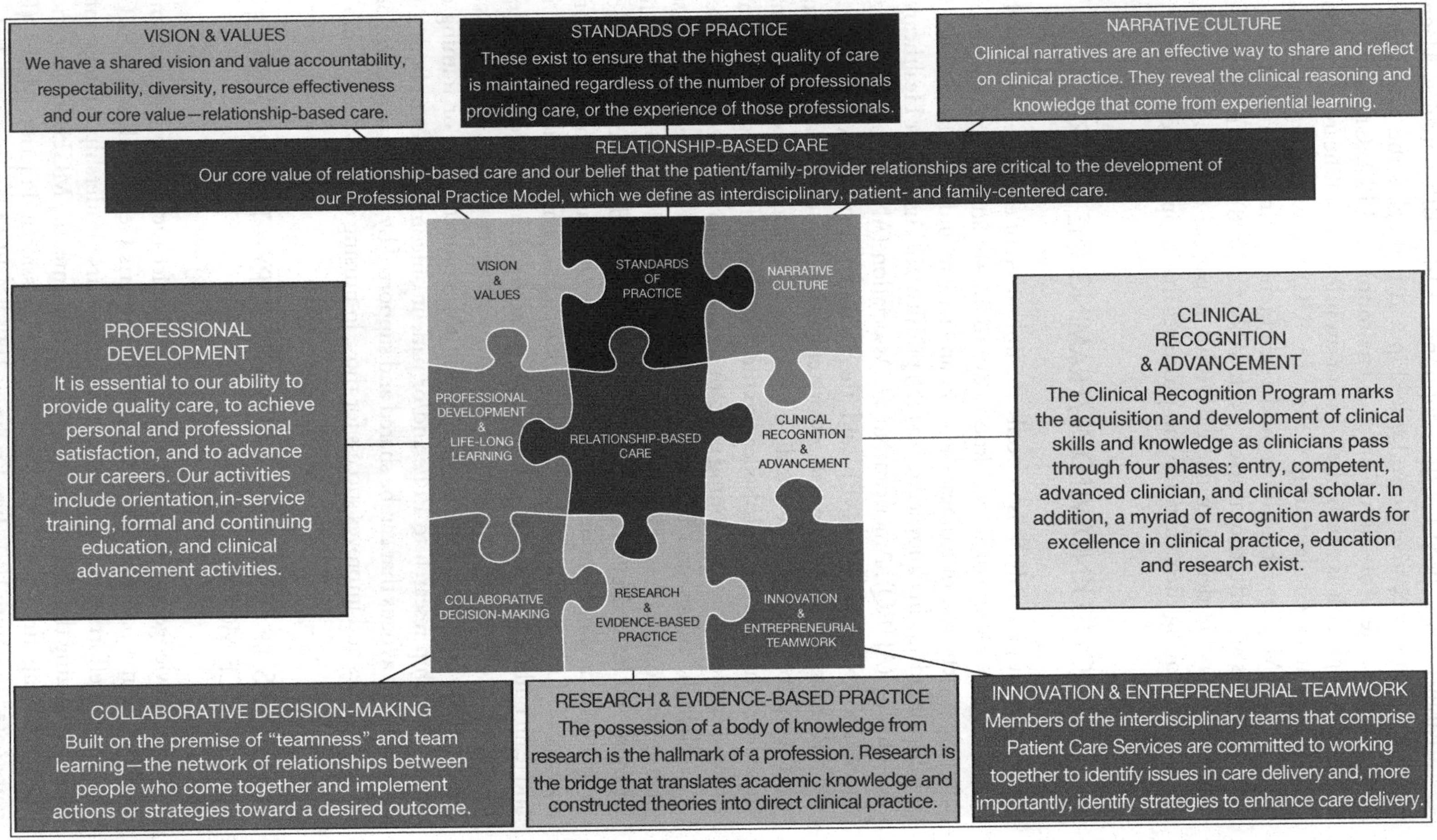
VISION & VALUES
We have a shared vision and value accountability, respectability, diversity, resource effectiveness and our core value—relationship-based care.
STANDARDS OF PRACTICE
These exist to ensure that the highest quality of care is maintained regardless of the number of professionals providing care, or the experience of those professionals.
NARRATIVE CULTURE
Clinical narratives are an effective way to share and reflect on clinical practice. They reveal the clinical reasoning and knowledge that come from experiential learning.
RELATIONSHIP-BASED CARE
Our core value of relationship-based care and our belief that the patient/family-provider relationships are critical to the development of our Professional Practice Model, which we define as interdisciplinary, patient- and family-centered care.
PROFESSIONAL DEVELOPMENT
It is essential to our ability to provide quality care, to achieve personal and professional satisfaction, and to advance our careers. Our activities include orientation,in-service training, formal and continuing education, and clinical advancement activities.
VISION & VALUES
STANDARDS OF PRACTICE
NARRATIVE CULTURE
PROFESSIONAL DEVELOPMENT & LIFE-LONG LEARNING
RELATIONSHIP-BASED CARE
CLINICAL RECOGNITION & ADVANCEMENT
COLLABORATIVE DECISION-MAKING
RESEARCH & EVIDENCE-BASED PRACTICE
INNOVATION & ENTREPRENEURIAL TEAMWORK
CLINICAL RECOGNITION & ADVANCEMENT
The Clinical Recognition Program marks the acquisition and development of clinical skills and knowledge as clinicians pass through four phases: entry, competent, advanced clinician, and clinical scholar. In addition, a myriad of recognition awards for excellence in clinical practice, education and research exist.
COLLABORATIVE DECISION-MAKING
Built on the premise of "teamness" and team learning—the network of relationships between people who come together and implement actions or strategies toward a desired outcome.
RESEARCH & EVIDENCE-BASED PRACTICE
The possession of a body of knowledge from research is the hallmark of a profession. Research is the bridge that translates academic knowledge and constructed theories into direct clinical practice.
INNOVATION & ENTREPRENEURIAL TEAMWORK
Members of the interdisciplinary teams that comprise Patient Care Services are committed to working together to identify issues in care delivery and, more importantly, identify strategies to enhance care delivery.

FIGURE 10.1 Massachusetts General Hospital—professional practice model.

and practical framework that provides nurses with an articulate, knowledge-based justification for practice of the profession. Developed and disseminated in 1996 and revised in 2007 and 2015, the MGH PPM is grounded in values and beliefs that embrace patient-centered care in partnership with the nurse and other providers of care within the patient care environment.

With a well-designed PPM framework, nurses feel connected within the context of their relationships to the patient, their own practice, the roles of other providers in contributing to the plan, other nurses, and the institution. Framework and structure support the nurse in planning, managing, and adapting to change, and they facilitate the identification of goals and strategies to improve outcomes. Articulation of a model for the nursing professionals within an organization provides a critical mass of energy to support resources, strength, and visibility within an often-complex structure. Routinely evaluating clinicians' perceptions of that practice model provides invaluable information toward the betterment of both the organization and patient care (Ives Erickson & Ditomassi, 2011).

■ PATIENT CARE DELIVERY MODEL

Flowing from the PPM is the articulation of a Patient Care Delivery Model (Figure 10.2). As a natural outgrowth of strategic planning was the decision to integrate relationship-based care at the heart of the delivery model.

The six aims of the IOM are sharing the center of the model by ensuring that care is patient- and family centered, safe, efficient, effective, timely, and equitable. The aims are the pillars of the care delivery model. Domains of practice speak to the importance of "doing for" and "being with" the patient to create an environment for healing and optimal care delivery. Empirical outcomes are how we measure the impact of our work which links back to leadership and the utilization of EBP. The four components are vital to ensuring effectiveness of care delivery and influence of the leader.

■ EVALUATING THE PPE

Furthering this agenda, the Staff Perceptions of Professional Practice Environment (SPPPE) survey instrument, comprised of the Professional Practice Work Environment Inventory (PPWEI; Ives Erickson, Duffy, Ditomassi, & Jones, 2017), a derivative of the PPE scale (Ives Erickson et al., 2004) and Revised Professional Practice Environment (RPPE) scale (Ives Erickson, Duffy, Ditomassi, & Jones, 2009) was developed as a mechanism for evaluating and informing leaders as to opportunities to improve the care delivery practice environment. This instrument was based on the work of the initial Magnet study (McClure, Poulin, Sovie, & Wandelt, 1983), which began the research associating positive practice environments to better patient outcomes. The PPWEI provides an assessment of nine organizational characteristics determined to be important to clinician satisfaction. These consist of autonomy and control over

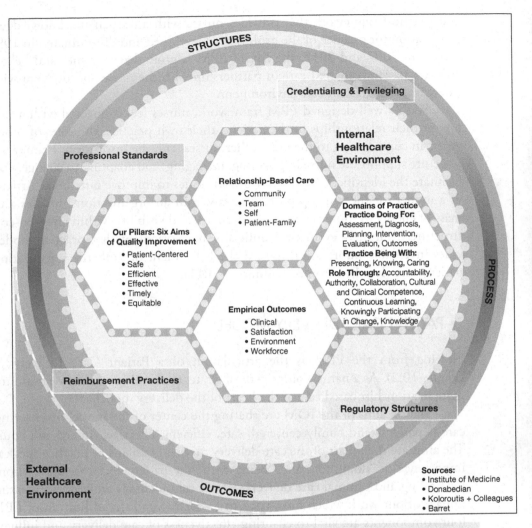

FIGURE 10.2 Massachusetts General Hospital—patient care delivery model.

practice; communication about patients; cultural sensitivity; handling disagreement and conflict; staff relations with physicians, staff, and hospital groups; sufficient staff, time, and resources for quality patient care; supportive leadership; teamwork; and work motivation. Through annual administration of the PPWEI, a greater understanding of organizational concepts that enhance clinical practice can be achieved.

■ DEVELOPING A CLIMATE OF INCLUSION

Adding to the knowledge development thread surrounding the PPE is the ongoing research focused on understanding the diversity of an organization's workforce and fostering a climate in which culturally competent and culturally sensitive care is delivered. The delivery of culturally competent care and the nurses' abilities as leaders to create an environment to meet the individual needs of our patients in a sensitive, healing, and respectful way must be a commitment of nurse leaders. If cultural diversity is to be viewed with an eye to the future, a shift in personal perspectives and values is necessary, whereby cultural competence cannot simply be about tolerance, as tolerance is a position of neutrality (Washington, Ives Erickson, & Ditomassi, 2004). To meet this commitment, executive nurse leaders must strengthen their awareness, knowledge, and skills surrounding cultural concepts and ensure that these are shared and integrated into clinical practice as a mechanism to improve both the care of patients and the PPE in which clinicians work.

■ EXECUTIVE NURSE LEADERSHIP AND THE PRACTICE ENVIRONMENT

Parallel to the practice environment enhancement research, MGH also began to emphasize looking at the "source" of organizational executive nurse leadership. As part of Ives Erickson's Robert Wood Johnson Executive Nurse Fellowship, a national survey of chief nurses was conducted to identify the skills needed to position nurse executives for success in an integrated delivery system (IDS) environment structure. Survey respondents include chief nurses of single-hospital facilities and leaders of multifacility IDSs. The 182 respondents identified critical skills needed to perform effectively at the IDS level, which are identified in Figure 10.3 and include

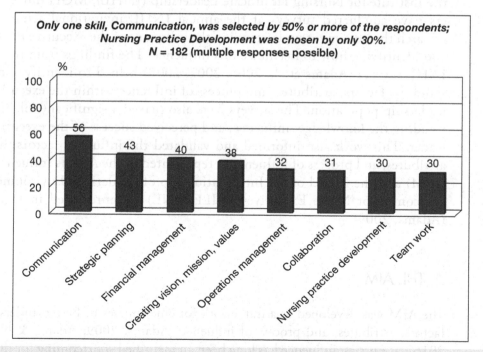

FIGURE 10.3 Top skills necessary for success as CNO in IDS.

CNO, chief nursing officer; IDS, integrated delivery system.

the following: communication; strategic planning; financial management; creating vision, mission, and values; operations management; collaboration; nursing practice development; and teamwork (Ives Erickson, 2002). Analysis of qualitative responses revealed that different skills specific to the IDS were emphasized, yet, interestingly, all were closely related to other independently identified standards, such as PPE/RPPE scales mentioned previously (Ives Erickson et al., 2004, 2009) and to the core competencies of nurse executive practice (business skills, knowledge of the healthcare environment, leadership skills, professionalism, and relationship building) as defined by AONE (2011).

■ EXECUTIVE NURSE LEADERSHIP INFLUENCE

Building on Ives Erickson's work, Adams, Duffy, and Clifford (2006) suggested that the approximately 5,000 chief nurses in the United States (Health Forum, 2006) serve as the gatekeepers for the advancement of the majority of the 3.6 million nurses practicing in the United States (ANA, 2017), yet were not maximizing influence in comparison with their C-suite counterparts (Adams et al., 2006, 2007), leaving us with the question, "Having gotten to that table, now what?"

Thus, from 2005 to 2008, in collaboration with Joyce C. Clifford, CEO of the Institute for Nursing Healthcare Leadership (INHL), MGH nurse researchers have conducted surveys at the annual INHL invitational seminars. This research thread aims at understanding the influence of the executive nurse leader and identifying how to maximize this influence. The findings from the series of INHL surveys (Adams et al., 2006, 2007, 2008) helped to identify and understand the factors, attributes, and process of influence within the executive nurse leadership population. The surveys have also played a significant role in understanding the knowledge, influence, and perceived success of the executive nurse leader. This work also informed and validated the influence factors, influence attributes, and process of influence as represented in the Adams Influence Model (AIM) and the Model of the Interrelationship of Leadership Environments and Outcomes for Nurse Executives (MILE ONE) as represented in Figure 10.4 (Adams, 2009).

■ THE AIM

The AIM was developed as a framework for chief nurses to better understand the factors, attributes, and process of influence (Adams, 2009; Adams & Natarajan, 2016), as nursing influence has long been an identified shortcoming for the profession (Godden, 1995; Robert Wood Johnson Foundation, 2010). It guides executive nurse leaders in their practice through the recognition of five primary influence

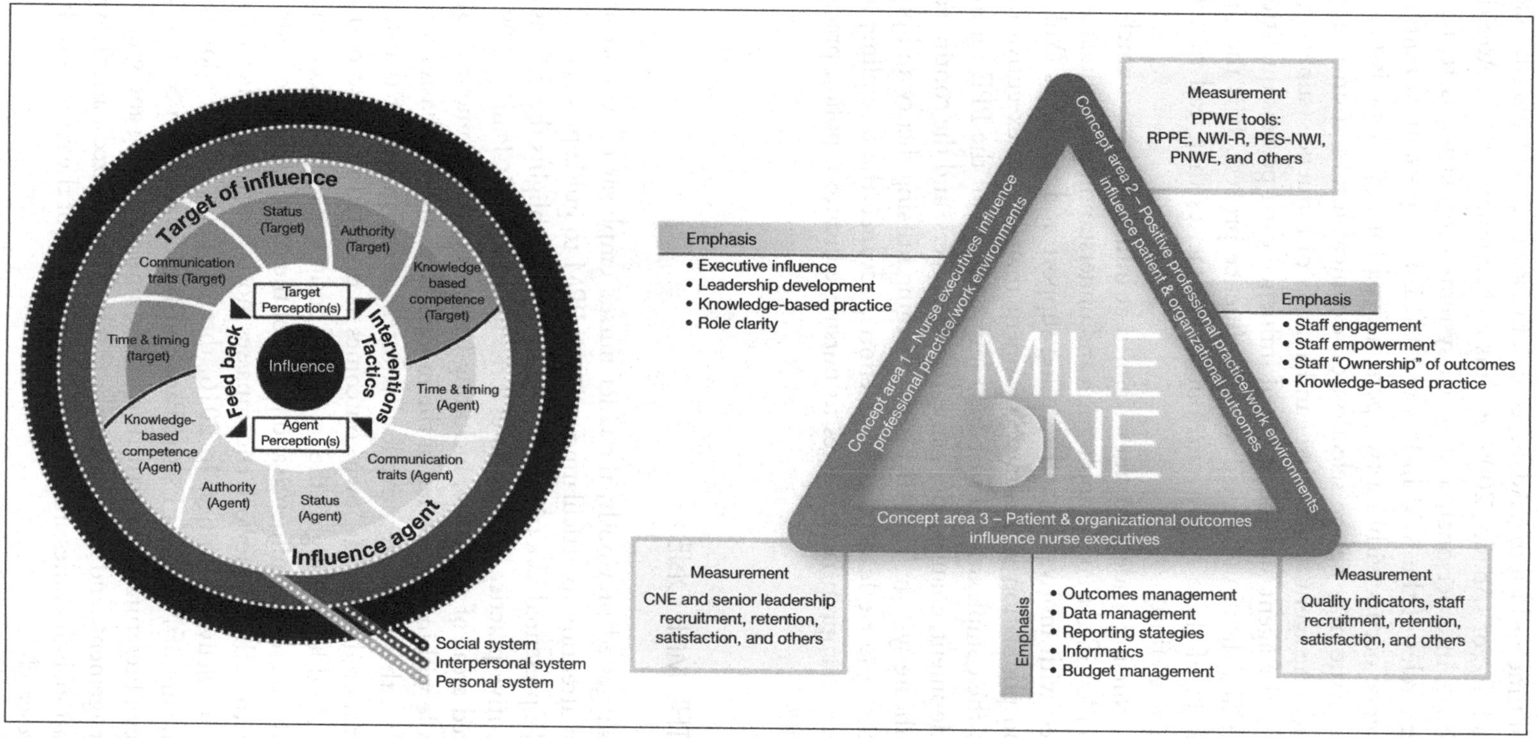
Target of influence
Status (Target)
Authority (Target)
Knowledge based competence (Target)
Communication traits (Target)
Time & timing (target)
Target Perception(s)
Feed back
Influence
Interventions Tactics
Agent Perception(s)
Time & timing (Agent)
Knowledge-based competence (Agent)
Communication traits (Agent)
Authority (Agent)
Status (Agent)
Influence agent
Social system
Interpersonal system
Personal system
Measurement
PPWE tools:
RPPE, NWI-R, PES-NWI, PNWE, and others
Emphasis
• Executive influence
• Leadership development
• Knowledge-based practice
• Role clarity
Concept area 1 – Nurse executives influence professional practice/work environments
Concept area 2 – Positive professional practice/work environments influence patient & organizational outcomes
MILE ONE
Emphasis
• Staff engagement
• Staff empowerment
• Staff "Ownership" of outcomes
• Knowledge-based practice
Concept area 3 – Patient & organizational outcomes influence nurse executives
Measurement
CNE and senior leadership recruitment, retention, satisfaction, and others
Emphasis
• Outcomes management
• Data management
• Reporting stategies
• Informatics
• Budget management
Measurement
Quality indicators, staff recruitment, retention, satisfaction, and others

FIGURE 10.4 **Adams influence model and model of the interrelationship of leadership, environments, and outcomes for nurse executives.**

CNE, chief nursing executives; NWI-R; PES-NWI; PNWE; PPWE, professional practice work environment; RPPE, revised professional practice environment factors (authority, communication traits, knowledge-based competence, status, and use of time and timing; Adams & Ives Erickson, 2011) and the associated attributes of each factor (Adams, 2009; Adams & Nataraian, 2016). Additionally, while the personal, interpersonal, and social systems interrelate, as represented within the outer circles of the AIM in Figure 10.4, it is important to note that interpersonal influence occurs within a two-person dyad for any single issue. As an example, a single issue may be the selection of a clinical information system. A dyad could include the agent (chief nurse) and a target of influence (superior, peer, or subordinate). The agent and the target of influence each possess qualities, characteristics, and skills that can be used in the influence process. It is the understanding and titration of these factors, attributes, and tactics that lead to achieved or missed influence efforts.

Nursing leadership studies aimed at influence are extremely important. It has been identified that the application and understanding of influence begins with those tasked with motivating and securing support and resources (Yukl & Falbe, 1990). In no population is this more pertinent than within executive nursing leadership, with the complexities of sustained improvement of the PPE through the workforce development, changes to organizational budgets, and the continued evolution of our healthcare system. The AIM is an emerging nursing theory and provides a guide for executive nurse leaders to focus efforts, advance the discipline, and more broadly influence appropriate changes to nursing education, policy, practice, research, and theory.

■ THE MILE ONE

As suggested previously, the chief nurse's emphasis of practice is the PPE. Paying keen attention to articulating a shared PPM to guide practice is the key. The MILE ONE presented as a triangle in Figure 10.4 highlights the PPE as the focus of nurse executive practice (Adams, Ives Erickson, Jones, & Paulo, 2009). It provides suggested areas of emphasis, including leadership development, KBP, and clarification of role within the first leg of the model. With the emphasis on the development of a PPE, the nurse executive leader fosters an environment that leads to an engaged, empowered staff that "own" outcomes as depicted in the second leg of the triangle. The third leg highlights the impact of positive patient and organizational outcomes on the increased influence and power of the nurse executive leader in his or her role. Together, this framework encompasses most, if not all, EBP/KBP projects that occur in care delivery settings. In 2016, the MILE ONE was adopted as the American Academy of Nursing's Expert Panel on Building Health System Excellence. It provides a literature-based structure toward understanding and guiding nurse executive, management, and staff nurse efforts toward optimized patient, workforce and organizational outcomes and was developed as part of the review for this general program of research.

■ PRACTICE ENVIRONMENT CONCEPTUAL FRAMEWORK— INTEGRATING CONCEPTS

Also in this vein, and in concert with the AIM and MILE ONE, Ives Erickson (2011, 2013) developed the practice environment conceptual framework (PECF) as represented in Figure 10.5. The PECF provides a framework for leadership influence of professional practice within organizations and demonstrates a relationship that can influence or can be leveraged to advance the PPE. The framework is intended to integrate ideas, philosophy, emerging evidence, and changes in the dynamic world of healthcare and nursing.

A critical success factor of the chief nurse is the ability to scan the environment and detect signals to inform strategic and tactical decision making. This consistent evaluation of the PPE is core to understanding the impact of changes to the increasingly complex healthcare delivery system. Identifying approaches for accommodating this complexity is a key step in improving the quality of patient care and in retaining nurses in the workforce. Barrett's (2010) work suggests that knowingly participating in change by being aware of what you choose to do, feeling free to do it, and acting intentionally should be guiding principles of chief nurse practice and should be a part of how the chief nurse encourages the interdisciplinary team to sort through clinical problems at the bedside. The use of a theoretical approach with exquisite leadership skill represents an important aspect of how a chief nurse might begin to measure, implement, and enhance an evidence-based approach to improving the PPE (Ives Erickson, 2013).

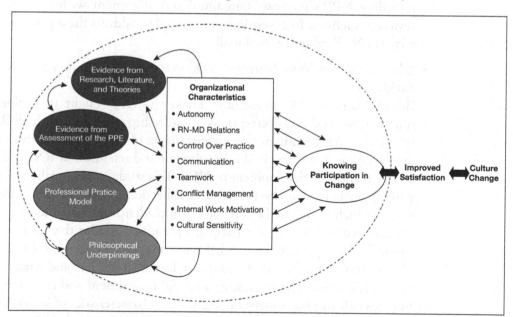

FIGURE 10.5 Dynamic interactions within a PPE model.

PPE, professional practice environment.

■ ENGAGING IN KNOWLEDGE AND EVIDENCE DEVELOPMENT

Active engagement of nurse executive leaders in research is paramount. Transformational leaders are committed to promoting new knowledge, innovation, and performance improvement. Integrating new knowledge and evidence into leadership practice is a continuous practice. Examples of nurse executive leadership studies follow.

- *Nursing Peer Review (NPR) Perceptions and Practice*
  Whitney, Haag-Heitman, Chisholm, and Gale's (2016) study sought to understand chief nurse executive perceptions of NPR and current NPR practice in their organizations to provide insights and recommendations for the path forward to a robust NPR approach nationally. The researchers noted that NPR is a key component of professional nursing practice focused on self-regulation and improving quality and safety. Despite its known benefits, NPR is not broadly disseminated, and how it is currently used and perceived is not well understood. A causal-comparison study design using a 25-question, web-based survey was administered to collect data variables. The results showed that chief nurse executives perceived NPR as important in improving quality and safety, however, its prevalence was low. Chief nurse executives also report NPR practices are not aligned with the ANA NPR guidelines. Results suggest that knowledge gaps exist regarding NPR's purpose, outcomes, and alignment with the ANA peer review guidelines. Interventions are needed to address these gaps to further advance NPR adoption nationally.

- *Characteristics of Nurse Directors (NDs) that Contribute to Registered Nurse Satisfaction*
  Burke, Flanagan, Ditomassi, and Hickey (2017) sought to explore staff nurses (RNs) and NDs perceptions of leadership on units with high RN satisfaction scores. Identifying the characteristics of NDs that contribute to RN satisfaction is important in the recruitment and retention of RNs and in the selection and role development of NDs. This study used a qualitative design with appreciative inquiry-guided data collection. Nine RNs and nine NDs met the inclusion criteria and each group identified four themes. Results showed that RN and ND participants identified similar themes representative of leadership attributes and behaviors that contribute to RN satisfaction (Figure 10.6). It is imperative for nurse leaders to understand what contributes to RN satisfaction to ensure successful recruitment and retention. These findings enhance the understanding of what characteristics of leadership RNs value in their NDs. NDs are vital members of nursing leadership, and, given the complexity of the role, it is important to identify the key attributes that contribute to their success.

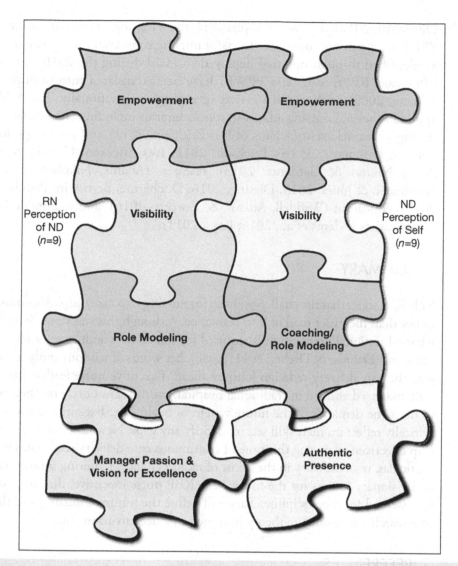

FIGURE 10.6 Nurse director and registered nurse themes.

■ ADVANCING AN AGENDA FOR EXECUTIVE NURSE LEADERS

This chapter highlights the importance and value of an executive nurse leader perspective and provides a description of what many identify as a program of research. Admittedly, there are many additional nursing research endeavors and for EBP/KBP projects underway within one organization, most if not all ongoing improvement efforts can be linked to this general administrative-focused thread in one way or another. The specific work highlighted here continues to be utilized in research and practice and has expanded significantly in the literature. Our work around the PPE as an emphasis for the nurse executive leader has served as a basis for a twinning relationship between Shanghai Haushan Hospital in China and MGH as a mechanism to advance learning across organizations and cultures (Ives Erickson, Hong, &

Ditomassi, 2012). The work emphasizing the adoption of the core components of a PPE fosters autonomous and successful nursing care, even during disaster situations as identified through our staff deployed to Haiti during the 2010 earthquake. The PPE scale, RPPE scale, and PPWEI have been translated into multiple languages (Chang, 2009), with use in a variety of settings internationally. The AIM has been applied to several nursing administration scenarios including chief nurse application during a sentinel event (Adams & Ives Erickson, 2011), influencing policy (Adams, Chisari, Ditomassi, & Ives Erickson, 2011; Ives Erickson, Colton, & Ditomassi, 2015; Nikitas & Gardener, 2013), research (Adams, Nikolaev, Ives Erickson, Ditomassi, & Jones, 2013; Diesing, 2016; Ducharme, Bernstein, Padula, & Adams, 2017), education (Waddell, Adams, & Fawcett, 2016), and as a guide for aspiring nurse leaders (Adams et al., 2016; Keys, 2011).

■ SUMMARY

Sally Reel states that the challenge ahead for nursing is to take the path of most resistance rather than the easier road of least resistance. Although this was stated in the context of what educational preparation is required for nurses to "conduct research versus utilize research" (Dahnke & Dreher, 2011, p. xiii), her words of wisdom apply to how to navigate the care delivery redesign journey ahead. Executive nurse leaders having successfully managed and led in traditional hospital settings cannot rely on their past skill set to meet the demands of the future system of healthcare. Executive nurse leaders must critically reflect on their skill sets to identify any gaps. New skills are needed for leadership effectiveness during this time of continuous care delivery redesign. Healthcare, in particular, is an industry in the midst of radical change, requiring innovative, adaptive, and visionary leaders for the future. The KBP nurse executive, director, and manager are essential for the discipline. They will define the future of nursing and the direction of research and assimilate theory into their practice environment.

■ REFERENCES

Adams, J. M. (2009). *The Adams Influence Model (AIM): Understanding the factors, attributes and process of achieving influence.* Saarbrücken, Germany: VDM Verlag.

Adams, J. M., Chatman Bryant, D., Deupree, J., Miyamoto, S., & Shillam, C. (2016). *White paper leadership influence self-assessment (LISA): Helping leaders optimize their potential for transformational change.* Robert Wood Johnson Foundation Executive Nurse Fellows Action Learning Team Final Report.

Adams, J. M., Chisari, R. G., Ditomassi, M., & Ives Erickson, J. (2011). Understanding and influencing policy: An imperative to the contemporary nurse leader. *Voice of Nursing Leadership*, 9(4), 4–7.

Adams, J. M., Duffy, M. E., & Clifford, J. C. (2006). *Knowledge and influence of the nurse leader: A survey of participants from the 2005 conference.* Boston, MA: Institute for Nursing Healthcare Leadership.

Adams, J. M., & Ives Erickson, J. (2011). Applying the Adams influence model (AIM) in nurse executive practice. *Journal of Nursing Administration, 41*(4), 186–192.

Adams, J. M., Ives Erickson, J., Duffy, M. E., Jones, D. A., Aspell Adams, A., & Clifford, J. C. (2007). *Knowledge and influence of the nurse leader: A survey of participants from the 2006 conference.* Boston, MA: Institute for Nursing Healthcare Leadership.

Adams, J. M., Ives Erickson, J., Jones, D. A., & Paulo, L. (2009). An evidence based structure for transformative nurse executive practice: The Model of the Interrelationship of Leadership, Environments & Outcomes for Nurse Executives (MILE ONE). *Nursing Administration Quarterly, 33*(4), 280–287.

Adams, J. M., & Natarajan, S. (2016). Understanding Nursing Influence: Development of the Adams Influence Model using practice, research, and theory. *Advances in Nursing Science, 39*(3), E40–E56.

Adams, J. M., Nikolaev, N., Ives Erickson, J., Ditomassi, M., & Jones, D. A. (2013). Identification of the psychometric properties of the leadership influence over professional practice environment scale. *Journal of Nursing Administration, 43*(5), 258–265.

Adams, J. M., Paulo, L., Meraz-Gottfried, L., Aspell Adams, A., Ives Erickson, J., Jones, D. A., & Clifford, J. C. (2008). *Success measures for the nurse leader: A survey of participants from the 2007 INHL conference.* Boston, MA: The Institute for Nursing Healthcare Leadership.

American Nurses Credentialing Center. (2008). *A new model for ANCC's magnet recognition program.* Retrieved from http://www.nursecredentialing.org

American Organization of Nurse Executives. (2011). *The AONE nurse executive competencies.* Chicago, IL: Author. Retrieved http://www.aone.org/resources/nurse-leader -competencies.shtml

Barrett, E. A. M. (2010). Power as knowing participation in change: What's new and what's next. *Nursing Science Quarterly, 23*(1), 47–54.

Burke, D., Flanagan, J., Ditomassi, M., & Hickey, P. (2017). Characteristics of nurse directors that contribute to registered nurse satisfaction. *Journal of Nursing Administration, 47*(4), 219–225.

Chang, C. C. (2009). *Development and evaluation of psychometric properties of the Chinese version of the Professional Practice Environment Scale in Taiwan.* Unpublished doctoral dissertation, Boston College, Boston, MA.

Dahnke, M. D., & Dreher, H. M. (2011). *Philosophy of science for nursing practice: Concepts and application* (p. xiii). New York, NY: Springer Publishing.

Diesing, G. (2016). Nurse leaders' authority, access to resources play large role in patient outcomes, study finds. Retrieved from http://www.hhnmag.com/articles/7091-nurse -leaders-authority-access-to-resource-plays-large-role-in-patient-outcomes-study-finds# .Vwtk1OIA0VY.mailto

Ducharme, M., Bernstein, J., Padula, M., & Adams, J. M. (2017). Leader influence, the professional practice environment, and nurse engagement in essential nursing practice. *Journal of Nursing Administration, 47*(7/8), 367–375. doi:10.1097/NNA.0000000000000497

Godden, J. (1995). Victorian influences on the development of nursing. In G. Gray & R. Pratt (Eds.), *Scholarship in the discipline of nursing* (pp. 243–258). Melbourne, Australia: Churchill Livingstone.

Health Forum. (2006). *AHA guide to the health care field.* Chicago, IL: Health Forum LLC.

Institute of Medicine. (2001). *Crossing the quality chasm: A new health system for the 21st century.* Washington, DC: National Academies Press.

Ives Erickson, J. (1996). *MGH Professional Practice Model, caring headlines.* Boston: Massachusetts General Hospital.

Ives Erickson, J. (2002). Chief nurse executive role in integrated delivery systems: Initial impressions from a national survey of chief nursing officers. The Robert Wood Johnson Foundation Executive Nurse Fellows Program.

Ives Erickson, J. (2011). *Nurses' perceptions of the professional practice environment across health-care settings.* DNP Capstone Project. Boston Massachusetts General Hospital Institute of Health Professions.

Ives Erickson, J. (2013). Influencing professional practice at the bedside. In J. Ives Erickson, D. Jones, & M. Ditomassi (Eds.), *Fostering nurse-led care* (pp. 1–19). Indianapolis, IN; Sigma Theta Tau.

Ives Erickson, J., Colton, D., & Ditomassi, M. (2015). Activating the advocacy plan. In R. M. Patton, M. L. Zalon, & R. Ludwick R (Eds.), *Nurses making policy from bedside to boardroom* (pp. 277–316). New York, NY: Springer Publishing.

Ives Erickson, J., & Ditomassi, M. (2011). Professional practice model: Strategies for translating models into practice. *Nursing Clinics of North America, 46*(1), 35–44.

Ives Erickson, J., Duffy, M. E., Ditomassi, M., & Jones, D. (2009). Psychometric evaluation of the revised professional practice environment (RPPE) scale. *Journal of Nursing Administration, 39*(5), 236–243.

Ives Erickson, J., Duffy, M. E., Ditomassi, M., & Jones, D. (2017). Development and psychometric evaluation of the professional practice work environment inventory. *Journal of Nursing Administration, 47*(5), 259–265.

Ives Erickson, J., Duffy, M. E., Gibbons, M. P., Fitzmaurice, J., Ditomassi, M., & Jones, D. A. (2004). Development and psychometric evaluation of the professional practice environment (PPE) scale. *Journal of Nursing Scholarship, 36*(3), 279–285.

Ives Erickson, J., Hong, J., & Ditomassi, M. (2012). Promoting a culture of professional practice through a twinning relationship. *Journal of Nursing Administration, 42*(2), 117–122.

Keys, Y. (2011). Perspectives on executive relationships—Influence. *Journal of Nursing Administration, 41*(9), 347–349.

McClure, M. L., Poulin, M. A., Sovie, M. D., & Wandelt, M. (1983). *Magnet hospitals: Attraction and retention of professional nurses.* Washington, DC: American Nurses Publishing.

Nikitas, D. M., & Gardner, D. (2013). Healthcare policy and politics: The risk and reward for public health nurses. In D. M. Nikitas, D. J. Middaugh, & N. Aries (Eds.), *Public policy and politics for nurses and other healthcare professionals: Advocacy and action* (pp. 201–216). Sudbury, MA: Jones & Bartlett.

Robert Wood Johnson Foundation. (2010). *Nursing leadership from bedside to boardroom: Opinion leaders' perceptions.* Retrieved from https://www.rwjf.org/en/library/research/2010/01/nursing-leadership-from-bedside-to-boardroom.html

Roy, C. (2007). Nursing knowledge development and clinical practice. In S. C. Roy & D. A. Jones (Eds.), *Advances in nursing knowledge and the challenge for transforming practice* (pp. 3–38). New York, NY: Springer Publishing.

Sackett, D. L., Straus, S. E., Richardson, W. S., Rosenberg, W., & Haynes, R. B. (2000). *Evidence-based medicine. How to practice and teach EBM* (2nd ed.). New York, NY: Churchill Livingstone.

Shortell, S. M., Gillies, R. R., & Devers, K. J. (1995). Reinventing the American hospital. *Milbank Quarterly, 73*(2), 131–160.

Waddell, A., Adams, J. M., & Fawcett, J. (2016). Thoughts about health policy content in baccalaureate nursing education. *Nursing Science Quarterly, 29*(4), 340–344.

Washington, D., Ives Erickson, J., & Ditomassi, M. (2004). Mentoring the minority nurse leader of tomorrow. *Nursing Administration Quarterly, 28*(3), 165–169.

Whitney, K., Haag-Heitman, B., Chisholm, M., & Gale, S. (2016). Nursing peer review perceptions and practices: A survey of chief nurse executives. *Journal of Nursing Administration, 46*(10), 541–548.

Yukl, G., & Falbe, C. M. (1990). Influence tactics and objectives in upward, downward, and lateral influence attempts. *Journal of Applied Psychology, 75*, 132–140.

Finding Our Voices: Defining Ourselves

JUDITH WEBB AND LEAH MCKINNON-HOWE

■ FINDING OUR VOICES

When we speak of finding our voices as doctor of nursing practice (DNP)-prepared nurses, what do we mean? Who speaks for us and what do they say? As a recently inaugurated degree, the first voices were those of the foremothers and fathers of the DNP. Those who framed the first DNP programs were primarily PhD-prepared nurses. They advocated for the development of the degree, designed educational preparation, established initial standards, and more. As the numbers of DNP graduates grew, the authority of experience brought more clarity to the voices. Increasingly, the voices of the DNP are DNP-prepared nurses themselves. We began to differentiate ourselves from PhD-prepared colleagues, and we further enhanced the distinctions of the degree. Our non-DNP professional colleagues and educators of DNP students continue to speak in support of us. The voice of the DNP can be heard as a chorus of multiple voices. We are a diverse group of advanced practice nurses and allies from various cultures, ethnicities, ages, genders, specialties, backgrounds, educational programs, and levels of experience. Although we are grounded in common standards, each voice that speaks for DNP-prepared nurses has a unique perspective. In this chapter, we aim to illuminate the rising voices of DNP-prepared nurses in education, policy, and practice.

■ DEFINING OURSELVES WITHIN NURSING EDUCATION

DNP AS A DISRUPTIVE INNOVATION IN NURSING EDUCATION

Educational institutions adopted the newest degree for advanced practice nursing in the first decade of the 21st century. The innovation of a clinical practice degree for advanced practice was neither novel nor without struggle. The emergence of the DNP degree within advanced practice nursing education is consistent with the phenomenon of disruptive innovation, a term coined by Clayton Christensen (2017) to describe organizational responses to significant changes. Blakeney, Carleton, McCarthy, and Coakley (2009) and others applied the disruptive innovation process to nursing. Blakeney described the impact of creative new transformations on healthcare environments and systems.

As DNP programs opened across the country, some looked to adopt common standards. Other programs took innovative approaches. These differences created national dialogue and debate about the relative strengths and weaknesses of the varying perspectives. There were differences in the degree title, the definition of clinical experiences, the nature and scope of culminating capstone projects, and the place of educators, administrators, and informaticists within DNP tracks. There were many voices, internal and external to the discipline, stating opinions about the use of the title "doctor." There were concerns that the DNP would siphon nurses away from PhD programs. Disruptive and critical voices gave rise to constructive innovation for an advanced clinical practice doctorate. Standardization of terminology along with nature and scope of programs evolved. PhD program enrollments remained stable, and many DNP-prepared nurses are using the title of the earned educational degree, "Doctor," clarifying in professional roles the difference between nurse and physician.

STAGES OF DEVELOPMENT IN DNP NURSING EDUCATION: EVOLUTION AND REVOLUTION

Nursing education progressed at an uneven pace toward the advanced academic degree of the DNP. Historically, nursing education has been marked by periods of steady growth interspersed with times of upheaval. These stages of growth and periods of evolution and revolution are typical in disciplines as they develop. The ebbs and flows of DNP progression can be examined within nursing education paradigms and have been influenced by business, social sciences, and feminist philosophies.

Greiner (1998/n.d.) described the growth and developmental stages of businesses and organizations. He defined organizational growth and development as having periods of revolution and evolution. The concepts of evolution and revolution are applicable to nursing education as well. Nursing education has experienced long and steady periods of evolution punctuated by changing paradigms or revolution. The revolution phases brought rapid change and growth, while the evolution phases were marked by steady progress. Florence Nightingale started an initial revolutionary period by formalizing nurses training in London in 1860 (Stanley & Sherratt, 2010). Nursing education then experienced a steady period of evolution in hospital-based diploma programs around the world. Significant changes occurred when nurses entered university-based degree programs, including associate degree and baccalaureate degree programs.

Advanced practice nursing programs activated new periods of revolution. Nurse anesthetists, nurse practitioners (NPs), nurse midwives and clinical nurse specialists, nurse executives, and nurse informaticists experienced periods of growth from training models to graduate degrees. Nurse anesthetists, after practicing for over 150 years, changed the educational and certification standards in 1998 to require a minimum of a master's degree. In 2007, nurse anesthetists became the first advanced nursing practice program to pass a resolution to require doctoral education for entry to practice by 2025 (American Association of Nurse Anesthetists, n.d.). NP education initiated a period of revolution. When Loretta Ford developed the NP role in 1965, she described characteristics of revolution as resistance from both within and outside nursing. On the 15th anniversary of the first NP program, Dr. Ford reflected on the unexpected resistance from her colleagues in nursing education, including criticism for partnering with a physician and charges of teaching content which was previously the domain of medicine (Ford, 2015).

Certificate and apprentice NP programs grew and ultimately became graduate degree programs. The same is true for clinical nurse specialists who evolved as expert nurses through mentorship in practice and then formalized the role into a graduate educational program (National Association of Clinical Nurse Specialists, n.d.-a, n.d.-b, n.d.-c). As technology advanced, informatics has infused nursing education. As healthcare systems grew in complexity, nurses took leadership and sought advanced education to promote systematic change as nurse informaticists, nurse leaders, and executives.

Prior to the DNP, advanced practice nurses enrolled in doctoral programs in education and philosophy, such as the EdD and PhD. Some focused on original research, but many were studying clinical practice problems. The development of the DNP as a clinical practice doctorate was a much-needed and revolutionary stage for advanced practice nursing. This upheaval cultivated fertile ground for intense and sometimes contentious disputes among the various nursing degrees. Questions about the clinical practice doctorate in nursing raised important issues and often led to refinement and modification. DNP advocates found both criticism and support outside the silo of nursing with other clinical practice degrees, such as physical therapy, medicine, and pharmacy.

DEVELOPING AGENCY: SPEAKING FOR OURSELVES

Over time, DNP education began to produce a chorus of voices of DNP-prepared nurses themselves. As the cohort of DNP graduates increased, they began to develop agency and self-efficacy as nurses with clinical practice expertise. Bandura (1977) defined self-efficacy as the belief that individuals' capabilities could produce designated levels of performance, and ultimately, exercise influence over events that affect their lives. He further observed that individuals develop greater agency when they see others like themselves succeed through effort (Bandura, 1986). DNP-prepared nurses demonstrated achievements in clinical practice and inspired others to take on similar challenges.

■ PIVOTAL MOMENTS IN DNP EDUCATION

BOLD STEP BY AACN TO REQUIRE DNP BY 2015

In 2004, the American Association of Colleges of Nursing (AACN) took a bold step by voting to make the DNP the entry level for advanced nursing practice by 2015. The AACN, an organization primarily comprised of nursing school deans and executives, sets standards for nursing educational programs across the country. The rationale for this historic vote endorsing the DNP for entry to advanced practice nursing was threefold:

1. Current master's-level educational programs for advanced practice nursing carried credit loads equivalent to doctoral degrees in other healthcare professions.
2. The doctorate represents the highest level of nursing clinical practice.
3. Changing healthcare systems require the highest level of scientific knowledge (AACN, 2004a, 2004b).

The AACN followed the mandate with a task force to draft the "Essentials of Doctoral Education for Advanced Nursing Practice" (AACN, 2006). The essentials emphasized the differences between the PhD and the DNP by highlighting the research-focus of the PhD and the practice-focus of the DNP. These distinctions broadened the division between the research-focused doctorate and practice-focused doctorate. Research for the generation of new knowledge was shifted to PhDs and application of research was assigned to the DNP (AACN, 2010). This position of absolute dichotomy was later disputed and clarified, recognizing the reality of overlapping foci and the value of collaboration between PhD and DNP nurses (Murphy, Staffileno, & Carlson, 2015).

VARIATION AMONG PROGRAMS IN EARLY DEVELOPMENT

The first decade of DNP programs was marked by accelerated change and vast variation. Programs conferred multiple degrees, including DNP, ND, and DrNP. The scope of the final deliverables varied and were called multiple names such as capstone, dissertation, or scholarly project. Faculty and mentors were referred to as readers, committees, advisors, and more. These discrepancies evolved due to rapid growth of DNP programs; however, consistency was needed to promote greater acceptance of the DNP.

Consistency regarding the degree title arose through the accrediting organization, the Commission on Collegiate Nursing Education (CCNE), and AACN. The CCNE sets the standard for uniformity of the degree title as DNP by asserting that only programs that conferred the DNP would be accredited (CCNE, 2005). This resulted in swift conformity among developing programs. Then CCNE began the process of evaluating and accrediting programs. MGH Institute of Health Professions in Boston, MA was the first DNP program nationally accredited on

November 5, 2008. West Virginia University was accredited 5 days later, followed by Columbia University in the same month (CCNE, n.d.). DNP programs were gaining credibility.

In 2015, the AACN established a task force charged with eliminating confusing terminology and variation in programs. After evaluating the DNP track record for a decade, AACN published a white paper delineating recommendation for greater standardization. The final scholarly product would be called the DNP Project. Additionally, terminology was recommended for the faculty and mentors who guide DNP projects. The term "DNP Project Team" was widely adopted to differentiate from other doctoral programs. The white paper also brought clarity to the scope of advanced clinical practice to include individuals, populations, and provision of indirect care. This change sanctioned the inclusion of nurse executives, leaders, and informaticists. Further clarification was affirmed regarding nurse educators. Neither the DNP nor the PhD degree prepared graduates to become nurse educators. Additional preparation in the art and science of education should be obtained by nurse educators (AACN, 2015).

BARRIERS TO ADOPTION OF THE DNP

The AACN commissioned a study in 2014 to evaluate barriers and facilitators to full adoption of the DNP. The study, known as the RAND report, investigated progress toward adoption of the DNP and factors that impeded or facilitated this change (Auerbach et al., 2015). There had been resistance to the mandate to move to the DNP for entry to practice, and this mandate was retracted. The RAND report focused on the four advanced practice registered nurse (APRN) roles. The study did not examine advanced practice roles at the aggregate, systems, or organizational levels.

The RAND report established that, while the number of DNP programs had steadily increased in the decade since the 2004 AACN directive, schools of nursing had varied in their adoption of the DNP. Most schools (57%) offering an MS degree for APRNs had added the MS to DNP track. Others had added both the BS to DNP and the MS to DNP. Some early adopters had discontinued the MS program in favor of a BSN to DNP option, while a few schools had chosen not to offer the DNP at all. Barriers to adoption of the DNP were more onerous in larger universities that posed challenging institutional regulations. Other barriers were cost, faculty resources, adequate clinical sites, availability of preceptors, and the workload of managing final projects.

Facilitators of DNP program development were enthusiastic leadership from clinical sites as well as champions among faculty and academic leadership. The changing landscape of healthcare was identified as a facilitator for the preparation of advanced practice nurses. The Institute of Medicine's (IOM) *Future of Nursing* report had further propelled doctoral programs, calling for increased educational preparation at the baccalaureate and doubling of doctoral-prepared nurses (IOM, 2010).

■ DNP IN ACADEMIA

FACULTY ROLES FOR DNP-PREPARED NURSES

The demand for increased enrollments in all nursing programs is hampered by a shortage of qualified faculty (AACN, 2014; National League for Nursing, 2014). Schools of nursing have consistently experienced a shortage of doctoral-prepared faculty, often leaving faculty positions unfilled and admissions restricted. Prior to the DNP, PhD-prepared nurses filled faculty positions. Following the 2004 directive by the AACN to mandate the DNP by 2015, the number of DNP graduates grew rapidly and surpassed the number of PhD graduates. Schools of nursing were compelled to consider filling vacant faculty positions with DNP-prepared nurses. Nursing leaders held and voiced conflicting views about DNP-prepared faculty joining the ranks of the academies (Meleis & Dracup, 2005). The faculty role had been established for the PhD graduate. Objectors made the point that DNP programs did not prepare graduates for the educator role. While accurate, the same is true for PhD programs. It is important to recognize that, similarly, other non-nursing practice doctorates do not prepare graduates in education without additional coursework. Both DNP and PhD graduates need additional coursework to prepare them for effective teaching (AACN, 2015). The DNP degree along with education elective courses or education leadership options effectively prepares faculty in areas of educational theory, assessment, evaluation, curriculum development, and classroom and online learning (Danzey, Fitzpatrick, Garbutt, Rafferty, & Zychowicz, 2011; Dreifuerst et al., 2016).

Among DNP graduates, approximately one-third to one-half have plans to pursue a career in teaching (Dreifuerst et al., 2016; Fang & Bednash, 2017). Many current faculties, urged to complete a doctorate, are teaching while co-enrolled in DNP programs. Some estimates are upward of two-thirds of DNP-prepared nurses have a full-time or part-time teaching position (Dreifuerst et al., 2016). Graduates express confidence in clinical teaching, implementing evidence-based practice, and interest in impacting patient care (Dreifuerst et al., 2016). Disadvantages of the teaching role are lower salary and a perception of inferior status of teachers compared to those in clinical practice (Dreifuerst et al., 2016).

TENURE STATUS FOR DNP-PREPARED FACULTY

Tenure status for faculty is specific to an institution and is intended to provide job security and academic freedom without fear of retribution. Some institutions do not grant tenure. There is no consistency across the country regarding DNP and tenure. Traditionally, tenure was granted when a faculty member had completed substantial funded research. Many institutions have promotion and tenure criteria that were created based on the PhD and give preference to funded research-focused scholarship (Agger, Oermann, & Lynn, 2014; Danzey et al., 2011; Honig, Smolowitz, & Larson, 2013; Nicholes & Dyer, 2012).

DNP SCHOLARSHIP

Scholarship is a central component of a faculty role. To expand the discussion of advancement and promotion for DNP-prepared faculty, the definition of scholarship needs to be clarified. Boyer's definition of scholarship could be used as criteria for promotion and tenure of DNP faculty. The four areas of scholarship according to Boyer are (a) scholarship of discovery, (b) scholarship of teaching, (c) scholarship of practice, and (d) scholarship of integration (Boyer, 1990).

Some leaders in education have promoted a polarized view of scholarship with the research-focused PhD and the practice-focused DNP on opposite sides of a clear divide. Research has little benefit until it is applied or translated into practice, yet the average research-practice time lag is 17 years (Morris, Wooding, & Grant, 2011). There are rising voices that see a more collaborative model and an expansive interpretation of the potential of DNP-prepared scholars. The emergence of the DNP has propelled nursing education in the direction of closing the theory-practice gap (AACN, 2017; Agger et al., 2014; Benner, Sutphen, Leonard, & Day, 2010; Honig et al., 2013). The term "generation of new knowledge," formerly sequestered in the wheelhouse of the PhD alone, was expanded by the AACN in 2015.

> Graduates of both research- and practice-focused doctoral programs are prepared to *generate new knowledge*. Research-focused graduates are prepared to generate knowledge through rigorous research and statistical methodologies that may be broadly applicable or generalizable to diverse populations and systems and inform health policy and practice. Practice-focused graduates are prepared to generate new knowledge through innovation of practice change, the translation of evidence, and the implementation of quality improvement processes in specific practice settings, systems, or with specific populations to improve health or health outcomes. (AACN, 2017, pp. 8–9)

DNP-prepared faculty can help address critical workforce issues in schools of nursing. As more DNP graduates pursue careers in academic settings, it is essential to acknowledge the strengths that they contribute to a faculty and offer opportunities for development in education as needed. Criteria for rank, promotion, and tenure should be modernized to include career paths for DNP-prepared faculty.

Residencies and Fellowships

The clinical practice doctorate in nursing does not require a residency or a fellowship, however, some residency programs for NPs are beginning across the country. Residency, a term most-closely associated with medicine, is a postgraduate training program that typically provides additional clinical experience. Fellowships, also postgraduate programs, usually provide specialist training. Medical residencies receive significant financial support from Medicare and Medicaid to provide graduate medical education (Eden, Berwick, & Wilensky, 2014). Physicians are under no obligation when they enter practice to provide care to Medicaid or Medicare patients.

These public funds are not available for NP residencies. Multiple outcomes studies have demonstrated that new graduate NPs have competency to practice after passing national certification exams. DNP graduates differ in focus, including direct care to individuals, populations, and systems. DNP students vary widely in clinical experience, many having had years of experience prior to the DNP. Although some voices have called for a required NP residency, evidence speaks loudly for optional postgraduate programs. Requiring residencies could create barriers to practice for advanced practice nurses (Nurse Practitioner Roundtable, 2014). In a world where there are significant physician shortages, workforce issues can and will not be solved by investing in a single group of healthcare providers. The DNP-prepared nurse must advocate for parity in the allocation of dollars appropriated for APRN education, education that promotes meaningful educational experiences that create value for the workplace during the APRNs education, not after graduation.

◼ DNP POLICY

The United States spends more on healthcare per capita than any other industrialized nation, yet consistently ranks lower than most on key measures of health and healthcare access and quality. Our healthcare system will continue to face challenges as a new administration and the 115th Congress jockey to overhaul the healthcare system. It is imperative that forward-thinking leaders from healthcare, business, finance, government, and technology work together to inform the development of health and social policies that promote a culture of health (Ladden, 2017; Robert Wood Johnson Foundation [RWJF], n.d.). Heiman and Artiga (2015) cite that although healthcare is essential to health, research demonstrates that it is a relatively weak determinant of health, with increased recognition that achieving health equity and improving population health will require broader approaches that address economic, environmental, and social factors that influence health. There has been a growing movement in the public health community to take a "Health in All Policies" approach to improve population health, acknowledging the importance of social determinants of health (Heiman & Artiga, 2015). "Health in All Policies" is defined as a "collaborative approach to improving the health of all people by incorporating health considerations into decision-making across sectors and policy areas" (Rudolph, Caplan, Ben-Moshe, & Dillon, 2013, p. 6).

THE VOICE OF THE DNP IN HEALTH POLICY

The AACN's DNP Essential V: *Health Care Policy for Advocacy in Health Care* (2006) represents one of eight foundational competencies that transcend the DNP's clinical focus, specialty, or advanced practice role and is aligned with the American Nurses Association's (ANA) definition of nursing, which encompasses advocacy in the care of individuals, families, groups, communities, and populations

(AACN, 2006; ANA, n.d.). The AACN Task Force on the Implementation of the DNP further clarified and restated the definition of advanced practice nursing as

> any form of nursing intervention that influences healthcare outcomes for individuals or populations, including the provision of direct care or management of care for individual patients or management of care populations, and the provision of indirect care such as nursing administration, executive leadership, health policy, informatics, and population health. (AACN, 2015, p. 1)

DNP-prepared advanced practice nurses give voice to the profession and the patients that they serve by influencing legislative and health policy initiatives that ensure access to high quality, equitable, and affordable healthcare and fulfill the Institute for Healthcare Improvement's (IHI) Triple Aim: improving the health of populations, reducing the cost of healthcare, and improving the patient experience (IHI, 2017).

Recognizing the importance and value of coalition building, the DNP fosters interprofessional relationships, appreciating that "no single profession working alone, can meet the complex needs of patients and communities" (Altman, Butler, & Shern, 2015, p. 3). DNPs must know who is representing their voice in the policy realm and assist in crafting policies where, in musical terms, their individual voice becomes part of a larger choir. At a minimum, the DNP must support the work of professional nursing organizations that represent the voice of nursing and advanced practice through individual membership in the professional nursing organization that is best aligned with their practice. Beyond individual membership, the DNP-prepared nurse will ideally take a more active leadership role in professional organizations in addition to serving on committees, boards, and task forces that improve healthcare delivery and outcomes at the state, national, and international levels (AACN, 2006).

STAKEHOLDERS AND POLICY PRIORITIES

Professional organizations representing the voice of nursing and organized medicine have defined core principles and priorities that guide their healthcare reform advocacy efforts. Truly meaningful healthcare reform will rely on a shared vision for a healthcare system that is sustainable and meets the healthcare needs of the nation. A comprehensive review of state-based stakeholders is beyond the scope of this chapter. A broader look at the national landscape provides a basis for comparison and finding common ground. Ober and Wilkie outline the policy agendas for the organizations representing the voice of professional nursing and advanced practice nursing in Chapter 18. Collectively, there is significant overlap of the policy priorities of the national nursing organizations, which seek to address meaningful healthcare reform initiatives that promote universal access to affordable healthcare, modernize state licensure laws, remove barriers that restrict practice, and fund a sustainable healthcare workforce. National physician organizations embrace a similar agenda and promote expanded access and coverage of healthcare services, providing greater cost transparency throughout the healthcare system and reducing regulatory burdens that detract from patient care and increase costs (American Medical Association, 2017a, 2017b). The DNP-prepared nurse with advanced training in organizations, systems, and aggregate care can promote unity among discordant voices by contributing to policy development that achieves harmony and helps Americans to build healthier communities and a healthy future.

FINDING COMMON GROUND

Several themes emerge from the policy and advocacy agendas of the respective nursing and medical associations with the following areas of shared concern:

- Expanding coverage and access to affordable healthcare
- Promoting of consumer choice
- Reducing regulatory burdens to streamline care and reduce costs through administrative simplification
- Careful consideration of the impact of "repeal and replace" efforts to maintain coverage and protections created by the Patient Protection and Affordable Care Act
- Insurance and payment reform
- Stable funding for workforce development
- Leveraging health information technology to reduce healthcare costs and improve healthcare quality

Many of the concerns surrounding access to care, promoting consumer choice, and reducing regulatory burdens to streamline care and reduce healthcare costs could be achieved by removing barriers to APRN practice at the state and national levels. Unnecessary regulatory and legislative requirements, such as physician supervision, are costly and at odds with efforts to design a more effective healthcare system (ANA, 2016).

The 2010 IOM report *The Future of Nursing* put forth a set of recommendations that addressed the crucial role of nurses in the rapidly changing world of healthcare reform and provided a road map for policy initiatives that would strengthen the role and voice of nursing in healthcare redesign (IOM, 2011). The RWJF convened a task force to assess the progress in implementing the report's recommendations and the changes in the field of nursing since the release of *The Future of Nursing Report*. The committee found that although significant strides have been made in many aspects of the work, several areas, including removing barriers to practice and care, collaborating and leading, workforce data, and promoting diversity in the nursing profession, require further work (Altman et al., 2015). These areas are particularly relevant to the DNP who is prepared and positioned to take a leadership role in advancing this work.

REMOVAL OF PRACTICE BARRIERS

Despite a growing body of evidence that APRN-provided care in states with full practice authority is comparable to the care provided in states with physician oversight, barriers to practice exist in many states, imposing unnecessary practice restrictions and impeding patients' access to high-quality and affordable care. The RWJF

Charting Nursing's Future brief titled *The Case for Removing Barriers to APRN Practice* highlights the debate around the regulation of APRN practice and the highly variable laws and regulations that restrict patients' access to APRN services, which are dependent upon the state, APRN role, and employment setting. The barriers restricting the practice of APRNs include restrictive Centers for Medicare and Medicaid Services (CMS) guidelines, oversight of APRN prescribing practices, statutorily mandated collaborative practice agreements, on-site supervision requirements, and dual oversight by state Boards of Medicine and Boards of Nursing. These restrictions do not contribute to patient safety and may also give patients and policy makers the false impression that physicians must oversee APRN decision making (RWJF, 2017b).

Restrictive "transition to practice" regulations in some "full practice" states challenge the role competence of the APRN (clinical competence following preparation at the graduate level, graduation and national certification) by requiring a transition period ranging from 1,000 hours to 3 years. Oversight requirements may include the use of collaborative practice agreements, physician approved protocols for Schedule II controlled substance prescribing, or when seeking autonomous prescriptive practice. There is no evidence to substantiate the need for additional postlicensure supervision of APRN practice beyond current certification and educational standards (ANA, 2016). Widespread adoption of the National Council of State Boards of Nursing's (NCSBN) Consensus Model for APRN Regulation would achieve uniformity in APRN regulation in all states, eliminate the need for "transition to practice" requirements, remove obstacles to portability in licensure, and potentially increase access to care (NCSBN, n.d.).

The DNP-prepared advanced practice nurse has increased knowledge of healthcare policy, healthcare systems, healthcare finance and regulations, and their impact on clinical practice. By serving on state boards of nursing and advisory committees with health policy decision makers, the DNP advanced practice nurse can reduce barriers to practice, thereby increasing access to APRN-provided care, filling critical provider gaps, and improving the health of the nation.

Barriers imposed by state practice acts, regulations from the CMS, and federal statutes continue to restrict APRN practice, resulting in increased healthcare costs, decreased access to care, and disruption in practice innovation (RWJF, 2017). Healthcare institutions further reinforce these barriers by creating polices that dictate who will be allowed to practice within their organizations. It is not uncommon for institutional policies guiding APRN practice to lag behind changes in statute, unnecessarily restricting APRN practice. DNP-prepared nurse executives can play a pivotal role in shaping institutional polices that maximize the contribution of APRNs within their organizations by aligning practice policies with state statutes that allow them to practice to the fullest extent of their licensure and clinical experience.

REIMBURSEMENT

Third-party payers exert their own form of influence by dictating who will be paid to deliver services and how much they will be reimbursed. The DNP is uniquely qualified to articulate the role and value of nursing and the contributions of the APRN.

Insurance regulations will continue to evolve and change as payers and purchasers of healthcare embrace value-based purchasing and pay for performance strategies that improve the cost-effectiveness and quality of care while delivering a larger return on invested healthcare dollars (ANA, 2010). Nursing administrators, nurse informaticists, and APRNs will influence or be financially impacted by Pay for Quality incentives and reimbursement. The ANA offers 10 Pay for Quality Principles that will prepare the DNP for discussions related to Pay for Quality and ensure adequate representation at the local, state, and national levels (ANA, 2010).

The DNP must continue to forge relationships with policy makers to advance legislation at the state and federal levels. Also critically important is the need to expand the DNP's circle of influence by working with a diverse group of stakeholders including the broader nursing community, other health profession groups, health systems, consumer groups, and third-party payers to remove practice restrictions and increase interprofessional collaboration (Altman et al., 2015).

■ DNP PRACTICE

A DEGREE, NOT A ROLE

The DNP is widely recognized as one of the profession's two terminal degrees; it is *not* a role and therefore does not define the DNP in practice. The advanced education and skills attained by those seeking preparation at the highest level of nursing practice have a strong impact upon practice and may influence changes in role as a result of obtaining the DNP degree. The degree, however, was not intended to expand the scope of advanced practice or prepare nurses for new roles but to contemporize competencies that prepare nurses engaged in advanced practice to be leaders in direct and indirect patient care activities that influence patient and organizational outcomes in an increasingly complex healthcare environment (AACN, 2015; Ahmed & O'Dell, 2013).

WHERE WILL PRACTICE TAKE US? WHAT IS OUR ROLE?

A recent study by Udlis and Mancuso (2015) explored nurses' perception of the role of the DNP-prepared nurse and sought to identify areas of ambiguity in understanding the roles that DNP-prepared nurses fulfill. They found that, although nurses clearly support the DNP degree with a focus on the improvement of healthcare outcomes through leadership roles in policy, health organizations, interprofessionalism, and translation of evidence into practice, multiple areas of confusion regarding the role of the DNP-prepared nurse within academia, research, and scholarship exist. The role(s) of the DNP-prepared nurse and the distinctions of the DNP degree are embedded in practice. Enhanced leadership skills and the application of evidence-based practice effect healthcare system change that improves healthcare delivery and patient outcomes. We must provide clarity and give voice to the distinctive and vital contributions of the DNP-prepared nurse through scholarly dissemination of this work (Udlis & Mancuso, 2015). Broom, Riner, and Allam (2013) and Redman, Pressler, Furspan, and Potempa (2015) examined the publication practices of DNP-prepared nurses and trends of the scholarship being published. The majority of DNP authored and coauthored publications focused on clinical practice and education with a positive trend in interdisciplinary scholarship with colleagues with a mix of academic degrees (Broome, Riner, & Allam, 2013; Redman et al., 2015). The DNP-prepared nurse's role in leading healthcare change, impact on population health, and contributions to translating evidence into practice must be documented through publication in peer-reviewed journals due to the lack of a centralized repository for scholarly products at this time (Redman et al., 2015). It will be difficult to fully articulate the role(s) of the doctoral-prepared APN without analyzing outcomes data, trends in practice, and impact on health outcomes.

FINDING A VOICE IN A CHANGING PRACTICE ENVIRONMENT

The effects of changes to the Affordable Care Act on access to healthcare and coverage of services have yet to play out, but the fact remains that an aging America with increasingly complex healthcare needs will continue to grow and increase healthcare utilization. Changes in the healthcare industry and workforce trends are being driven by consumer preferences and a shift in payment from volume-based (fee for service) care to value-based payments that reward appropriate utilization of resources and preventive care. There has been tremendous growth in the convenient care market including retail clinics, urgent care centers, and freestanding emergency departments, largely staffed by APRNs. Hospital consolidations, expansion of major medical groups and systems, and a shift towards population health management are changing how care is delivered. Interdisciplinary teams are being called upon to respond to the complex needs of patients, addressing social determinants of health to control cost and increase care quality (Merritt Hawkins, 2017).

A 2017 Merritt Hawkins survey on physician and advanced practitioner recruiting reflects an increased demand for NP services, ranking fourth as the most recruited category. NPs and physician assistants (PAs) when combined ranked third, trailing only family physicians and psychiatrists, and moved up from 11th in 2016 (Merritt Hawkins, 2017). Physician shortages will increase the need for a robust primary care work force and the demand for APRNs due to their prominent role in team-based care. The aforementioned survey illustrates a model of the *Composition of the Primary Care Led Team* that is led by three chief officers: chief integration officer, chief population health officer, and chief transformation officer. The team, in rank order, is comprised of a family medicine physician, a general internist, a nursing care manager, a PA, an NP, a community resource specialist, a social worker, a care coordinator, and a grand aide (Merritt Hawkins, 2017 p. 24). Historically, medical school curricula have not typically focused on leadership, thus, it should not be assumed that the physician is the logical or best choice for team leader. DNP-prepared APNs are well prepared to lead interdisciplinary teams due to enhanced leadership skills and knowledge of health systems, population management, evidence-based practice, and informatics. They will challenge the notion that the physician is best suited to serve as the "captain of the ship."

■ CONCLUSION

In this chapter, we echoed the rising voices of DNP-prepared nurses in education, policy, and practice. The course of DNP education has been marked by periods of growth and upheaval. Standards have evolved to build greater consistency across programs. The landscape of healthcare has changed dramatically during the same period and created increasing waves of policy change. DNP-prepared advanced practice nurses are reaching greater autonomy in practice environments and continue to pursue roles in which they can practice to the fullest extent of their education. As DNP-prepared nurses have increased in number and grown in self-efficacy, they have increasingly become the voices of the degree. Attainment of the DNP degree brings with it a responsibility to mentor and develop the next generation of practice scholars and nursing leaders who will optimize and change the health of the nation. DNP-prepared nurses must take their rightful place in academia and celebrate and embrace the synergistic attributes of the DNP- and PhD-prepared nurses. We must bridge the gap between the bench and bedside by investing valuable resources in care that is rooted in evidence, while testing and refining interventions that guide best practices and produce excellent outcomes. We must position ourselves as leaders in government, organizations, and healthcare systems, and effect change by representing the unique voice of nursing. "Nursing is a progressive art such that to stand still is to go backwards" (Florence Nightingale, n.d.).

■ REFERENCES

Agger, C., Oermann, M., & Lynn, M. (2014). Hiring and incorporating doctor of nursing practice-prepared nurse faculty into academic nursing programs. *Journal of Nursing Education, 53*(8), 439–448.

Ahmed, S. W., & O'Dell, D. G. (2013). DNPs: Finding our voices and defining ourselves. In S. W. Ahmed, L. C. Andrist, S. M. Davis, & V. J. Fuller (Eds.), *DNP education, practice and policy* (pp. 233–243). New York, NY: Springer Publishing.

Altman, S., Butler, A., & Shern, L. (2015, December). *Assessing progress on the Institute of Medicine report* The future of nursing. Retrieved from http://www.nationalacademies .org/hmd/~/media/Files/Report%20Files/2015/AssessingFON_releaseslides/Nursing -Report-in-brief.pdf

American Association of Colleges of Nursing. (2004a). *AACN adopts a new vision for the future of nursing education and practice*. Retrieved from http://www.aacn.nche.edu/news/ articles/2004/dnp-release

American Association of Colleges of Nursing. (2004b). *AACN position statement on the practice doctorate in nursing*. Washington, DC: Author. Retrieved from http://www.aacnnursing .org/Portals/42/News/Position-Statements/DNP.pdf

American Association of Colleges of Nursing. (2006). *The essentials of doctoral education for advanced practice nursing*. Retrieved from http://www.aacnnursing.org/Portals/42/ Publications/DNPEssentials.pdf

American Association of Colleges of Nursing. (2010). *The research-focused doctoral program in nursing: Pathways to excellence*. Washington, DC: Author. Retrieved from http://www .aacnnursing.org/Portals/42/Publications/PhDPosition.pdf

American Association of Colleges of Nursing. (2014). *Nurse faculty shortage fact sheet.* Retrieved from https://kaiserhealthnews.files.wordpress.com/2012/08/facultyshortagefs.pdf

American Association of Colleges of Nursing. (2015). *The doctor of nursing practice: Current issues and clarifying recommendations.* Retrieved from http://www.aacnnursing.org/ Portals/42/DNP/DNP-Implementation.pdf?ver=2017-08-01-105830-517

American Association of Colleges of Nursing. (2017). *Defining scholarship: Draft position statement May 23, 2017.* Retrieved from http://www.aacnnursing.org/LinkClick.aspx?file ticket=CmntDakuz5c%3D&portalid=42

American Association of Nurse Anesthetists. (n.d.). AANA announces support of doctorate for entry into nurse anesthesia practice by 2025. Retrieved from https://sharepoint.aana .com/newsandjournal/News/Pages/092007-AANA-Announces-Support-of-Doctorate -for-Entry-into-Nurse-Anesthesia-Practice-by-2025.aspx

American Medical Association. (2017a). AMA vision on health reform. Retrieved from https://www.ama-assn.org/ama-health-reform-vision

American Medical Association. (2017b). *2017 AMA legislative and regulatory dashboard.* Retrieved from https://www.ama-assn.org/sites/default/files/media-browser/public/ government/advocacy/2017-ama-advocacy-dashboard.pdf

American Nurses Association. (n.d.). *What is nursing?* Retrieved from http://www .nursingworld.org/EspeciallyForYou/What-is-Nursing

American Nurses Association. (2010). *ANA's principles of pay for quality.* Retrieved from http://www.nursingworld.org/MainMenuCategories/ThePracticeofProfessionalNursing/ NursingStandards/ANAPrinciples/ANA-Principles-for-Pay-for-Quality.pdf

American Nurses Association. (2016, May). *ANA's principles for advanced prac- tice registered nurse full practice authority.* Retrieved from http://nursingworld .org/MainMenuCategories/ThePracticeofProfessionalNursing/NursingStandards/ ANAPrinciples/Principles-for-APRN-Full-Practice-Authority.pdf

Auerbach, D. I., Martsolf, G., Pearson, M., Taylor, E., Zaydman, M., Muchow, A., . . . Lee, Y. (2015). *The DNP by 2015: A study of the institutional, political, and professional issues that facilitate or impede establishing a post-baccalaureate doctor of nursing practice program.* Santa Monica, CA: RAND Corporation. Retrieved from https://www.rand.org/pubs/research_ reports/RR730.html

Bandura, A. (1977). Self-efficacy: Toward a unifying theory of behavioral change. *Psychological Review, 84*(2), 191–215.

Bandura, A. (1986). *Social foundations of thought and action: A social cognitive theory.* Englewood Cliffs, NJ: Prentice Hall.

Benner, P., Sutphen, M., Leonard, V., & Day, L. (2010). *Educating nurses: A call for radical transformation.* San Francisco, CA: Jossey-Bass.

Blakeney, B., Carleton, P., McCarthy, C., & Coakley, E., (2009). Unlocking the power of innovation. *Online Journal of Issues in Nursing, 14*(2), Manuscript 1. doi:10.3912/OJIN. Vol14No02Man01

Boyer, E. (1990). *Scholarship reconsidered: Priorities for the professorate.* Princeton, NJ: The Carnegie Foundation for the Advancement of Teaching.

Broome, M. E., Riner, M. E., & Allam, E. S. (2013). Scholarly publication practices of doctor of nursing practice-prepared nurses. *Journal of Nursing Education, 52*(8), 429–434.

Christensen, C. (2017). Disruptive innovation: Key concepts. Retrieved from http://www
.claytonchristensen.com/key-concepts

Commission on Collegiate Nursing Education. (n.d.). CCNE-accredited doctor of nursing practice programs. Retrieved from http://directory.ccnecommunity.org/reports/
rptAccreditedPrograms_New.asp?sort=institution&sProgramType=3

Commission on Collegiate Nursing Education. (2005). Commission on Collegiate Nursing
Education moves to consider for accreditation only practice doctorates with the DNP
degree title. Retrieved from www.aacn.nche.edu/ccne-accreditation

Danzey, E., Fitzpatrick, J., Garbutt, S., Rafferty, M., & Zychowicz, M. (2011). The doctor
of nursing practice and nursing education: Highlights, potential, and promise. *Journal of
Professional Nursing, 27*(5), 311–314.

Dreifuerst, K., McNelis, A., Weaver, M., Broome, M. Draucker, C., & Fedko, A. (2016).
Exploring the pursuit of doctoral education by nurses seeking or intending to stay in
faculty roles. *Journal of Professional Nursing, 32*(3), 201–212.

Eden, J., Berwick, D., & Wilensky, G. (Eds.). (2014). *Graduate medical education that meets
the nation's health needs.* Washington, DC: National Academies Press.

Fang, D., & Bednash, G. (2017). Identifying barriers and facilitators to future nurse faculty
careers for DNP students. *Journal of Professional Nursing, 3*(1), 56–67. doi:10.1016/
j.profnurs.2016.05.008

Florence Nightingale. (n.d.). *AZQuotes.com.* Retrieved from http://www.azquotes.com/
author/10825-Florence_Nightingale

Ford, L. C. (2015). Reflections on 50 years of change. *Journal of the American Association of
Nurse Practitioners, 27*(6), 294–295.

Greiner, L. (n.d.). Evolution and revolution as organizations grow. *Harvard Business Review.*
Retrieved from https://hbr.org/1998/05/evolution-and-revolution-as-organizations
-grow (Original work published 1998)

Heiman, H. J., & Artiga, S. (2015, November). Beyond health care: The role of social
determinants in promoting health and health equity. Retrieved from http://www.kff
.org/disparities-policy/issue-brief/beyond-health-care-the-role-of-social-determinants
-in-promoting-health-and-health-equity

Honig, J., Smolowitz, J., & Larson, E. (2013). Building framework for nursing scholarship:
Guidelines for appointment and promotion. *Journal of Professional Nursing, 29,* 359–369.

Institute for Health Improvement. (2017). The IHI triple aim. Retrieved from http://www
.ihi.org/Engage/Initiatives/TripleAim/Pages/default.aspx

Institute of Medicine. (2010). *The future of nursing: Leading change, advancing health.*
Washington, DC: US Government Printing Office.

Ladden, M. D. (Ed.). (2017, March). The case for removing barriers to APRN practice.
Charting Nursing's Future, (30). Retrieved from http://www.rwjf.org/content/dam/farm/
reports/issue_briefs/2017/rwjf435543

Meleis, A., & Dracup, K. (2005). The case against the DNP: History, timing, substance, and
marginalization. *Online Journal of Issues in Nursing, 10*(3), Manuscript 2. doi:10.3912/
OJIN.Vol10No03Man02

Merritt Hawkins. (2017). 2017 review of physician and advanced practitioner recruiting
incentives. Retrieved from https://www.merritthawkins.com/uploadedFiles/Merritt
Hawkins/Pdf/2017_Physician_Incentive_Review_Merritt_Hawkins.pdf

Morris, Z., Wooding, S., & Grant, J. (2011). The answer is 17 years, what is the question:
Understanding time lags in translational research. *Journal of the Royal Society of Medicine,
104*(12), 510–520. doi:10.1258/jrsm.2011.110180

Murphy, M., Staffileno, B., & Carlson, E. (2015). Collaboration among DNP and PhD-prepared nurses: Opportunity to drive positive change. *Journal of Professional Nursing, 31*, 388–394.

National Association of Clinical Nurse Specialists. (n.d.-a). Mission and goals. Retrieved from http://nacns.org/about-us/mission-and-goals

National Association of Clinical Nurse Specialists. (n.d.-b). 2016–2018 public policy agenda. Retrieved from http://nacns.org/advocacy-policy/public-policy-agenda

National Association of Clinical Nurse Specialists. (n.d.-c). What is a CNS? Retrieved from http://nacns.org/about-us/what-is-a-cns

National Council of State Boards of Nursing. (n.d.). APRN consensus model. Retrieved from https://www.ncsbn.org/aprn-consensus.htm

National League for Nursing. (2014). *NLN nurse educator shortage fact sheet.* Retrieved from http://www.nln.org/docs/default-source/advocacy-public-policy/nurse-faculty-shortage -fact-sheet-pdf.pdf?sfvrsn=0

Nicholes, R. H., & Dyer, J. (2012). Is eligibility for tenure possible for the doctor of nursing practice-prepared faculty? *Journal of Professional Nursing, 28*, 13–17.

Nurse Practitioner Roundtable. (2014). *Nurse practitioner perspective on education and post-graduate training.* Retrieved from http://c.ymcdn.com/sites/nonpf.site-ym.com/ resource/resmgr/Docs/NPRoundtableStatementPostGra.pdf

Redman, R. W., Pressler, S. J., Furspan, P., & Potempa, K. (2015). Nurses in the United States with a practice doctorate: Implications for leading in the current context of health care. *Nursing Outlook, 63*(2), 124–129.

Robert Wood Johnson Foundation. (n.d.). *Health systems.* Retrieved from http://www.rwjf .org/en/our-focus-areas/focus-areas/health-systems.html

Rudolph, L., Caplan, J., Ben-Moshe, K., & Dillon, L. (2013). *Health in all policies: A guide for state and local governments.* Washington, DC and Oakland, CA: American Public Health Association and Public Health Institute. Retrieved from https://www.apha.org/~/ media/files/pdf/factsheets/health_inall_policies_guide_169pages.ashx

Stanley, D., & Sherratt, A. (2010). Lamp light on leadership: Clinical leadership and Florence Nightingale. *Journal of Nursing Management, 18*, 115–121.

Udlis, K. A., & Mancuso, J. M. (2015). Perceptions of the role of the doctor of nursing practice-prepared nurse: Clarity or confusion. *Journal of Professional Nursing, 30*(4), 274–283. doi:10.1016/j.profnurs.2015.01.004

SECTION FOUR

The Scholarship of Practice

VALERIE J. FULLER

All health professionals should be educated to deliver patient-centered care as members of an interdisciplinary team, emphasizing evidence-based practice, quality improvement approaches, and informatics.
> Institute of Medicine, *Crossing the Quality Chasm* (2001)

Doctor of nursing practice (DNP) graduates are expected to function as leaders within increasingly complex healthcare systems. Inherent to this role will be the ability to critically appraise and translate best evidence for patients, systems, and organizations; integrate and implement health information technology; and measure outcomes to improve patient care.

Section IV reviews the core essentials of outcomes measurement, health information technology, and evidence-based practice. These interrelated concepts are woven throughout the DNP essentials and serve as the foundation for DNP practice. Additionally, this section serves as an example of DNP- and PhD-prepared nurses working together to generate new knowledge in the pursuit of best practice.

Evidence-Based Practice: The Scholarship Behind the Practice

VALERIE FULLER, DEBRA GILLESPIE, AND DEBRA KRAMLICH

Knowledge is of no value unless you put it into practice.
—Anton Chekhov

Evidence-based practice (EBP) is the cornerstone of the doctor of nursing practice's (DNP's) role. It represents the practitioners' commitment to use all means possible to locate the best (most effective) evidence for any given problem and at all points of planning and contact with clients (Fischer, 2009). In Chapter 4, Drs. Crabtree and Andrist define the role of clinical nurse scholars in generating scientific evidence for practice and the translation of this evidence into practice to achieve optimal health outcomes. In Chapter 5, Drs. Sipe and Andrist review the steps of developing an evidence-based doctor of nursing practice (DNP) project, starting with the formulation of a burning question through to its development, implementation, evaluation, and dissemination. We continue to build on this concept in Chapter 13 by providing a general overview of EBP, including a nursing framework for EBP, challenges to its use, and implementation of EBP in the clinical setting.

■ EBP AND THE DNP

It is a well-known and troubling statistic that it takes one to two decades for original research to be put into routine clinical practice (Agency for Healthcare Research and Quality [AHRQ], 2001). Thus, the translation of research findings into sustainable improvements for clinical practice and patient outcomes remains a substantial obstacle to improving the quality of healthcare (AHRQ, 2001). This separation or knowledge "gap" between research and clinical practice has been well documented in two landmark reports from the Institute of Medicine: *Crossing the Quality Chasm: A New Health System for the 21st Century* (2001) and *Health Professions Education: A Bridge to Quality* (2003). Both reports emphasize the need for additional education in EBP for all healthcare professionals.

In 2004, the American Association of Colleges of Nursing (AACN) released their position statement on the DNP and recommended that the content of such programs include analytic methodologies related to the evaluation of practice and the application of evidence for practice (AACN, 2004). This was later incorporated in the AACN's *Essentials of Doctoral Education for Advanced Nursing Practice* as Essential III: Clinical Scholarship and Analytical Methods for Evidence-Based Practice (AACN, 2006). This essential stresses the need for DNP graduates to translate research into practice in order to improve practice and outcomes of care. Specifically, the AACN recommends that DNP programs prepare graduates to

1. Use analytic methods to critically appraise existing literature and other evidence to determine and implement the best evidence for practice.
2. Design and implement processes to evaluate outcomes of practice, practice patterns, and systems of care within a practice setting, healthcare organization, or community against national benchmarks to determine variances in practice outcomes and population trends.
3. Design, direct, and evaluate quality improvement (QI) methodologies to promote safe, timely, effective, efficient, equitable, and patient-centered care.
4. Apply relevant findings to develop practice guidelines and improve practice and the practice environment.
5. Use information technology and research methods appropriately to
   • Collect appropriate and accurate dates to generate evidence for nursing
   • Inform and guide the design of databases that generate meaningful evidence for nursing practice
   • Analyze data from practice
   • Design evidence-based interventions
   • Predict and analyze outcomes
   • Examine patterns of behavior and outcomes
   • Identify gaps in evidence for practice
6. Function as practice specialist or consultant in collaborative knowledge-generating research.
7. Disseminate findings from EBP and research to improve healthcare outcomes (AACN, 2006, p. 12).

More recently, the AACN released its *Current Issues and Clarifying Recommendations* statement on the DNP. They continue to stress that practice-focused doctoral programs should be heavily focused on practice that is innovative, evidence-based, and reflects the application of credible research findings (AACN, 2015, p. 2). Similarly, in her 2016 editorial "The Doctor of Nursing Practice Degree: Evidence-Based Practice Expert," Melnyk stresses the need for DNP programs to prepare students extensively in EBP with a focus on how to translate the evidence being generated by PhD-prepared nurses into clinical practice and policy in order to improve healthcare quality and patient outcomes (p. 183).

There are currently over 303 DNP programs nationwide with another 124 programs in the planning stages (AACN, 2017). With this meteoric rise in programs, it is essential that educational curriculums support DNP students to become EBP leaders and provide the knowledge and skill set needed to translate evidence into practice (Singleton, 2017).

■ EBP, QI, AND NURSING RESEARCH

Numerous synonyms exist for EBP—evidence-based medicine, evidence-based nursing, evidence-based healthcare, and others. Likewise, there exists an abundance of EBP definitions. Broadly defined, EBP is the integration of best research evidence with clinical expertise and patient values (Institute of Medicine [IOM], 2001; Sackett, Rosenberg, Gray, Haynes, & Richardson, 1996).

Defining what EBP is and is not is an important first step in understanding the concept of evidence. EBP is not nursing research, research utilization, QI, or translational science; while these terms are inextricably linked, there are distinct differences. For example, an EBP project can lead to a research study or a QI project (Beyea & Slattery, 2006). One of the most important distinctions between QI and research lies within the intent. QI intends to improve systems and processes with the goal of improving outcomes. The intention of research is to generate new knowledge, with the results being generalizable to a larger population (Newhouse, Pettit, Poe, & Rocco, 2006). We have defined these terms in the next section in order to provide additional understanding and context for their use in the literature.

DEFINITIONS OF RESEARCH UTILIZATION, NURSING RESEARCH, QI, AND TRANSLATION SCIENCE

Research utilization is the process of using research findings to improve patient care. According to Titler (2002), it involves dissemination of scientific knowledge, study critique, synthesis of research findings, determination of the applicability of findings, developing a research-based practice standard, implementation of the standard, and evaluation. This term is most closely linked to EBP and is often considered a subset of EBP (Cullen, Titler, & Belding-Schmitt, 2009).

Polit and Beck (2008) define *nursing research* as systematic inquiry designed to develop trustworthy evidence about issues of importance to the nursing profession. Nursing research involves the application of a methodology (quantitative or qualitative) to investigate a phenomenon of interest in order to develop, refine, or extend nursing knowledge (Bond, n.d.; Polit & Beck, 2008; Titler, 2002).

QI utilizes a system to monitor and evaluate the quality and appropriateness of care (outcomes) based on EBP and research (Bond, n.d.). Often, QI projects involve solving a problem in a particular setting as opposed to attempting to generalize across all settings and populations (Beyea & Slattery, 2006).

Translation science (also called translational research) is another term often confused with EBP. Translation science is a unique field of research focused on testing the interventions that enhance the uptake and use of evidence to improve patient outcomes and population health and to determine what implementation strategies work for whom, in what settings, and why (Titler, 2014).

■ HISTORY OF EBP

While not widely recognized in the literature, Florence Nightingale is considered by some as the true founder of improving patient outcomes through the use of evidence. Nightingale frequently collected and analyzed data to make improvements in patient care. In her book *Notes on Nursing*, Nightingale describes experimenting with bathing patients with cold water without soap, cold water with soap, and hot water with soap to determine which works best for patients' cleanliness (Nightingale, 1969). Despite this, most of the literature traces the roots of evidence-based medicine (EBM) back to Archie Cochrane in the 1970s. While the term *evidence-based medicine* was not fully adopted until the 1990s, Cochrane believed that due to a hospital's limited resources, clinical decisions should be made only on procedures that had proven to be the most effective (Mackey & Bassendowski, 2017). While Cochrane valued the results of randomized clinical trials as a means for decision making, others have placed a higher value on patient preferences as part of the evidence equation and preferred the term *evidence-based practice*.

EBM and EBP have shifted decision making from an authoritative approach to an objective, scientific, and outcome-based approach. EBM has been criticized for having an experimental perspective on research, a strong "clinical trials" orientation, and therefore defines evidence in quantitative terms and largely ignores qualitative and hermeneutic forms of evidence showcasing the philosophical differences between medicine and nursing (French, 1999). In this view, the evidence answers the question "can it work" without being concerned with "how it works" or "is it worth it?" (Canadian Health Services Research Foundation [CHSRF], 2005). Evidence-based nursing is defined as "integration of the best evidence available, nursing expertise, and the values and preferences of the individuals, families and communities who are served" (Sigma Theta Tau International, 2005, p. 69). Regardless of terminology, the premises of EBP include actual scientific-based clinical practices rather than practices based upon tradition, a focus on individualized care, valuing the contribution of clinical expertise, and incorporating patients' expectations into the plan of care (Hudson, Duke, Haas, & Varnell, 2008).

In 2005, the CHSRF conducted a systematic review to examine the concept of evidence by those who produce evidence and those who make decisions based on evidence. They determined that evidence defined as a science is valued by methodological tests and information gained through rigorous processes and procedures defined as scientific. When evidence is defined colloquially, it becomes valued as it relates to context sensitive applications specific to the circumstances in which it is applied. Therefore, evidence is uncertain, complex, dynamic, and rarely complete, adding to the challenges to negotiate and adopt a common definition for translation into practice (CHSRF, 2005).

Following the definition of evidence, the scientific evidence must be integrated with the patient and family preferences along with nurses' explicit and tacit knowledge. The actual role that patients play in their decision making has not yet been formalized, but it is essential that healthcare practitioners acknowledge patients' choices (Chummun & Tiran, 2008).

Research by Benner, Tanner, and Chesla (1996) demonstrated that nurses come to clinical situations and decision making inherently with a sense of what is good and right. These values are often unspoken and unrecognized but profoundly influence nurses' decision making. In addition, clinical judgments are extremely complex, often made under very stressful situations, in fractions of a minute and with other staff who may have competing interests (Tanner, 2006). Nurses may be reluctant to embrace the EBP/research paradigm, not understanding the research language and EBP concepts; however, they do collectively seek to provide the best care to their patients.

The paradigm of translational research has seen remarkable uptake in a short period of time with national organizations around the world endorsing research translation as a means for applying scientific evidence into practice. This can be reflected by the National Institutes of Health (NIH) forming centers for translational research and developing the Clinical and Translational Science Award (Woolf, 2008).

Although specific terminology may differ slightly, the terms research translation and translational research may be used interchangeably; however, they, in fact, have differing meanings (Davidson, 2011). "Research translation is the process whereby knowledge is passed anywhere along the translational pathway from basic science at one end to improved community-based health outcomes at the other end . . ." (Davidson, 2011, p. 910). To add to the confusion, the terms knowledge transfer, knowledge translation, knowledge exchange, research utilization, diffusion, and implementation are often used synonymously (Logan & Graham, 2004).

Given that the definition of EBP is the integration of evidence from rigorous scientific experiments with clinical expertise and patient preferences, the Multisystem Model of Knowledge Translation and Integration (MKIT) has purposely chosen to use the term *knowledge translation* as a more generalized concept describing the uptake of all forms of knowledge, not just results of scientific experiments to the practice environment.

USE OF THE MKIT TO EMPLOY EBP

A model is a schematic description that takes essential components of a process and attempts to explain the relationships between them (Wolf & Greenhouse, 2007). Models serve as a map illustrating to the user how to get from one point to another. With the acceleration of the EBP paradigm, many new research utilization and EBP models to assist practitioners have been developed (Table 12.1). Each of these models has strengths and limitations, is designed for individual or organizational use, is linear or unidirectional, is difficult for novice evidence users to understand, does not have an algorithm that is easy to follow, and focuses on empirical knowledge alone and ignores the importance of practitioners' tacit knowledge.

The process for innovation is often quite complex and cannot be reduced to a simple, linear model (Van de Ven, Polley, Garud, & Venkataraman, 2008). Quality and safety literature processes, such as plan–do–study act (PDSA), have implicit ongoing interconnections (Thor et al., 2004). Action research incorporates spirals of learning, doing, and reflection that are well recognized with embedded ongoing cyclical processes (Titchen & Manley, 2006). Cyclical process patterns are not new to innovations.

Traditional models of research have separated research and practice into distinct domains, thereby expanding the existing significant division between theorists and practitioners. Rycroft-Malone and Bucknall (2010) suggest that the application of frameworks and models to research can make a difference in our understanding of the processes involved and the outcomes that result. The MKIT addresses linear systems thinking and is supported with a well-established conceptual framework (Palmer & Kramlich, 2011). Unlike other translation models, the MKIT process begins with reflection. The cyclical process of the MKIT is ongoing and includes reflection, action, and monitoring of outcomes and reflection. Tacit knowledge integrated with scientific evidence and patients' values can be catapulted by the formation of communities of practice (CoP), allowing for the sharing of knowledge and expertise for better patient care. This fundamental component of true knowledge translation begins with creating opportunities for interaction between both the evidence creators and users.

There is emerging literature recognizing the importance that practitioners' tacit knowledge is grossly undervalued. The MKIT model, supported by CoP, integrates explicit and tacit knowledge as well as scientific evidence to practice. The application of the MKIT for the integration of knowledge management and clinical process improvements also allows for a higher performing organization.

Operating within the theoretical framework of CoP (Wenger, McDermott, & Snyder, 2002), the MKIT is circular rather than unidirectional with reflective inquiry, knowledge seeking/generation, integration, implementation, evaluation, mentoring, and reflective inquiry. Anthropologists Jean Lave and Etienne Wenger coined the term CoP while studying apprenticeship as a learning model. CoP are defined as, "Groups of people who share a concern, a set of problems, or a passion about a topic, and who deepen their knowledge and expertise in this area by interacting on an ongoing basis" (Wenger et al., 2002, p. 4). CoP begin when a group of people who are committed to a common domain of interest focus on sharing "best" practices and creating knowledge and resources to advance their practice.

The processes of the MKIT are straightforward for the knowledge seeker evaluating practice through searching, creating, integrating, and translating new evidence into practice by forming strategic partnerships employing a microsystem or "bottom up" approach to identifying and resolving problems with an interdisciplinary group of frontline workers to sustain the solution. The advanced practice registered nurse (APRN) will engage in reflective practice upon challenging clinical situations that lead to forming a clinical question. This reflection will guide the literature search and development of a researchable question. Based on the results of the literature search, the APRN will then decide to develop policies and protocols to move the evidence into practice or develop a research study to generate evidence if little is found. After implementing the changes in practice, it is imperative to monitor the patient outcomes. The MKIT encourages pilot testing with a small group of clinicians and patients to demonstrate the feasibility of the change in practice (Palmer & Kramlich, 2011). If outcomes are favorable from a pilot test, change could then be made in practice in other units with other like populations and monitored over time to determine its impact on the environment, staff, costs, and the patient and family. The APRN should disseminate the results of the changes in practice either by presentations and/or publications for others to elicit the knowledge for their organizations and to advance the state of the science. All of the steps occur within the micro, meso, and macro organizational levels, and it is imperative that the APRN engage key stakeholders, change agents, and early adopters in the process in order to successfully implement change.

A multitude of issues and factors come together to identify the complexity and scope of patient safety and quality care, as well as the necessity for intricate strategies to create change within healthcare systems and processes of care. APRNs typically take care of many patients during their day, each with conflicting, yet simultaneous needs. Increasing patient acuity, decreasing length of hospital stay, and mandated governmental regulations have contributed to the complexity of clinical practice challenging APRNs today. In using EBP by employing the easy to use MKIT, the APRN is in the forefront of engaging in initiatives to continually improve quality by striving for excellence (Hughes, 2008).

TABLE 12.1 Research Translation and EBP Models

Research Translation and EBP Models	Authors	Year
Stetler Model	Stetler and Marram	1976 Revised 1994, 2001
CURN Model	Horsley, Crane, Crabtree, and Wood	1983
Ottawa Model	Logan and Graham	1998 Revised 2004
Rosswurm and Larrabee Model	Rosswurn and Larrabee	1999

(continued)

TABLE 12.1 Research Translation and EBP Models (*continued*)

Research Translation and EBP Models	Authors	Year
Iowa Model	Titler, Kleiber, Steelman, Rakel, Budreau, Everett, Buckwalter, Tripp-Reimer, and Goode	2001 Revised 2017
ACE Star Model of Knowledge Transformation	Stevens	2004
PARIHS Model	Rycroft-Malone	2004
Johns Hopkins Model	Newhouse, Dearhold, Poe, Pugh, and White	2005
MKIT	Palmer and Kramlich	2011
ARCC	Melnyk and Fineout-Overholt	2011

ACE, Academic Center for Excellence; ARCC, Advancing Research and Clinical Practice through Close Collaboration; CURN, The Conduct and Utilization of Research in Nursing; EPB, evidence-based practice; MKIT, Multisystem Model of Knowledge Integration and Translation; PARIHS, Promoting Action on Research Implementation in Health Services; TRIP, turning research into practice.

■ EBP EXEMPLARS

If you are still feeling uncertain of your ability to engage in EBP, you are not alone. Novice EBP users often wonder how to get started, where to find the evidence, how to implement the evidence, and whether such implementation will yield the expected outcome. The following are several examples of EBP projects conducted by frontline staff that may inspire confidence and emphasize the myriad ways DNPs can promote EBP.

PEDIATRIC PAIN ASSESSMENT

A staff nurse working in the pediatric intensive care unit (PICU) felt dissatisfied with the scales used for assessment of pain in children in the institution. There were too many scales (four, to be exact!), several were complicated and difficult to use, and none were appropriate or had been validated in the PICU population. Concurrently, the patient satisfaction scores regarding pain management in children were below benchmark, and chart audits showed poor compliance with pain assessment documentation. This nurse had recently been introduced to the FLACC (Face, Legs, Activity, Cry, Consolability) Scale (Merkel, Voepel-Lewis, Shayevitz, & Malviya, 1997), which seemed like a more appropriate scale for the patient population and was consistent with other 0 to 10 scales. A thorough critical analysis of the literature revealed that pain management did not improve following staff education. Implementation of a valid, objective pain assessment and documentation tool appropriate for the patient population did seem to improve pain management, as did improved documentation. Staff surveys regarding knowledge of pain assessment and documentation policies and best practices and chart audits were conducted. Education about the FLACC scale, pediatric pain assessment, and the pain documentation policy was then provided to all staff in the form of a paper packet, a computer-based program, resource binders, and staff mentors. Charts were again audited one month and four months posteducation to assess for change in documentation. Postimplementation surveys were also administered to assess for change in knowledge. Documentation of pain using objective criteria, patient satisfaction with pain management, and staff satisfaction with the pain scales available all improved following implementation of the FLACC scale. Institutional policy was changed to replace several of the previously used pain scales with the FLACC scale.

FAMILY PRESENCE DURING RESUSCITATION

Nurses and physicians in the intensive care units were experiencing more requests for family presence during resuscitation. With no policy, guidelines, or additional support staff, the experiences of staff and families were not always positive. One staff nurse with personal experience of being denied family presence during the resuscitation of a loved one pursued the implementation of a guideline to support families and staff during such events. The literature was rich with evidence to support the practice, numerous professional nursing and medical associations endorsed the practice, and a published guideline to assist in presenting the option for family presence existed. There were still many obstacles to simply implementing such a guideline, including firmly entrenched beliefs, fears, and misperceptions. Using the MKIT, the staff nurse performed a critical analysis of the literature, formed a multidisciplinary team, and methodically worked to gain consensus for development of a guideline to support families during resuscitation of their loved one, whether or not bedside presence was requested or allowed. The guideline has been successfully implemented for nearly 10 years, with improved family and staff satisfaction as a result. Revisions to the guideline have been made to accommodate changes in staffing patterns and organizational processes, in consultation with the original nurse champion, with no disruption in patient and family care.

DETECTING DETERIORATION IN CHILDREN

It has been well documented that signs of clinical deterioration may be apparent hours before cardiac arrest in acutely ill patients, and early detection may prevent adverse outcomes (Monaghan, 2005; Parshuram, Hutchison, & Middaugh, 2009). One of the attending pediatric intensivists expressed concern about anecdotal cases of missed early signs of deterioration and suggested implementation of the Pediatric Early Warning Score (Monaghan, 2005). This was met with little interest, and it seemed the proposal had hit a brick wall. A staff nurse then conducted a chart audit of children who had been transferred from the pediatric inpatient unit to the PICU over the previous 18 months and found that of 161 unexpected transfers there were 33 missed opportunities for early detection and intervention, including several cardiorespiratory arrests. This evidence was brought forward to nursing and physician leadership, which renewed interest in implementation of an early detection of deterioration scoring system. Concurrently, the institution was approached by developers of the Bedside Pediatric Early Warning System (BPEWS) to collaborate on validation of this scale (Parshuram et al., 2009). This partnership resulted in a significant reduction in adverse outcomes in the year following implementation: more than 80% reduction in cardiorespiratory arrest events; 2.5-fold increase in the number of rapid response team evaluations per patient day; 3.5-fold increase in the number of rapid response team evaluations that resulted in avoidance of an unplanned transfer to the PICU; and a 60% reduction in the deterioration events per patient day. The initiative was then successfully moved forward by advanced practice pediatric nurses on the unit. The tool has been embedded in the institution's electronic health record with accompanying case-matched recommendations for intervention and continues to positively impact length of stay and overall mortality.

FALL AND INJURY RISK ASSESSMENT IN CHILDREN

As part of The Joint Commission's 2005 National Safety Goals, acute care facilities are required to implement a fall prevention program and evaluate its effectiveness. Fall prevention programs have proven to be an effective intervention for the adult and geriatric populations; screening tools have been developed, tested, and deemed reliable and valid. Conversely, development of a fall prevention instrument for pediatrics has proven to be challenging. Recognizing the need to choose a pediatric fall risk assessment instrument that would be appropriate for the patient population and acceptable to staff, a team that included several staff nurses and an experienced staff nurse research mentor conducted a study investigating the reliability, specificity, and sensitivity of five pediatric fall scale instruments (Harvey, Kramlich, Chapman, Parker, & Blades, 2010). Findings indicated that while almost all of the instruments showed acceptable reliability and sensitivity, specificity for all five scales was lacking. Furthermore, the study demonstrated that none of the five instruments adequately assessed risk of injury from falls. Pediatric nurses involved in this study expressed great concern regarding a patient's risk of injury from a fall and indicated it should be a priority when assessing a child. Much of the published pediatric fall-related literature focused on the development and testing of screening instruments and the implementation of fall prevention programs. There were no studies that investigated nursing perceptions of pediatric falls. Bedside pediatric nurses play a significant role in protecting their patients against falls and are frequently the individuals responsible for reporting a fall occurrence. Because of those concerns, staff felt it would be important to clearly and accurately define a reportable fall before implementation of a pediatric fall and injury risk assessment tool and prevention program. Therefore, an exploratory study of pediatric healthcare practitioners' perceptions of a reportable fall occurrence was conducted to help define a reportable pediatric fall and inform development of a prevention program (Kramlich & Dende, 2016). Based on staff-identified factors, the Humpty Dumpty Fall Scale, a screening tool with acceptable sensitivity and specificity and parameters that included most factors identified by the focus group participants, was adopted and integrated into the electronic medical record. Staff was actively involved in the development of definitions, selection of tools, and identification of next steps toward a comprehensive fall reduction program for their patients. Staff engagement in the process increased the likelihood of successful, sustained practice change and successful endorsement by the organization (Palmer & Kramlich, 2011).

■ ADDITIONAL RESOURCES FOR EBP

Table 12.2 provides a list of additional resources for EBP.

TABLE 12.2   Evidence-Based Practice Websites

Website Name	Website Address
Introduction to Evidence-Based Practice from Duke and University of North Carolina	http://guides.mclibrary.duke.edu/ebmtutorial
Agency for Healthcare Research and Quality	www.ahrq.gov
World Confederation for Physical Therapy	http://www.wcpt.org/node/29661
TRIP Database	https://www.tripdatabase.com
Bandolier	http://www.bandolier.org.uk/index.html
National Guideline Clearinghouse	https://www.guideline.gov
Johns Hopkins Evidence-Based Practice Center	http://www.jhsph.edu/research/centers-and-institutes/johns-hopkins-evidence-based-practice-center/index.html
Academy of Medical–Surgical Nurses	https://www.amsn.org/practice-resources/evidence-based-practice
Institute for Healthcare Improvement	http://www.ihi.org/Pages/default.aspx
Registered Nurses' Association of Ontario	http://rnao.ca/bpg
Veterans Administration/Department of Defense	https://www.healthquality.va.gov
Center for Evidence-Based Medicine at Oxford University	http://www.cebm.net
The Cochrane Collaboration	http://www.cochrane.org
Virginia Henderson Global Nursing e-Repository	http://www.nursinglibrary.org/vhl
Nursing Center Evidence-Based Practice Network	http://www.nursingcenter.com/evidencebasedpracticenetwork/home
University of Washington Health Sciences Library APRN/DNP Toolkit	http://hsl.uw.edu/toolkits/dnp
University of Kansas SUMSearch 2	http://sumsearch.org

APRN, advanced practice registered nurse; DNP, doctor of nursing practice; TRIP, turning research into practice.

■ SUMMARY

EBP is a process that enables clinicians to seek out best practices and determine if and how these practices can be incorporated into patient care (Poe & White, 2010). The DNP-prepared nurse is uniquely prepared to synthesize clinical expertise with EBP to improve patient outcomes, provide clinical leadership, and transform healthcare.

■ REFERENCES

Agency for Healthcare Research and Quality. (2001). *Translating research into practice (TRIP)-II fact sheet*. Retrieved from http://www.ahrq.gov/research/trip2fac.htm

American Association of Colleges of Nursing. (2004). *AACN position statement on the practice doctorate in nursing*. Washington, DC: Author. Retrieved from http://www.aacnnursing.org/DNP/Position-Statement

American Association of Colleges of Nursing. (2006). *The essentials of doctoral education for advanced practice nursing*. Retrieved from http://www.aacnnursing.org/Portals/42/Publications/DNPEssentials.pdf

American Association of Colleges of Nursing. (2015). *The doctor of nursing practice: Current issues and clarifying recommendations*. Washington, DC: Author. Retrieved from http://www.aacnnursing.org/Portals/42/DNP/DNP-Implementation.pdf?ver=2017-08-01-105830-517

American Association of Colleges of Nursing. (2017, June). DNP fact sheet. Retrieved from http://www.aacnnursing.org/News-Information/Fact-Sheets/DNP-Fact-Sheet

Benner, P., Tanner, C., & Chesla, C. (1996). *Expertise in nursing practice: A possible role for the consultant nurse*. New York, NY: Springer Publishing.

Beyea, S. C., & Slattery, M. J. (2006). *Evidence-based practice in nursing: A guide to successful implementation*. Retrieved from http://www.hcmarketplace.com/supplemental/3737_browse.pdf

Bond, S. (n.d.) Evidence-based practice: What's in it for you? Retrieved from http://slideplayer.com/slide/4536218

Canadian Health Services Research Foundation. (2005). *Conceptualizing and combining evidence for health system guidance*. Retrieved from http://www.cfhi-fcass.ca/migrated/pdf/insightAction/evidence_e.pdf

Chummun, H., & Tiran, D. (2008). Increasing research evidence in practice: A possible role for the consultant nurse. *Journal of Nursing Management, 16*(3), 327–333.

Cullen, L., Titler, M. G., & Belding-Schmitt, M. (2009). *Online webcourse: Evidence-based practice*. Retrieved from www.uihealthcare.org/otherservices.aspx?id=225170

Davidson, A. (2011). Translations research: What does it mean? *Anesthesiology, 115*(5), 909–911.

Fischer, J. (2009). Evidence-based practice. In J. Fischer (Ed.), *Toward evidence-based practice: Variations on a theme* (pp. 451–468). Chicago, IL: Lyceum Books.

French, P. (1999). The development of evidence-based nursing. *Journal of Advanced Nursing, 29*(1), 72–78.

Harvey, K., Kramlich, D., Chapman, J., Parker, J., & Blades, E. (2010). Exploring and evaluating five pediatric falls assessment instruments and injury risk indicators: An ambispective study in a tertiary care setting. *Journal of Nursing Management, 18*(5), 531–541.

Horsley, J., Crane, J., Crabtree, M., & Wood, D. (1983). *Using research to improve nursing practice: A guide*. New York, NY: W. B. Saunders.

Hudson, K., Duke, G., Haas, B., & Varnell, G. (2008). Navigating the evidence-based practice maze. *Journal of Nursing Management, 16*(4), 409–416.

Hughes, R. G. (Ed.). (2008). *Patient safety and quality: An evidence-based handbook for nurses*. Rockville, MD: Agency for Healthcare Research and Quality.

Institute of Medicine. (2001). *Crossing the quality chasm: A new health system for the 21st century*. Washington, DC: National Academies Press.

Institute of Medicine. (2003). *Health professions education: A bridge to quality*. Washington, DC: National Academies Press.

Kramlich, D. L., & Dende, D. (2016). Development of a pediatric fall risk and injury reduction program. *Pediatric Nursing, 42*, 77–82.

Logan, J., & Graham, I. (1998). Toward a comprehensive interdisciplinary model of health care research use. *Scientific Community, 20*(2), 227–246.

Mackey, A., & Bassendowski, S. (2017). The history of evidence-based practice in nursing education and practice. *Journal of Professional Nursing, 33*(1), 51–55.

Melnyk, B. M., & Fineout-Overholt, E. (Eds.). (2011). *Evidence-based practice in nursing & healthcare* (2nd ed.). Philadelphia, PA: Wolters Kluwer Health/Lippincott Williams & Wilkins.

Merkel, S. I., Voepel-Lewis, T., Shayevitz, J. R., & Malviya, S. (1997). The FLACC: A behavioral scale for scoring postoperative pain in young children. *Pediatric Nursing, 23*(3), 293–297.

Monaghan, A. (2005). Detecting and managing deterioration in children. *Paediatric Nursing, 17*(1), 32–35.

Newhouse, R. P., Pettit, J. C., Poe, S., & Rocco, L. (2006). The slippery slope: Differentiating between quality improvement and research. *Journal of Nursing Administration, 36*(4), 211–219.

Nightingale, Florence. (1969). *Notes on nursing: What it is, and what it is not*. New York, NY: Dover Publications

Palmer, D., & Kramlich, D. (2011). An introduction to the multi-system model of knowledge integration and translation. *Advances in Nursing Science, 34*(1), 29–38. doi:10.1097/ANS.0b013e318209439f

Parshuram, C. S., Hutchison, J., & Middaugh, K. (2009). Development and initial validation of the bedside paediatric early warning system score. *Critical Care, 13*(4), R135.

Poe, S. S., & White, K. M. (2010). *Johns Hopkins nursing evidence-based practice: Implementation and translation*. Indianapolis, IN: Sigma Theta Tau International.

Polit, D. F., & Beck, C. T. (2008). *Nursing research: Generating and assessing evidence for nursing practice* (8th ed.). Philadelphia, PA: Wolters Kluwer/Lippincott Williams & Wilkins.

Rosswurm, M., & Larrabee, J. (1999). A model for change to evidence-based practice. *Image—Journal of Nursing Scholarship, 31*, 317–322.

Rycroft-Malone, J. (2004). The PARISH framework: A framework for guiding the implementation of evidence-based practice. *Journal of Nursing Care Quality, 19*(4), 297–304.

Rycroft-Malone, J., & Bucknall, T. (2010). Using theory and frameworks to facilitate the implementation of evidence into practice. *Worldviews on Evidence-Based Nursing, 7*(2), 57–58.

Sackett, D. L., Rosenberg, W. M., Gray, J. A., Haynes, R. B., & Richardson, W. S. (1996). Evidence based medicine: What it is and what it isn't. *British Medical Journal, 312*, 71–72.

Sigma Theta Tau International Honor Society of Nursing. (2005). Evidence-based nursing position statement. Retrieved from http://www.sigmanursing.org/why-sigma/about -sigma/position-statements-and-resource-papers/evidence-based-nursing-position -statement

Singleton, J. (2017, October). Evidence-based practice beliefs and implementation in doctor of nursing practice students. *Worldviews on Evidence-Based Nursing, 14*(5), 412–418. doi:10.1111/wvn.12228

Stetler, C. (2001). Updating the Stetler Model of research utilization to facilitate evidence-based practice. *Nursing Outlook, 49*, 272–278.

Stetler, C.B., & Marram, G. (1976). Evaluating research findings for applicability in practice. *Nursing Outlook, 24*, 559–563.

Stevens, K. (2004). ACE Star Model of EBP: Knowledge Transformation. San Antonio: Academic Center for Evidence-based Practice/The University of Texas Health Science Center at San Antonio. Retrieved from http://nursing.uthscsa.edu/onrs/starmodel

Tanner, C. A. (2006). Thinking like a nurse: A research based-model of clinical judgment in nursing. *Journal of Nursing Education, 45*(6), 204–211.

Thor, J. L., Wittlov, K., Herrlin, B., Brommels, M., Svensson, O., Skar, J., & Ovretveit, J. (2004). Learning helpers: How they facilitated improvement and improved facilitation-lessons from a hospital-wide quality improvement initiative. *Quality Management in Health Care, 13*(1), 60–74.

Titchen, A., & Manley, K. (2006). Spiraling towards transformational action research: Philosophical and practical journeys. *Educational Action Research, 14*(3), 333–356.

Titler, M. G. (2002). *Toolkit for promoting evidence-based practice.* Iowa City: The University of Iowa Hospital and Clinics, Department of Nursing Services and Patient Care.

Titler, M. G. (2014). Overview of evidence-based practice and translation science. *Nursing Clinics of North America, 49*(3), 269–274.

Titler, M. G., Kleiber, C., Steelman, V., Rakel, B. A., Budreau, G., Everett, L. Q., . . . Goode, C. J. (2001). The Iowa Model of evidence-based practice to promote quality care. *Critical Care Nursing Clinics of North America, 13*(4), 497–509.

Van de Ven, A. H., Polley, D. E., Garud, R., & Venkataraman, S. (2008). *The innovation journey.* New York, NY: Oxford University Press.

Wenger, E., McDermott, R., & Snyder, W. M. (2002). *Cultivating communities of practice: A guide to managing knowledge.* Boston, MA: Harvard Business School Press.

Wolf, G. A., & Greenhouse, P. K. (2007). Blueprint for design: Creating models that direct change. *Journal of Nursing Administration, 37*(9), 381–387.

Woolf, S. (2008). The meaning of translational research and why it matters. *Journal of the American Medical Association, 299*(2), 211–213.

CHAPTER THIRTEEN

The Scholarship Supporting Leadership, Organizations, and Systems

MARJORIE S. WIGGINS AND KRISTINA HYRKÄS

The importance of evidence-based practice (EBP) has been recognized since the early 1990s, and the scholarship behind organizations, systems, and identification of different media to bridge the research–practice divide has been gaining more attention and popularity, meanwhile nurses and nurse leaders' involvement in clinical scholarship has also become increasingly active. Traditionally, clinical nurses (BSN/baccalaureate-level education) have been considered as the "consumers" of knowledge (i.e., EBP), the advanced practice nurses (master's-level education) as catalysts for practice improvements (i.e., quality improvement [QI]), and nurse researcher (PhD/doctor of nursing practice [DNP] education) as producers of new knowledge. The reality is, however, that nurses and nurse leaders' traditional "roles" and engagement in scholarly activities have been expanding as research evidence, systematic reviews, and evidence-based guidelines and bundles are produced at an increasing rate, and nursing research is growing in response to increasing emphasis on EBP (Carter, Mastro, Vose, Rivera, & Larson, 2017; Curtis, Fry, Shaban, & Considine, 2016; Parkosewich, 2013; Ubbink, Guyatt, & Vermeulan, 2013). Yet, despite the recognized benefits of EBP (i.e., reduced variation and costs; improved quality, safety, patient outcomes), a wide gap has remained between the emergence of research findings and their application to practice in the 21st century; EBP and utilization of research findings have been surprisingly slow despite considerable efforts by the scientific community and investment of funds and resources in healthcare settings (Melnyk, Gallagher-Ford, Long, & Fineout-Overholt, 2014; see also Dogherty, Harrison, Graham, Vandyk, & Keeping-Burke, 2013). The literature shows that in the field of nursing EBP awareness, adoption and implementation, the bodies of knowledge and research utilization, as well as managerial support, are still developing (Kim, Stichler, Ecoff, Gallo, & Davidson, 2017; Melnyk, Fineout-Overholt, Gallagher-Ford, & Kaplan, 2012; Melnyk, Gallagher-Ford, Troseth, & Szalacha, 2016; Ubbink et al., 2013).

In today's fast-changing and complex healthcare environment it is natural and an expectation that bedside clinicians change their assumptions and long-standing practices based on new evidence supporting something better. However, it is more difficult to move an entire organization and, in turn, an entire healthcare system toward the same evidence-based way of thinking and behaving (Centrella-Nigro et al., 2015; Curtis et al., 2016). In the same way that nursing practice needs to constantly change, the organizations within healthcare need to evolve and become continuously learning healthcare systems to meet the changing needs of the patients, populations, and the communities which they serve by actively bringing research-based knowledge into practice and promoting its utilization to improve the quality, cost-effectiveness, and safety of healthcare delivery and service outcomes (Curtis et al., 2016; M. Smith, Saunders, Stuckhardt, & McGinnis, 2013).

Nurses' active involvement in clinical scholarship is necessary to advance the nursing profession and improve patient outcomes. Scholarship is also an essential component of enabling evidence-based nursing (EBN) and the development of best practice standards. However, there is no comprehensive definition of scholarship in the literature from practicing nurses (Wilkes, Mannix, & Jackson, 2013). Various terms have been used to refer to scholarly activities, for example, EBP, quality assurance, QI, research utilization, translational research, implementation science, or some combination of these. The lack of definitional clarity, inconsistent use of terminology, and the separation of EBP, QI, and research into mutually exclusive categories may sometimes cause confusion to nursing scholars. Also, lines between EBP, QI, and research often can be blurry. In the late 1990s, the Sigma Theta Tau International Clinical Scholarship Task Force defined clinical nursing scholarship comprehensively as:

> An approach that enables evidence-based nursing and development of best practices to meet the needs of clients efficiently and effectively. It requires the identification of desired outcomes; the use of systematic observation and scientifically based methods to identify and solve clinical problems; the substantiation of practice and clinical decisions with reference to scientific principles, current research, consensus-based guidelines, quality improvement data and other forms of evidence; the evaluation, documentation and dissemination of outcomes and improvements in practice and the use of clinical knowledge and expertise to anticipate trends, predict needs, create effective clinical products and services, and manage outcomes. (1999, p. 4)

Clinical scholarship refers to nurses' participation in activities that improve patient care, advance the nursing profession, and contribute to new knowledge. The definition is broad and thus clinical scholarships in nursing occur along a continuum of EBP, QI, and research activities with varying degrees of interdependence and synergy in improving patient care (Carter et al., 2017). The spectrum of activities in practice is wide, and thus understanding the similarities and differences between

EBP, QI, and research is important to be familiar with, as is identifying work that requires a plan to protect the rights and safety of human subjects, and approval from the institutional review board (IRB; Baker et al., 2014; Carter et al., 2017).

The difficulty of getting healthcare professionals to implement EBP and consistently use products of research in their practice, for example, in a form of a protocol or a bundle, has been an ongoing, almost intractable challenge. Regardless of the increasing quantities of high-quality evidence for the past 20 years, the slow uptake to adopt evidence persists (Appleby Roskell, & Daly, 2015). However, today we know more about successful implementation of EBP and healthcare professionals' intentions toward using research and products of research in clinical practice. Successful implementation of evidence-based care seems to be affected by factors such as quality (i.e., scientific robustness) of the evidence; pragmatism; complexity and difficulties to implement evidence in practice; professional consensus, influence of peers, and patients' preferences; context that is receptive to change with sympathetic cultures, strong leadership, and appropriate monitoring and feedback systems; and appropriate change facilitation strategies with input from skilled external and internal facilitators (Appleby et al., 2015; Rycroft-Malone, 2004).

This chapter focuses on EBP from the organizational and systems perspective and evidence-based management and administration from the decision makers' perspective. It includes information about major professional organizations and policy-making bodies emphasizing EBP and how their perspectives have evolved. It also discusses the context and models of EBP, transformational leadership, and organizational change theories. Next, the focus moves to infrastructure and how it may support EBP and research. Readiness for change and strategies to promote and increase EBP readiness are discussed from different perspectives, such as theoretical aspects of diffusion of innovations. Finally, the chapter explores how EBP has evolved and its interprofessional future.

■ MAJOR PROFESSIONAL ORGANIZATIONS' AND POLICY-MAKING BODIES' EMPHASIS ON EBP

More than a decade ago, three major professional and health organizations and policy-making bodies started to emphasize the importance of EBP and research: (a) the Institute of Medicine (IOM; Greiner & Knebel, 2003), (b) The Joint Commission (2003), and (c) the American Nurses Credentialing Center (ANCC; Greiner & Knebel, 2003).

Between 2003 and 2004, the IOM published two essential reports: *Keeping Patients Safe: Transforming the Work Environment of Nurses* and *Health Professions Education: A Bridge to Quality.* The first report identified RNs' important role in providing safe patient care and also outlined systems and structures needed to provide such care (Page, 2004). The second report focusing on education ascertained five core competencies (i.e., EBP, informatics, patient-centered care, QI, and teamwork and collaboration) and asserted that all healthcare professionals should be educated to deliver ". . . patient-centered care as members of an inter-professional team, emphasizing EBP, quality improvement and informatics" (Greiner & Knebel, 2003). The IOM has recommended that by the year 2020, 90% of all clinical decisions should be supported by accurate, timely, and up-to-date clinical information that is based on the best available evidence (Olsen, Aisner, & McGinnis, 2007). A more recent report, *The Future of Nursing: Leading Change, Advancing Health*, acknowledged nurses' unique opportunity with their direct patient care role to implement EBP and improve patient care outcomes, placing an economic value on their actions. This report also recognized the necessity of EBP as a competency for nurses and that increasing the proportion of the workforce with BSNs from the current 50% to 80% by 2020 will help to prepare a workforce competent in such areas as EBP (IOM, 2011). The need for a research base has been articulated in this report as well, as it identifies healthcare as complicated and requiring research and EBP for the delivery of high-quality care.

In the early 2000s, The Joint Commission started to provide resources for implementation of EBP, including *Putting Evidence to Work* (2003) that focuses on concepts, principles, and techniques of EBP and tools for appraising evidence. It also offered examples of starting or improving EBP programs, and supplied tools and templates for incorporating patients' values in shared decision making (The Joint Commission, 2003). The Joint Commission has fully recognized the benefits of EBP and requires, for example, that disease-specific certifications be based on national standards, effective use of evidence-based clinical practice guidelines, and performance measurement and improvement. Today, The Joint Commission has also made the "Nursing Reference Center" available online, which is a resource that provides evidence-based information for point of care (e.g., evidence-based care sheets, patient education handouts), and easy access for nurses to the most current information to provide the best care possible to their patients (health.ebsco.com/products/nursing-reference-center; see also: The Joint Commission International, 2016; www.jointcommission.org).

In nursing, one of the most influential organizations is the ANCC, a subsidiary of the American Nurses Association. The ANCC's Magnet Recognition Program® recognizes healthcare organizations that provide the very best in-patient care and is the gold standard for nursing practice. Hospitals acknowledged with the status are expected to foster and utilize EBP as part of the evidence-driven empirical Magnet model composed of transformational leadership, structural empowerment, exemplary professional practice, and new knowledge, innovations, and improvements. The Magnet Recognition Program relies heavily on current evidence, the use of best practices, and the ability to demonstrate high-quality outcomes, and thus these organizations are also expected to demonstrate expertise in research, data acquisition, analysis, and application of findings (ANCC, 2014; Lavin, 2013). Organizations that achieve Magnet status possess established and evolving programs related to EBP and have resources in place to support the advancement of EBP and research in all clinical settings (ANCC, 2014). Empirical evidence is available today demonstrating that Magnet hospitals promote organizational EBP and research culture, including infrastructure and resources (Johantgen et al., 2017; McLaughlin, Speroni, Kelly,

Guzzetta, & Desale, 2013; Kelly, Turner, Gabel Speroni, McLaughlin, & Guzzetta, 2013). The evidence is showing, for example, that in Magnet and Pathway to Excellence designated hospitals, compared to non-Magnet facilities, EBP is implemented more consistently, fewer EBP barriers are reported, availability of EBP experts is higher, organizational culture supports EBP, routine EBP education is offered, and EBP efforts are routinely recognized; shared governance allows nurses to have input into practice and to work closely with nursing leadership to promote change (McHugh et al., 2013; Melnyk et al., 2012; see also Lang, Wyer, & Haynes, 2007).

■ CONTEXT AND EBP

In has been recognized in the literature that context/organizational context is a critical element to successful implementation and sustainability of EBP (Gallagher-Ford, 2014a, 2014b; Melnyk et al., 2014; Rycroft-Malone et al., 2011). Context has been addressed in a majority of the implementation models and frameworks and it has been defined often as the specific environment in which implementation, utilization, and creation of evidence may take place. It includes, for example, leadership, organizational culture, and measurement or evaluation. Context interacts, influences, modifies, and facilitates, or it can constrain, implementation. As an overarching concept, context comprises not just a physical location but also roles, interactions, and relationships at multiple levels (e.g., individual/micro-, environmental, organizational/meso-, environmental/macro-, and cultural levels) (see, e.g., Gallagher-Ford, 2014a, 2014b; Gallagher-Ford, 2015; May, Johnson, & Finch, 2016; Pfadenhauer et al., 2017; Rycroft-Malone et al., 2011; Stetler, Ritchie, Rycroft-Malone, & Charns, 2014).

Interest in organizational features of EBP and context started in the late 1990s. Over the years, for example, Kitson and colleagues (Kitson, Harvey, & McCormack, 1998; Kitson & Harvey, 2016; McCormack et al., 2002; Rycroft-Malone et al., 2002; Rycroft-Malone et al., 2004; Rycroft-Malone et al., 2013; Rycroft-Malone et al., 2015) have conducted pioneering studies on the concept of context demonstrating that factors, such as leadership, organizational context, and facilitation, influence knowledge translation and implementation. It is noted, however, that leadership alone is unlikely to be effective for EBP implementation without attention to organizational context for change; the characteristics of leaders and organization are both important for promoting EBP use (Aarons, Ehrhart, Farahnak, & Hurlburt, 2015). The discussion is focused first on an overview of EBP models and research utilization, followed by leadership perspective on EBP.

■ MODELS OF EBP AND RESEARCH UTILIZATION

Models of EBP, research dissemination, and utilization started to emerge in the late 1970s.[1] The first models developed by Stetler and Marram (1976) and Funk, Champagne, Wiese, and Tornquist (1989) were important milestones historically because these started a "new era" in nursing by de-emphasizing rituals and traditions, as well as raising awareness about the importance of applying research findings in nursing practice.

Today, there are a few EBP models available both for individual practitioners and organizations. Most EBP models are process models and outline the steps of EBP or sequences conducting an EBP project (e.g., the Johns Hopkins Nursing Evidence-Based Practice Model, the Iowa Model of Evidence-Based Practice to Promote Quality Care, the Model of Evidence-Based Practice Change, and the ACE Star Model of Knowledge Translation) and some models are system-wide, organizational assessment models (e.g., the Advancing Research and Clinical Practice through Close Collaboration [ARCC]) (Melnyk, Fineout-Overholt, Giggleman, & Choy, 2017). The models represent, at least, four thematic areas: (a) EBP, research utilization, and knowledge transformation processes; (b) strategic/organizational change theory to promote uptake and adoption of new knowledge; and (c) knowledge exchange and synthesis for application and inquiry; and (d) designing and interpreting dissemination research (Mitchell, Fisher, Hastings, Silverman, & Wallen, 2010).

The models have been developed to help conceptualize multifaceted processes of evidence translation and move evidence into practice: it is anticipated that the use of a model leads to a systematic approach to EBP, guides the design and implementation of approaches strengthening evidence-based decision making, prevents incomplete implementation, promotes timely evaluation, and maximizes use of time and resources (Curtis et al., 2016; Gawlinski & Rutledge, 2008; Stevens & Ovretveit, 2013). Since their development, many of these models, including their interventions/strategies, have been examined, but empirical evidence on their sustainability and long-term outcomes demonstrating increased use of EBP is still often lacking and little is known about the long-term effects of the proposed strategies (Warren, Montgomery, & Friedman, 2016; see also Melnyk et al., 2017). Major changes have evolved in healthcare since the 1970s, including an explosion of synthesized evidence, national and international initiatives promoting adoption of EBP, enhanced interprofessional collaboration, widespread use of electronic databases, emergence of implementation science, pay for performance, and enhanced patient engagement. These changes have prompted a need for reevaluation and revision of the models (Iowa Model Collaborative, 2017; see also Melnyk et al., 2017). Review of every available model today and how these have been revised and tested is beyond the scope of this chapter. Instead, it is more pragmatic to focus on processes that help organizations choose models of EBP.

Because there are several EBP models available, the selection and adoption process of a model for an organization is an important decision. An example of this process utilizing a systematic approach has been described by Schaffer, Sandau, and Diedrick (2012), Newhouse and Johnson (2009), Gawlinski and Rutledge (2008), and Mohide and Coker (2005). The first step for selecting a model is to establish a structure or forum (e.g., use of an existing nursing research committee, formation of an EBP council, or appointment of a task force) in which discussions can occur about various EBP models, their advantages and disadvantages, and their applicability to organizational needs. The second step is to review and systematically evaluate a selection of the models. Gawlinski and Rutledge (2008) suggest focusing on (a) the history and development of the EBP model; (b) any revisions of the model over time; (c) overall concepts in the EBP model, process, and flow of the model; and (d) publications describing how the model has guided EBP changes in other facilities. Mohide and Coker (2005) emphasize that there seem to be, in fact, three important core criteria for evaluation: clarity and conciseness, comprehensiveness, and ease of use by direct care nurses. Along these lines, Newhouse and Johnson (2009) developed three criteria that were found particularly relevant in a Magnet hospital for the needs of nurses in practice to compare, contrast, and eventually select the model best fit for their organization. The criteria were the following: the model should (a) facilitate the work required for completing an EBP project, (b) have an educational component that helps nurses to critique and assess the strengths and quality of the evidence, (c) guide the process of implementing practice changes, and (d) potentially be implemented across specialty practice areas. Schaffer et al. (2012) have used these criteria for an evaluation of the four most common EBP models (i.e., Iowa Model, Johns Hopkins Nursing Evidence-Based Practice Model, ARCC, and ACE Start Model of Knowledge Transformation) which provides valuable information for model selection. The final selection of a model should be based on a consideration of (a) how easy the EBP model is to understand and how it facilitates EBP projects and process; (b) direction and guidelines for evidence critique, the process of implementing a practice change, or conducting research; (c) the flow of steps in the model and whether this is similar to the flow of practice algorithms; and (d) decision points in the EBP model regarding opportunities for thoughtful reflection, decision making, and adoption across practice areas (Gawlinski & Rutledge, 2008; Schaffer et al., 2012). Once the model is chosen, the third and last step is its implementation and use within an organization.

Several strategies can be used for system-wide implementation that guarantee sustainability of the model, including strong leadership support; enhancement of individual clinician and healthcare leader knowledge and skills through education; cultivation of a context and culture that supports and aligns with the model; and development of healthcare leaders who can spearhead teams that integrate the model in an exciting vision, mission, and strategic goal. Further strategies can include adding content about the EBP model in preceptor development programs, orientation, nursing grand rounds, and incorporating it in education with clear expectations linking EBP competencies to annual skills and competency forums, performance appraisals, and clinical ladder promotion processes (Gawlinski & Rutledge, 2008; see also Melnyk et al., 2014, 2016).

■ LEADERSHIP PERSPECTIVE ON EBP

Transformational leadership is an approach that has been shown to have an impact on both practice changes in nursing and on the development of an organizational culture that is more receptive to progression, change, quality, and safety (see, e.g., Cheater et al., 2005; Jennings, Disch, & Senn, 2008; Shaw, 2005). Transformational leadership is also a core component of the Magnet model (ANCC, 2014). By definition, a transformational leader is one who develops the potential of others and seeks a relationship that is mutually beneficial toward creating a vision and reaching higher levels of performance together.

The importance of interdependent collaboration formed by transformational leaders and transformational leadership style, as described through the seminal work of Burns's (1978) theory of leadership and, later, Bass and Riggio's (2006) work, is closely aligned to the five exemplary leadership practices described by Kouzes and Posner (2007) called "Model the Way," "Inspire a Shared Vision," "Challenge the Process," "Enable Others to Act," and "Encourage the Heart." Transformational leaders are at their best when they engage in practices, are able to model the way, challenge the process, encourage the heart, inspire a shared vision, and enable others to act (Clavelle, Drenkard, Tullai-McGuinness, & Fitzpartick, 2012; Herman, Gish, & Rosenblum, 2015).

Kouzes and Posner started their work in the early 1980s when they conducted a research project that examined what people did when they felt they were at their personal best when leading others (Kouzes & Posner, 2007). Their leadership model was described in the best-selling book *The Leadership Challenge* (4th ed.), which was grounded in extensive research and found to be applicable in the United States, Europe, Asia, Australia, and elsewhere around the world. Kouzes and Posner conducted interviews of leaders at all levels and collected written case studies from personal best leadership practices in both public and private organizations. When research was repeated 20 years after the model was developed, the concepts and principles of the model remained unchanged (Kouzes & Posner, 2002). Supported by hundreds of external research studies and utilized by academics (e.g., Waite & McKinney, 2015) and organizational leaders (e.g., Clavelle, Drenkard, Tullai-McGuinness, & Fitzpartick, 2012; Herman et al., 2015; Ross, Fitzpatrick, Click, Krouse, & Clavelle, 2014), the model has been analyzed, tested, critiqued, and applied with repeated success and validation (Kouzes & Posner, 2000–2011). The Leadership Practices Inventory (LPI), a tool that is used to measure the five practices of exemplary leadership, was developed through a triangulation of qualitative and quantitative research methods and studies (Kouzes & Posner, 2000). Both self-report and observer forms of the LPI have been established (Kouzes & Posner, 2007). Under the key practices, the authors have identified 10 commitments of leadership that should be followed to be successful in using the model (Table 13.1).

Relationship is a key word in understanding this model. In fact, two of the most powerful statements in *The Leadership Challenge* are the last sentences of the book: "Leadership is not an affair of the head. Leadership is an affair of the heart" (Kouzes & Posner, 2002, p. 351). Kouzes and Posner are not the only contemporaries who feel leadership is about the heart. Others, for example, Turkel (2014), speak of love and leadership. She has discussed a paradigm shift from transformational leadership to contemporary transformational leadership. Transformational leadership emphasizes aspects such as skilled communication, collaboration, effective decision making, outcomes measures, financial management in terms of productivity, and strategic planning. Contemporary transformational leadership, on the other hand, emphasizes authentic leadership styles, relational caring, meaningful recognition, creativity, building trust, relationships, participative decision making, dialogue with time for reflection, and innovation. Turkel has invited leaders: "to reflect on the future and what transformational leadership would look like when nurse leaders make decisions based on love, caring and values" (p. 173).

TABLE 13.1 Five Practices of Exemplary Leadership and 10 Commitments of Leadership

Practice	Commitments
Model the way	1. Clarify values by finding your voice and affirming shared ideals
	2. Set an example by aligning actions with shared values
Inspire a shared vision	3. Envision the future by imagining exciting and ennobling possibilities
	4. Enlist others in a common vision by appealing to shared aspirations
Challenge the process	5. Search for opportunities by seizing the initiative and by looking outward for innovative ways to improve
	6. Experiment and take risks by constantly generating small wins and learning from experience
Enable others to act	7. Foster collaboration by building trust and facilitating relationships
	8. Strengthen others by increasing self-determination and developing competence
Encourage the heart	9. Recognize contributions by showing appreciation for individual excellence
	10. Celebrate the values and victories by creating a spirit of community

Source: Adapted from Kouzes, J. M., & Posner, B. Z. (2007). *The leadership challenge* (6th ed.). San Francisco, CA: Jossey–Bass.

■ ORGANIZATIONAL CHANGE THEORIES

Change theory or planned approaches to implement organizational shifts are often used in successful change initiatives (Shirey, 2013). There are at least five theories (e.g., Kurt Lewin's theory; Everett Rogers's Diffusion Theory; Chris Argyris and Donald Schon's Organizational Learning Theory; Edgar Schein's Theory of Organizational Culture; Andrew Pettigrew, Evan Ferlie, and Lorna Makee's Receptive Context Change Theory) describing organizational change, organizational dynamics and processes, and assumptions related to strategies and approaches to facilitate and manage change (Batras, Duff, & Smith, 2014). Many of these help to better understand the change process, define the leader's role, and why change participants are so often resistant to change.

An early and pioneering theory of change developed by Lewin in the late 1990s is widely used and also considered by scholars a valuable and much-needed approach to manage change (Burnes & Cooke, 2013). Lewin's theory describes change as a three-stage process. The first stage he called "unfreezing." It involves getting ready for change and it may begin, for example, with nurse leaders conducting a gap analysis illustrating discrepancies between the desired and current state/status quo. This stage involves selection of a solution/strategy and preparation for moving away from a current reality. It also requires identifying the factors for and against change. Successful change necessitates strengthening the driving forces and/or weakening the restraining forces. At this juncture, leaders need to bypass defense mechanisms to effectively manage resistance. In the second stage, "moving or transitioning," change or movement occurs. This necessitates creating a detailed plan of action and engaging people to try out the proposed change. The stage can be difficult because of the uncertainty and fear associated with change. The transition includes coaching to overcome fears and clear communication to avoid losing sight of the desired target. Leader's actions can facilitate movement at this stage, which may include persuading employees to agree that the status quo is not beneficial to them and encouraging them to view the problem from a new and improved reality. The third and final stage, called "refreezing," focuses on stabilizing the change so that it becomes embedded into existing systems, such as culture, policies, and practices. In refreezing the change, nurse leaders need to consider the driving forces facilitating change and counteract the restraining forces getting in the way of change. The dynamics of refreezing the new change produces a new equilibrium, which is sustained and recognized as the new norm or higher level of performance expectation (Batras et al., 2014; Shirey, 2013).

While Lewin's theory of planned change has strengths, it has certain limitations as well. The theory assists in avoiding the common pitfalls that thwart change initiative success and offers a framework to guide a sustainable change. The concepts also provide for a better understanding of how to design detailed action plans for change from the top down; the theory is versatile, practical, simple to use, and easy to understand. Lewin's theory represents one of the oldest, but still pertinent, change management models; there is much experience and literature available with this framework (Burnes & Cooke 2013; Shirey, 2013; see, e.g., Manchester, Gray-Miceli, & Metcalf, 2014). Some criticism focuses on suggesting that today's healthcare systems are complex, nonlinear, and dynamic; thus, change happens more quickly than Lewin's theory accommodates and it is often not possible to frame a practice from unfreezing, moving, and refreezing perspectives. Other critiques have claimed the theory for being too simplistic, driven from the top down and quaintly linear, and framed from a static perspective (Burnes & Cooke 2013; Shirey, 2013). Lewin's theory of planned change is one of many organizational change theories, and thus it is useful to consider various theories/models and how they resonate with the values and beliefs of the organization before choosing one.

■ INFRASTRUCTURE SUPPORTING EBP AND RESEARCH

An infrastructure supporting EBP and research is becoming increasingly important in hospital organizations for at least three reasons: (a) generation of new knowledge is a requirement for Magnet recognition and redesignation and thus hospitals taking this journey need a research and EBP infrastructure to infuse research and EBP into clinical practice; (b) research is increasingly conducted in hospital-based nursing research programs stimulated, in part, by requirements of Magnet designation; and (c) in the past, research has been conducted by academic, university-affiliated nursing faculty, but today staff at hospital organizations have the skills, knowledge, and education to conduct research as principal investigators (Johantgen et al., 2017; Kelly et al., 2013; McLaughlin, et al., 2013; Parkosewich, 2013).

Research and EBP infrastructures and use of resources can vary considerably in hospital organizations (Johantgen et al., 2017; Kelly et al., 2013; McLaughlin et al., 2013). A national survey, conducted in 2010, provides interesting and important bench-mark information regarding the hospital-based research programs. This extensive study examined nursing research program requirements, scholarly outcomes, and facilitators and hindrances associated with the conduct of RN-led research in Magnet and non-Magnet hospitals (Kelly et al., 2013; McLaughlin et al., 2013). Various structures supported nurse-led research, such as mentoring, training, and research proposal peer-review/approval. On average, an annual total of four research studies were initiated, four disseminated via podium or poster, one published, and two funded research studies (McLaughlin et al., 2013). The findings also describe facilitators and hindrances in 24 areas which reflected/mirrored each other. The presence of mentors was ranked highest in both Magnet and non-Magnet organizations as a facilitator or hindrance, respectively. Institutional leadership support for research was ranked the second highest facilitator or hindrance.

Nurses at the bedside are perfectly positioned to ask clinically relevant questions, and they can play an integral role in generation and dissemination of new knowledge through working with mentors, nurse leaders, and partners in academia. However, today nurses are often weighted down with a variety of competing priorities, and thus finding time and resources can becomes challenging (e.g., Hatfield et al., 2016) without a supporting infrastructure. A recent study illuminates the current infrastructure supporting nursing research in Magnet hospitals (n = 418, 59.6 % response rate) focusing on six domains: nursing research council, research department, research financial support, research internship/fellowship programs, research mentoring, and outcome metrics (Johantgen et al., 2017). More than half (74%) of the organizations had nursing research councils and a third had a research department; 58% reported that the hospital specified an annual budget for nursing research and personnel (e.g., research coordinator). More than a third had a formal research internship or fellowship program. The majority of the hospitals (96%) had research mentors available who were from a variety of sources and measured outcomes (e.g., publications, presentations). Differences were found, however, between teaching and nonteaching hospitals (e.g., interdisciplinary research council; mentoring infrastructure; budget; staff and budgeted positions for a research coordinator, administrative assistant, and statistician). Supporting clinical nurses' time away from the bedside was a challenge: nearly half (44%) reported that research was conducted within nurses' clinical hours or "own time" (40%) by necessity, often secondary to patient care priorities. It is reasonable to conclude that more targeted resources (i.e., time) are needed to fully integrate research into clinical practice.

A few challenges for involving clinical nurses in research have been reported, and thus information regarding the best practices to engage nurses in research is highly valuable (Scala, Price, & Day, 2016). Scala and colleagues identified from the literature the following five major themes: (a) access to infrastructure, (b) executive leadership support, (c) strategic priorities and relative interests, (d) educational tactics, and

(e) leveraging established networks and resources. More specifically, access to an established infrastructure supports and encourages nurses to pursue advanced education, connecting research with ongoing EBP and QI initiatives, offering mentorship and coaching, and making goals part of job descriptions and advancement. An infrastructure provides resources, support, and services such as a research office or institute (a central location for research); a nursing research council; onsite libraries; online access to articles; available biostatistician; support with data management; and access to grant funding. Executive leadership support contributes to the sustainability of a nursing research center and provides financial support to conduct research (e.g., fellowship budget, small grants, speaker honoraria, textbooks, and supplies). Strategic priorities and relevant interests implies the importance to be connected with greater organizational research activities, while relating research topics to patient care ensures that clinical staff feel empowered, enthusiastic, and stay invested in the study. Educational tactics refer to the necessity to provide clinical nurses with exposure to experiential learning with hands-on activities, tutorials, mentors, and workshops. Established educational programs, such as the clinical scholars' model, nursing research advancing practice program, or hosting a nursing research internship or fellowship, have been shown to be successful in clinical settings. Leveraging established networks and resources implies partnering and tapping into already established resources locally, in academia, and with established community groups such as professional associations' research networks and other hospital systems. Hospital organizations need to perform their own assessments to determine the potential best practices that promote clinical nurses' engagement in research; and nursing leadership can use these areas to structure a multifaceted approach and strategies to support these practices.

■ READINESS FOR CHANGE

Although a great emphasis has been placed on EBP implementation, organizations and individuals within the organizations need to systematically assess how ready their institution and its culture are for EBP; without a culture that fully supports EBP, evidence-based care is not likely to be sustained. *Environmental readiness* refers to the ability of the healthcare environment to respond to change and implement processes that can improve care. In other words, organizational readiness is a stage of psychological and behavioral preparedness for change. This requires having necessary knowledge, skills, resources, and support (Weiner, 2009). Organizational readiness for change refers often to organizational members' shared determination to implement change (i.e., change commitment) and shared belief in their collective capacity to do so (i.e., change efficacy). The readiness for change can vary depending on, for example, how much its members value the change, and it also entails collective behavior change/changes in the form of systems redesign (i.e., multiple, simultaneous changes in work flows, staffing, decision making, communication, and reward systems) (Weiner, 2009).

Organizational readiness is a critical precursor to successful implementation of (complex) changes in practice and sustaining change as a part of the culture. It has been speculated in the literature (J. R. Smith & Donze, 2010) that 50% of efforts for organizational change fail because organizational leaders have not established sufficient readiness for change. It is thus possible to argue that the best time to assess organizational readiness for change is before its implementation; therefore, the organizational leaders' roles are crucial. The role of a nurse leader has been clearly articulated in the literature. According to Gallagher-Ford (2014a, 2014b; see also Kim et al., 2017), nurse leaders, at all levels of an organization, are in significant and important positions in the success of EBP because they allocate the human and material resources that provide the context for the work environment and shape the culture for resource use. They can create a culture where EBP is valued and expected, where dialogue between administration and staff is prevalent, and opportunities for interprofessional collaboration are encouraged. Additionally, promotion and support of the development of practitioners' EBP knowledge and skills, the availability of resources, including access to EBP mentors, and adequate staffing and time to review and implement evidence and measure and evaluate outcomes are critical.

One of the most important steps and the first step from an organizational perspective is to assess the organizational context and readiness for EBP. This allows, for example, leaders to plan, pave the path for the right direction to promote adoption, and avoid or mitigate difficulties of implementation of EBP, which are also referred to as "change implementation failure" (Kaplan, Zeller, Damitio, Culbert, & Bayley, 2014). French et al. (2009) conducted a review of the literature and instruments in an attempt to answer the question "What can management theories offer to EBP?" The authors conducted a structured search in healthcare and management databases and focused on four domains: research utilization, research activity, knowledge management, and organizational learning. As a result, 30 measurement tools were identified and appraised. Eighteen instruments from the four domains were selected for a closer analysis. The instruments measured three organizational attributes (i.e., vision, leadership, and a learning culture) and four different types of knowledge stages (i.e., need, acquisition of new knowledge, knowledge sharing, and knowledge use). The authors concluded that these concepts measure the absorptive and receptive capacity of organizations. Weiner, Amick, and Lee (2008) have also conducted an extensive review of the literature in health services research focusing on the conceptualization and measurement of organizational readiness for change. The authors found 106 peer-reviewed articles and 43 instruments measuring the concept. The review revealed, among other things, that there were different perspectives to operationalize the concept and limited evidence of reliability and validity for many instruments.

Newhouse (2010) has presented an overview of the instruments to assess organizations' readiness for EBP in nursing. An interesting observation is that the Promoting Action on Research Implementation in Health Services (PARIHS) framework and its major concepts of evidence, facilitation, and context have been used as a foundation for three instruments: the Context Assessment Instrument (CAI), Alberta Context Tool (ACT), and Organizational Readiness to Change Assessment (ORCA). Each instrument measures the readiness of the work context for EBP specifically. The CAI contains 37 items and it measures five domains: collaborative practice, evidence-informed practice, respect for persons, practice boundaries, and evaluation

(McCormack, McCarthy, Wright, Slater, & Coffey, 2009). The second instrument, ACT, is composed of 56 items and the core dimensions include leadership, culture, evaluation, social capital, structural and electronic resources, formal and informal interactions, and organizational slack (Estabrooks, Squires, Cummings, Birdsell, & Norton, 2009; see also Squires et al., 2015). The third instrument, ORCA, contains 77 items and these measure three domains: evidence (i.e., research, clinical experience, and patient preference), context (i.e., leadership culture, staff culture, leadership behavior, measurement/leadership feedback, opinion leaders, and general resources), and facilitation (i.e., leadership practices, clinical champions, leadership implementation roles, implementation team roles, implementation plan, project communication, project progress tracking, project resources and context, and project evaluation) (Helfrich, Li, Sharp, & Sales, 2009). The ARCC is another model that is a foundation for an instrument assessing organizational culture and readiness for EBP implementation. The ARCC was first conceptualized as a mentorship framework to assist advanced practice nurses in implementing EBP. After further development, the model is intended to serve as a guide to advance system-wide implementation and sustainability of EBP. The first step in the ARCC model is an organizational assessment of the culture and readiness for EBP using the Organizational Culture Readiness for System-wide Integration of Evidence-Based Practice (OCRSIEP) scale so that EBP facilitators and barriers can be identified together with a plan to overcome them (Melnyk & Fineout-Overholt, 2002). The OCRSIEP has 25 items measured on a five-point Likert-type scale and it provides information about the organizational culture and readiness for EBP for system-wide integration of EBP (Fineout-Overholt & Melnyk, 2006; Melnyk, & Fineout-Overholt, 2015; Wallen et al., 2010).

■ NURSING READINESS FOR EBP

A call for greater clinical effectiveness (outcomes) started to require healthcare professionals to enhance their knowledge and skills by incorporating EBP into decision making and practice in the early 2000s (Mick, 2017). Also, at that time, the growing demands for quality and safety, as exerted by Joint Commission International and Magnet hospitals also further promoted EBP. In 2001, the IOM's quality chasm series suggested EBP as one of the core competencies for professional healthcare curricula; EBP was included in nursing curricula in 2003 (Mick, 2017; Ubbink et al., 2013).

Almost 20 years after its introduction, the EBP paradigm has been embraced by healthcare professionals including nurses, as an important means to improve quality of patient care, improve outcomes, and lower costs (Melnyk et al., 2016; Ubbink et al., 2013). Regardless of these benefits of EBP, its implementation has been increasing slowly. Pravikoff, Tanner, and Pierce (2005) surveyed 1,097 RNs across the United States to determine perceptions regarding nurses' readiness for EBP and their access to EBP resources. The conclusion at that time was that nurses were not yet ready to implement EBP mostly because of the perceived "lack of value to patient care." Nurses' daily information needs were substantial; given the demand for rapid decision making, nurses turned to a variety of sources: social interactions, peers and colleagues, practice experience, documents, and intrinsic knowledge (e.g., knowledge from school). Gaps in information literacy and computer skills, lack of access to resources, perceived lack of time and tools were considered major barriers. Almost 10 years later, Melnyk et al. (2012) conducted another survey to assess the state of perceptions of EBP among a random sample of 1,015 nurses in the United States. The results reported, among other things, that over half (53.6%) of the respondents agreed or strongly agreed that EBP was consistently implemented in their organization, but only 35% agreed or strongly agreed that their colleagues consistently implemented EBP. Almost half (46.4%) agreed or strongly agreed that findings from research studies were routinely implemented to improve patient outcomes in their institutions. However, 76% agreed or strongly agreed that it was important for them to get more education and skills building in EBP. In 2012, the conclusions were that nurses were "ready for" and value EBP, but all the earlier reported barriers to implement EBP persisted including lack of time, knowledge, mentors, colleagues (e.g., physician, fellow nurses, nurse leaders, and managers), and organizational support.

The results from two major national surveys described earlier (Melnyk et al., 2012; Pravikoff et al., 2005) measuring readiness for EBP mirror findings from many other studies (e.g., Stavor, Zedreck-Gonzaletz, & Hoffmann, 2017, Warren, McLaughlin, et al., 2016; M. Wilson et al., 2015; Yoder et al., 2014) reporting that nurses favor EBP yet struggle with similar barriers for implementation. A review of international literature in a sample of healthcare professionals from 17 countries, conducted by Ubbink et al. (2013), reported that those same types of barriers exist worldwide. According to findings of this systematic review, the general attitudes toward EBP are positive/welcoming, but only half of the clinical practices (MDs: median 52.6%, RNs: 44.9%) were considered evidence based; the majority (MDs/RNs: median 64%) considered that their EBP knowledge was insufficient; the most appropriate way to move forward EBP was thought to be evidence-based guidelines (median 68%; evidence summaries: median 39%) or critical appraisals (36%). However, clinical decision making was based on consulting textbooks and colleagues rather than by searching electronic databases. Several individual and organizational barriers, but also many facilitators for EBP implementation were summarized from the literature. The organizational barriers included lack of human and material resources and leadership support. The major reported facilitators to increase EBP were dedicated time to learn and practice EBP, leadership support, promotion and integration of EBP by all disciplines, communication and role modeling, and easily accessible sources of evidence such as guidelines and protocols. Additionally, characteristics of the leader, organization, and culture were considered vital and equally important for EBP implementation (Ubbink et al., 2013).

Nurse leaders' support is critical for the point-of-care staff to implement EBP. Little is still known today about leadership support to facilitate EBP, but it is possible to assume that their beliefs, level of implementation, and perceptions of a hospital's EBP organizational culture affect the provided support. In 2016, Melnyk and colleagues conducted a nationwide study ($N = 5,100$; 8% responded) throughout the United States exploring nurse leaders' (i.e., chief nursing officers [CNO] and chief nursing executives [CNE]) EBP beliefs, perceptions of their hospital's EBP organizational culture, level of implementation and hospital's performance metrics, how they prioritize EBP and the extent of investment in EBP. The CNOs' and CNEs' beliefs about the value of EBP were high, but implementation of EBP in the practice was relatively low. More than 50% believed that EBP is practiced "somewhat" or "not at all" in their organizations. Organizational culture and organizational readiness for EBP were moderately low as well; and slightly over half (52%) responded that within 6 months there had been "somewhat" or "not at all" progress toward EBP culture. More than one third of the hospitals were not meeting the National Database of Nursing Quality Indicators (NDNQI) performance metrics; and almost one third were above the national core measures benchmarks, such as falls and pressure ulcers. Although the respondents believed that EBP results in high-quality care, this was ranked as a low priority with little budget allocation. Only 3% of the respondents considered EBP as a priority. Over half of the respondents (72%) invested only 0% to 10% of the annual operating budget on building and sustaining EBP in their organizations.

Although healthcare professionals, including nurses and nurse leaders, hold positive attitudes toward EBP and the uptake of EBP is progressing, important barriers are still obstructing the full implementation of EBP in practice and causing a disconnect between the beliefs and actual bedside implementation (Ubbink et al., 2013). The use and self-reported implementation of EBP in clinical settings have slightly improved in nursing over the years (Duffy et al., 2015; Warren, Montgomery, & Friedman, 2016; Ubbink et al., 2013), but the progress has been slow regardless of substantial investment in resources (Yoder et al., 2014) and the use of multiple strategies targeted on individual, organizational, and leadership barriers to advance practice based on evidence (Warren, Montgomery, & Friedman, 2016; Melnyk et al., 2012; Yoder et al., 2014). There can be multiple reasons for this slow, low, but sustained progress, and thus it has been speculated that there is a need to revisit the current EBP expectations (Warren, Montgomery, & Friedman, 2016), or that perhaps the most frequently reported barriers are not the main reasons for poor implementation of EBP, but rather, it is a mindset of healthcare providers to perceive these as barriers (Ubbink et al., 2013).

■ STRATEGIES TO PROMOTE AND INCREASE EBP READINESS

Although nurses believe in the value of EBP, they do not routinely demonstrate it, and it is believed that the barriers to the use of EBP are a key factor in its low use. An approach that has been often used to promote and increase EBP implementation has emphasized identification of the barriers and tailoring strategies to address and/or overcome these (e.g., Kajermo et al., 2010; Kaplan et al., 2014; Melnyk et al., 2012; see also Upton, Upton, & Scurlock-Evans, 2014) as well as targeting resources and using intervention to promote and/or improve the known facilitators (EBP mentors, access to library services, supportive EBP context, etc.). Identification of different types of barriers has also served as an assessment of the educational needs, values, implementation, and knowledge of EBP in an attempt to develop and sustain an EBP culture. A number of tools, as shown in Table 13.2, have been developed and tested over two decades to assess and measure such concepts as EBP beliefs, attitudes, knowledge, barriers, and factors influencing EBP uptake and implementation and values. Table 13.2 is not comprehensive, but rather a selection from the literature.

TABLE 13.2 Examples of EBP Instruments Since 1991 to 2016

Year	Instrument	Subscales/Area of Interest	Author
1991	BARRIERS Scale	Characteristics: an adopter (nurse's research values, skills, and awareness), organization, innovation and organization	Funk, Champagne, Wiese, and Tornquist
1999	Perception of nurses attitude and knowledge skills	Level of knowledge of clinical effectiveness and EBP; attitudes toward EBP and clinical effectiveness; application of EBP; barriers and solutions	Upton
2003	KAP survey	(1) Identifying clinical problems, (2) establishing current best practice, (3) implementing research into practice, (4) administering research implementation, and (5) conducting	Eller, Kleber, and Wang
2004	Assessment of EBP knowledge	Beliefs and attitudes toward EBP; access to and use of evidence; understanding of terms associated with EBP; moving from opinion to evidence; barriers and facilitators to EBP	O'Donnell
2005	Readiness for nurses using EBP	Information need and information seeking; resource availability and use; barriers to EBP	Pravikoff, Tanner, and Pierce
2007	DEBP	Bases of practice knowledge; barriers to finding and reviewing evidence; barriers to changing practice on the basis of evidence; facilitation and support in changing practice; self-assessment of skills	Gerrish et al.
2008	EBP beliefs scale and EBP implementation scale	EBP beliefs: beliefs about the value of EBP and the ability to implement it; EBP implementation: extent to which EBP is implemented	Melnyk, Fineout-Overholt, and Mays
2008	Nurses' understanding and interpretation of EBP	Types of evidence influencing practice; sources of evidence; application of evidence; reasons for adopting EBP	Rolfe, Segrott, and Jordan
2009	Attitude and knowledge about EBP	Self-rated ability on conducting a search, searching electronic databases and critical appraisal	Waters, Rychetnik, and Barratt

(*continued*)

TABLE 13.2 Examples of EBP Instruments Since 1991 to 2016 (*continued*)

Year	Instrument	Subscales/Area of Interest	Author
2009	EBPSE scale	EBP self-efficacy (17 items; 1% to 100% response scale)	Tucker, Olson, and Frusti
2013	EBP-COQ	EBP: attitude, knowledge, and skills	Ruzafa-Martinez, Lopez-Iborra, Moreno-Casbas, and Madrigal-Torres
2011	EPIC scale	Belief in ability to implement EBP, known as EBP self-efficacy	Salbach and Jaglal
2014	EBP nursing leadership scale and EBP work environment scale	EBP Nursing Leadership Scale: staff nurses' perception of support provided by the nurse manager for EBP; EBP Work Environment Scale: organizational support for EBP	Pryse, McDaniel, and Schafer
2016	Quick-EBP-VIK	EBP—value (V), implementation (I), and knowledge (K)	Paul, Connor, McCabe, and Ziniel

DEBP, developing evidence-based practice; EBP, evidence-based practice; EBP-COQ, evidence-based practice evaluation competencies questionnaire; EBPSE, evidence-based practice self-efficacy; EPIC, evidence-based practice confidence; KAP, knowledge, attitudes, and practices.

Today, the literature is rich in describing a variety of strategies and interventions that have been tailored to improve and promote EBP implementation and addressing different individual (knowledge, skills, etc.) and/or organizational (leadership support, culture, inter- and intraprofessional collaboration, etc.) barriers (Table 13.3).

TABLE 13.3 EBP Interventions

EBP Intervention	Author(s)
Academic and hospital system partnerships	Centrella-Nigro et al. (2015); Rickbeil and Simones (2012); Whitmer, Auer, Beerman, and Weishaupt (2011)
Clinical nurse specialist support	Davidson and Brown (2014); Levin, Fineout-Overholt, Melnyk, Barnes, and Vetter (2011); Muller, McCauley, Harrington, Jablonski, and Strauss (2011); Wintersgill and Wheeler (2012)
Fellowships	Kim et al. (2017); Warren, McLaughlin, et al. (2016)
Formal classes and webinars	Balakas, Sparks, Steurer, and Bryant (2013); Black, Balneaves, Garossino, Puyat, and Qian (2015); Brown, Johnson, and Appling (2011); Kinney, Lima, McKeever, Twomey, and Newall (2012); Levin et al. (2011); Phillips et al. (2014); Ramos-Morcillo, Fernández-Salazar, Ruzafa-Martínez, & Del-Pino-Casado (2015); Rutledge and Skelton (2011); Whitmer et al. (2011); Wintersgill and Wheeler (2012); Yackel, Short, Lewis, Breckenridge-Sproat, and Turner (2013)

(*continued*)

TABLE 13.3 EBP Interventions (*continued*)

EBP Intervention	Author(s)
Grand rounds	Underhill, Roper, Diefert, Boucher, and Berry (2015)
Incorporation of EBP into a clinical advancement program	Whitmer et al. (2011)
Incorporation of EBP into job descriptions, annual competencies, performance appraisals, and nursing orientation	Burke, Johnson, and Bernsteiner (2017); Fisher, Cusack, Cox, Feigenbaum, and Wallen (2016); Melnyk et al. (2014); Whitmer et al. (2011)
Independent self-study	Pierson and Schuelke (2009)
Journal clubs	Kinney et al. (2012); Whitmer et al. (2011)
Librarian involvement	Crabtree, Brennan, Davis, and Coyle (2016); League et al. (2012); Wintersgill and Wheeler (2012)
Mentor	Magers (2014); Patterson, Mason, and Duncan (2017)
Online learning	Moore (2017); Ramos-Morcillo et al. (2015)
Online resources	League et al. (2012); Muller et al. (2011); Whitmer et al. (2011); Wintersgill and Wheeler (2012)
Selection of an EBP model	Brown et al. (2011); Levin et al. (2011); Whitmer et al. (2011)
Senior leader support	Muller et al. (2011); Whitmer et al. (2011); Wintersgill and Wheeler (2012)
Shared governance and clinical nurse council involvement	Brody, Barnes, Ruble, and Sakowski (2012); Brown et al. (2011); Kinney et al. (2012); Muller et al. (2011); Whitmer et al. (2011); Wintersgill and Wheeler (2012)

EBP, evidence-based practice.

EDUCATION

Educational intervention (e.g., EBP classes, online courses, webinars) is one of the most common strategies that have been offered to practicing nurses, and also to nursing leadership (i.e., frontline, middle, and senior leadership), in hospital organizations to increase their EBP knowledge and skills, or overcome the knowledge deficit they may have to successful implementation of EBP due to the lack of their educational preparation (e.g., Kaplan et al., 2014; Kim et al., 2017; Moore, 2017). Undergraduate nursing curriculum started to include EBP education in the early 2000s, and many organizations are including EBP education in their nurse residency programs, but nurses who have graduated prior to the major shift in professional education over the past 20 years may lack this educational preparation. A challenge that hospitals encounter today is the varying levels of education and clinical experience (Connor, Paul, McCabe, & Ziniel, 2017) and thus a collective group of nurses and nurse leaders who may lack the knowledge and skills needed to implement and maintain a culture of EBP due to the deficiency of their educational preparations (Melnyk et al., 2012; see also Aglen, 2016, Chappell, 2014).

Knowledge and skill deficits have very often been considered barriers to EBP implementation. Much of today's literature focuses on different education methods or a combination of methods to overcome those barriers (see, e.g., Moore, 2017). The evidence from many studies has shown, however, that the educational strategies have varied, as has the length of the implementation period and the measurement instruments (Phillips et al., 2014), so that the measured outcomes (e.g., EBP implementation) may have often remained smaller than expected (e.g., Kim et al., 2017). Despite continued research efforts, and investment of time and resources in EBP education, it has not been possible to determine, due to the quality of the reported evidence, the best and most efficient type and dose of educational interventions (Phillips et al., 2014; see also Kajermo et al., 2010).

MENTORS

Availability of EBP mentors, or a lack of mentors, has been identified as one of the key facilitators, or a critical barrier, to the EBP implementation (e.g., Day, Lindauer, Parks, & Scala, 2017; Melnyk et al., 2012; Kelly, et al., 2013). The EBP mentor's role is clearly described in the literature: it can start from identification and formulating a PICOT (**P**opulation/Patient Problem: *Who is your patient?* **I**ntervention: *What do you plan to do for the patient?* **C**omparison: *What is the alternative to your plan?* **O**utcome: *What outcome do you seek?* **T**ime: *What is the time frame?*) question with staff through dissemination and sustainment of practice by moving a project through higher levels of organizational committees while minimizing or navigating any potential barriers. An EBP mentor's role also includes team building, maintaining a level of engagement, setting a clear vision, communications promoting "buy-in," and empowering support (Magers, 2014; Patterson et al., 2017). Some evidence is available today showing that a structured mentor program could be effective in improving EBP knowledge, attitudes, skills, and confidence levels and organizational readiness in nurses (Spiva et al., 2017); but it has also been reported that mentorship does not necessarily increase engagement in EBP behaviors (Yost et al., 2015). However, the EBP mentor's role to build an organizational culture of EBP and implement evidence-based care has been confirmed in one study (Melnyk et al., 2017).

COMPETENCIES

In 2013, the IOM identified in the *Health Professions Education: A Bridge to Quality* report five core competencies that all healthcare professionals should learn: EBP, informatics, patient-centered care, QI, and teamwork and collaboration. The Quality and Safety Education for Nurses (QSEN) project was developed as a response to this report to identify additional nursing competencies. The QSEN competencies have been adopted in undergraduate and graduate curricula at schools of nursing nationwide in the United States and their integration into practice settings is increasing. The progression of EBP competencies have been described within a clinical advancement program with an assumption that clearly defined role expectations and enhance accountability, elevate and promote nursing practice, improve outcomes and quality care, and enhance position descriptions, performance evaluation, clinical recognition, and orientation and residency programs (Burke et al., 2017). Some evidence is available showing that development and integration of EBP competencies could facilitate implementation and sustainability of quality EBP care and culture (Fisher et al., 2016; Melnyk et al., 2014).

■ NURSING LEADERSHIP SUPPORT AND EBP

Making EBP an organization-wide reality is a challenging goal. Leadership has been recognized as an essential element in that process and literature supports that leaders have a critical role in implementation of EBP and promotion of innovations in healthcare settings (IOM, 2011). The role of "first-level leaders" (those supervising individuals providing direct services) is vital not just for organizational effectiveness but also for facilitating day-to-day EBP implementation (Aarons et al., 2015). However, little is known about the exact functions and role of first and various other levels of leadership in the successful institutionalization of EBP within an organization. Only a few studies have focused on leadership-related EBP behaviors and a few have focused on project-related EBP activity (e.g., use of guidelines) (Gifford et al., 2013; Morgeson, DeRue, & Karam, 2010). What is known, however, is that often first-level leaders may have been promoted based on clinical expertise with little support or training in effective leadership efforts such as EBP implementation (see also, e.g., Aarons et al., 2015; Warren, McLaughlin, et al., 2016). Leadership alone, however, is unlikely to be effective for EBP implementation without attention to organizational context for change; the characteristics of leaders and organization are both important for promotion of EBP use (Sandstrom, Borglin, Nilsson, & Willman, 2011).

"Leadership supporting EBP" has often been mentioned in the literature, but often leadership behaviors demonstrating support have not been specifically defined or explained. Stetler et al. (2014) have presented a conceptual framework of EBP leadership in an attempt to uncover what actions leaders at different levels and roles need to take to develop, enhance, and sustain EBP as a norm in an organization. The presented framework is composed of unique types of leadership themes and related behaviors that interact synergistically to form a pattern of overall EBP support. It is composed of three levels: functional, strategic, and cross-cutting behaviors. "Strategic leadership behaviors" are related to planning, organizing, and aligning, which demonstrate vision-focused and systems-oriented thinking. "Functional leadership behaviors" make the vision of "EBP as the norm" come alive. Six types of functional leadership behavior were described: (a) *inspiring* and including, (b) *intervening* actively and involving one's self in EBP, (c) *educating* and developing, (d) *role modeling*, (e) *monitoring*/providing feedback or seeking insights, and (f) *implementing* specific EBP projects. "Cross-cutting leadership behaviors" are composed of strategic thinking, communicating and building, and sustaining an EBP supportive culture (Figure 13.1).

The framework suggests that EBP supportive leadership is ongoing, strategic, vision-focused, and involves deliberative thinking and day-to-day behaviors that role model, reinforce, and live EBP. Although the framework needs further testing, it outlines and reinforces the dynamic nature of EBP supportive leader behaviors and

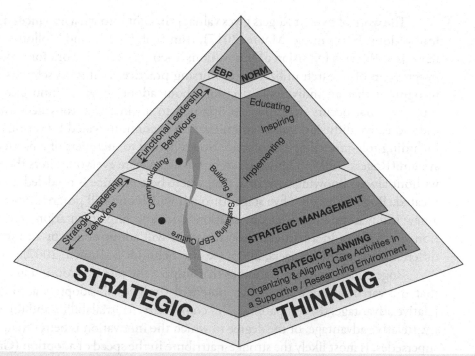

FIGURE 13.1 L-EBP, leadership behaviors supportive of EBP institutionalization.

EBP, evidence-based practice; L-EBP, leadership for evidence-based practice.

Source: Stetler, C., Ritchie, J., Rycroft-Malone, J., & Charns, M. (2014). Leadership for evidence-based practice: Strategic and functional behaviors for institutionalizing EBP. *Worldviews on Evidence-Based Nursing, 11*(4), 219–226.

illustrates the need for leaders to strategically and routinely use a range of integrated and transparent behaviors to achieve and sustain EBP as the norm.

■ DIFFUSION OF INNOVATIONS

New knowledge is coming into the profession on a daily basis but it is well known that tremendously long lag times continue to exist between the generation of research findings and their implementation and adoption in real-world clinical settings to improve care and outcomes (Melnyk et al., 2012, 2014). It has been speculated in the literature that, on average, it may take 17 years to move from research trials to clinical practice, which may or may not be true (Morris, Wooding, & Grant, 2011). The reality is, however, an "average" time lag of 17 years hides complexities that are relevant to policy and safety practice, and that time lag can vary depending on, for example, an innovation, results of a trial (4–5 years: positive results vs. 6–8 years: negative results), approvals for a new drug/device, safety testing, guideline preparation, and so forth (Hopewell, Clarke, Stewart, & Tierney, 2007; Morris et al., 2011).

The work of Everett Rogers gives valuable insight into what enhances diffusion of innovations. For example, Moore (2017), Kim et al. (2013), and Mollon et al. (2012) have used Rogers's Diffusion of Innovations Theory as a framework for explaining the progression of research utilization in nursing practice. Diffusion scholars have long recognized that an individual's decision about adoption of an innovation requires a process that occurs over time, as opposed to an instantaneous decision. During the successive diffusion stages, an innovation is communicated by various channels, including role-modeling best practice over a period to members of a particular social system (Rogers, 2003). Diffusion can be passive, where everyone alters their behavior without always knowing why, or active, where best practice is modeled and communicated. Rogers identifies five stages through which one will progress when adopting a new innovation: knowledge, persuasion, decision, implementation, and confirmation. Individuals in a particular social system will adopt or accept an innovation at different time points (Rogers, 2003; see also Schmidt & Brown, 2007).

Rogers has identified attributes that impact the rate of adoption and postulates that the variances are evaluated by potential (individual) adopters according to (a) relative advantage, (b) compatibility, (c) complexity, (d) trialability, and (e) observability. Relative advantage, or the degree to which the innovation is better than the idea it supersedes, is most likely the strongest attribute in the speed of adoption (Greenhalgh, Robert, Macfarlane, Bate, & Kyriakidou, 2004; Rogers, 2003). However, that may not be enough to adopt a new best practice if it is more costly or time-consuming. Compatibility is the degree to which an innovation is perceived as consistent with existing values, past experiences, and needs of potential adopters (Greenhalgh et al. 2004; Rogers, 2003). Complexity is another attribute. If an innovation is seen as difficult to understand or implement, it will be set aside by busy clinical practitioners who already have too many demands on their time. Trialability, the fourth attribute, offers the opportunity to experiment with an innovation on a limited basis to see its advantages and see how it fits into the context of the organization. Observability provides the opportunity for others to see the application of the innovation before they devote time and resources to adopting the innovation. Depending on the rate of adoption (i.e., relative speed/time at which participants adopt an innovation), Rogers has suggested a total of five categories of adopters: innovators, early adopters, early majority, late majority, and laggards. Diffusion scholars have also identified, among other things, the following as important elements of diffusion: (a) characteristics of organizations (e.g., tension for change, innovation-system fit, assessment of implications); (b) outer context (e.g., incentives and mandates, interorganizational norm setting, and networks), and (c) social systems (e.g., opinion leaders) (Greenhalgh et al., 2004). As described and discussed earlier, there are a few aspects and determinants that have an impact on the diffusion, dissemination, and implementation of innovations and should be carefully considered and addressed to facilitate and sustain these in practice.

Diffusion of Innovations Theory is widely used and cited, but it is important to discuss the criticism that has been presented as well. Why do innovations not spread, even if backed by strong evidence? One key criticism is called "pro-innovation bias." This implies that all innovation is "positive" and should be adopted. Linearity and the one-way information flow have been criticized as another weakness of the theory. The described five stages (i.e., knowledge, persuasion, decision, implementation, and confirmation) of an innovation and the information flows in complex systems/organization are not linear, but "messy," dynamic, and fluid. Complex organizations contain many different professional groups and there is no "single" decision point, but numerous decision points with contesting/competing contents by many people occurring over time. The sufficiency of robust scientific evidence is not always enough to change behaviors, but scientific "push" needs to be complemented by other strategies (e.g., feedback loops from users; recognition of affected outcomes). "Individual blame" bias puts an emphasis on an individual employee/employees not adopting and implementing an innovation. This bias may, however, lead an organization to overlook other important aspects of diffusion, such as managerial and technical/technological challenges. Innovations can vary from highly focused, "simple" (e.g., persuading clinicians to use a new treatment or drug) and rapidly progressing to broad, complex, and slowly progressing innovations including an interrelated set of changes, social components (e.g., a management strategy change), and corporate implications (Denis, Hébert, Langley, Lozeau, & Trottier, 2002; Ferlie, Fitzgerald, Wood, & Hawkins, 2005; Greenhalgh et al., 2004; see also Innis, Dryden-Palmer, Perreira, & Berta, 2015). The criticisms described earlier may explain a few barriers to the spread of innovations in complex, multiprofessional healthcare settings, and also help in choosing and developing strategies to overcome these challenges.

■ HOW HAS EBP EVOLVED AND WHAT IS NEXT?

Evidence-based medicine (EBM) was introduced in the early 1990s (Evidence-Based Medicine Working Group, 1992), whereas EBN approach, first called research utilization, began to develop in the 1970s (Titler, 1997). The emphasis on empirically supported treatments (i.e., EBP in psychology, i.e., EBPP) was starting to develop in psychology in the early 1990s (APA Presidential Task force on Evidence-Based Practice, 2006), and since the late 1990s, evidence-based social work practice (EBSWP) has been promoted, for example, by high-quality systematic reviews (Institute for the Advancement of Social Work Research, 2007). The development of the basis for EBPs for the healthcare-related professions mentioned earlier took place nearly two decades ago, and the evolution of EBPs within professions has continued to unfold until present (Satterfield et al., 2009). However, today multiple disciplines are invariably involved in solving increasingly complex patient health problems, making knowledge sharing across the disciplines foundational to effective care (see, e.g., Bridges, Davidson, Odegard, Maki, & Tomkowiak, 2011; Newhouse & Spring, 2010) and which also increase the need for interprofessional collaboration. Interprofessional collaboration is a process in which different professional groups work together, and it involves expertise and contributions that various healthcare professionals bring to patient care. Interprofessional collaboration and practices, when these are evidence based, can improve healthcare processes and outcomes (Zwarenstein Goldman, & Reeves, 2009).

Despite the assumption that healthcare provides work synergistically in practice, interprofessional collaboration involves difficulties, such as problematic power dynamics, lack of understanding of one's own and others' roles and responsibilities, and conflicts due to varied approaches/EBPs to patient care (Newhouse & Spring, 2010; Zwarenstein et al., 2009). Traditionally, the training of practitioners in the health professions has been more exclusive than inclusive (Newhouse & Spring, 2010), and their vocabulary, conceptual frameworks, and research methods (evidence) often differ as well, thereby impeding cross-disciplinary translation and research utilization (Satterfield et al., 2009).

Today, there is a widespread advocacy and increasing implementation of interprofessional education (IPE) that reflects the premise that IPE will contribute to developing healthcare providers with the skills and knowledge needed to work in a collaborative manner. IPE is defined as an education/intervention where the members of more than one health or social care profession learn interactively together for the explicit purpose of improving interprofessional collaboration and/or the health/well-being of patients/clients. The intent is that IPE breaks down professional silos while preparing healthcare providers to enter the workplace as members of the collaborative practice team (Reeves, Perrier, Goldman, Freeth, & Zwarenstein, 2013). In the future, IPE programs will be increasingly piloted, started, and evaluated in academic and hospital organizations (see, e.g., Bridges et al., 2011; B. Wilson, Austria, Banner, & Wilson, 2017) and instruments (e.g., Health Science-Evidence Based Practice Questionnaire; EBP Profile) will be increasingly available for evaluation of such programs (Fernández-Domínguez et al., 2017; McEvoy, Williams, & Olds, 2010).

■ SUMMARY

Literature on EBP for the way nurses provide and manage patient care has grown over the past few decades. Leaders can reap the benefit of new evidence that supports better practice, which results in more positive patient outcomes. Still, adopting EBP is difficult in environments such as healthcare. Today, hospitals are increasingly complex organizations requiring all healthcare professionals to use critical thinking skills, EBPs, and to develop and maintain clinical expertise for safe, high-quality patient care. Organizational context, infrastructure, and leadership can influence and support the scholarship behind organizations and systems. The role of leaders is key in creating an environment and context that facilitates the adoption and sustainability of EBP. Creating structures and providing resources that support clinical scholarship is the first critical step in the process. The second is to utilize theories and models that help facilitate and sustain EBP. Evidence-based leadership models, like Kouzes and Posner's model for transformational leadership, provide support and guidance for individuals to take organizations to a new level. Organizational change theories and methods to evaluate readiness for change are important to understand and help prepare for change. The future success of applying evidence to practice and in closing the evidence-to-practice gap lies in scholarship. The scientific and leadership knowledge embedded in the DNP curriculum helps ready DNPs to take a leading role in uniting disciplines to research new ways of improving care to increase health and well-being and improve the lives of those who are served by the healthcare system. Now, more than ever, this leadership is needed. The increasing presence of DNPs throughout the healthcare system can facilitate this important work that, to date, has been challenging since so many years.

■ NOTE

1. Estabrooks et al. (2006) published *A Guide to Knowledge Translation Theory*. (*Journal of Continuing Education in the Health Professions, 26*(1), 25–36). This guide includes helpful definitions regarding EBP concepts, models, and theories of knowledge translation.

■ REFERENCES

Aarons, G., Ehrhart, M., Farahnak, L., & Hurlburt, M. (2015). Leadership and organizational changes for implementation (LOCI): A randomized mixed method pilot study of a leadership and organization development intervention for evidence-based practice implementation. *Implementation Science BMC, 10*(11), 1–12.

Aglen, B. (2016). Pedagogical strategies to teach bachelors students evidence-based practices. *Nurse Education Today, 36*, 255–263.

American Nurses Credentialing Center. (2014). *Magnet application manual*. Silver Spring, MD: Author.

APA Presidential Task Force on Evidence-Based Practice. (2006). Evidence-base practice in psychology. *American Psychologist, 61*(4), 271–185.

Appleby, B., Roskell, C., & Daly, W. (2015). What are health care professionals' intentions towards using research and products of research in clinical practice? A systematic review and narrative synthesis. *NursingOpen, 3*(3), 125–139.

Baker, K., Clark, P., Henderson, D., Wolf, L., Carman, M., Manton, M., & Zavotsky L. (2014). Identifying the differences between quality improvement, evidence-based practice, and original research. *Journal of Emergency Nursing, 40*(2), 195–197.

Balakas, K., Sparks, L., Steurer, L., & Bryant, T. (2013). An outcome of evidence-based practice education: Sustained clinical decision-making among bedside nurses. *Journal of Pediatric Nursing, 28*(5), 479–485.

Bass, B., & Riggio, R. (2006). *Transformational leadership* (2nd ed.). New York, NY: Psychology Press.

Batras, D., Duff, C., & Smith, B. (2014). Organizational change theory: Implications for health promotion practice. *Health Promotion International, 31*(1), 231–241.

Black, A. T., Balneaves, L. G., Garossino, C., Puyat, J. H., & Qian, H. (2015). Promoting evidence-based practice through a research training program for point-of-care clinicians. *Journal of Nursing Administration, 45*(1), 14–20.

Bridges, D., Davidson, R., Odegard, P., Maki, I., & Tomkowiak, J. (2011). Interprofessional collaboration: Three best practice models of interprofessional education. *Medical Education Online, 16*, 6035.

Brody, A. A., Barnes, K., Ruble, C., & Sakowski, J. (2012). Evidence-based practice councils: Potential path to staff nurse empowerment and leadership growth. *Journal of Nursing Administration, 42*(1), 28–33.

Brown, C. R., Johnson, A. S., & Appling, S. E. (2011). A taste of nursing research. *Journal for Nurses in Staff Development, 27*(6), E1–E6.

Burke, K. G., Johnson, T., & Bernsteiner, J. (2017). Creating an evidence-based progression for clinical advancement programs. *American Journal of Nursing, 117*(5), 22–35.

Burnes, B., & Cooke, B. (2013). Kurt Lewin's field theory: A review and re-evaluation. *International Journal of Management Reviews, 12*(4), 408–425.

Burns, J. (1978). *Leadership*. New York, NY: Harper & Row.

Carter, E. J., Mastro, K., Vose, C., Rivera, R., & Larson, E. L. (2017). Clarifying the conundrum: Evidence-based practice, quality improvement or research? *Journal of Nursing Administration, 47*(5), 266–270.

Centrella-Nigro, A. M., Faber, K., Wiklinski, B., Bognar, L., Flynn, D. L., & LaForgia, M. (2015). Effective collaboration among Magnet hospitals: A win-win for nurses and institutions. *American Journal of Nursing, 115*(7), 50–54.

Chappell, K. (2014). The value of RN residency and fellowship programs for Magnet hospitals. *Journal of Nursing Administration, 44*(6), 313–314.

Cheater, F., Baker, R., Gillies, C., Hearnshaw, H., Flottorp, S., Robertson, N., . . . Oxman, A. D. (2005). Tailored interventions to overcome identified barriers to change: Effects on professional practice and health care outcomes. *Cochrane Database of Systematic Reviews*, Issue 3, CD005470. doi:10.1002/14651858.CD005470.

Clavelle, J. T., Drenkard, K., Tullai-McGuinness, S., & Fitzpartick, J. J. (2012). Transformational leadership practices of chief nursing officers in Magnet organizations. *Journal of Nursing Administration, 42*(4), 195–201.

Connor, L., Paul, F., McCabe, M., & Ziniel, S. (2017). Measuring nurses' value, implementation, and knowledge of evidence-based practice: Further psychometric testing of the Quick-EBP-VIK survey. *Worldviews on Evidence-Based Nursing, 14*(1), 10–21.

Crabtree, E., Brennan, E., Davis, A., & Coyle, A. (2016). Improving patient care through nursing engagement in evidence-based practice. *Worldviews on Evidence-Based Nursing, 13*(2), 172–175.

Curtis, K., Fry, M., Shaban, R. Z., & Considine, J. (2016). Translating research findings to clinical nursing practice. *Journal of Clinical Nursing, 26*, 862–872.

Davidson, J. E., & Brown, C. (2014). Evaluation of nurse engagement in evidence-based practice. *AACN Advanced Critical Care, 25*(1), 43–55.

Day, J., Lindauer, C., Parks, J., & Scala, E. (2017). Exploring the best practice of nursing research councils in Magnet organizations. *Journal of Nursing Administration, 47*(5), 253–258.

Denis, J. L., Hébert, Y., Langley, A., Lozeau, D., & Trottier, L. H. (2002). Explaining diffusion patterns for complex health care innovations. *Health Care Management Review, 27*(3), 60–73.

Dogherty, E., Harrison, M., Graham, I., Vandyk, A., & Keeping-Burke, L. (2013). Turning knowledge into action at the point-of-care: The collective experience of nurses facilitating the implementation of evidence-based practice. *Worldviews on Evidence-Based Nursing, 10*(3), 129–139.

Duffy, J., Culp, S., Yarberry, C., Stoupe, L., Sand-Jecklin, K., & Sparks Coburn, A. (2015). Nurses' research capacity and use of evidence in acute care: Baseline findings from a partnership study. *Journal of Nursing Administration, 45*(3), 158–164.

Eller, L., Kleber, E., & Wang, S. (2003). Research knowledge, attitudes and practices of health professionals. *Nursing Outlook, 51*(4), 165–170.

Estabrooks, C. A., Squires, J. E., Cummings, G. G., Birdsell, J. M., & Norton, P. G. (2009). Development and assessment of the Alberta context tool. *BMC Health Services Research, 9*(234), 1–12. doi:10.1186/1472–6963-9-234

Estabrooks, C. A., Thompson, D., Lovely, J., & Hofmeyer, A. (2006). A guide to knowledge translation theory. *Journal of Continuing Education in the Health Professions, 26*(1), 25–36.

Evidence-Based Medicine Working Group. (1992). Evidence-based medicine: A new approach to teaching the practice of medicine. *Journal of the American Medical Association, 142,* 2420–2425.

Ferlie, E., Fitzgerald, L., Wood, M., & Hawkins, C. (2005). The nonspread of innovations: The mediating role of professionals. *Academy of Management Journal, 48*(1), 117–134.

Fernández-Domínguez, J., de Pedro-Gómez, J., Morales-Asenico, M., Bennasar-Veny, M., Sastre-Fullana, P., & Sesé-Abda, A. (2017). Health services-evidence based practice questionnaire (HS-EBP) for measuring transprofessional evidence-based practice: Creation, development and psychometric validation. *PLOS ONE, 12*(5), e0177172. doi:10.1371/journal.pone.0177172

Fineout-Overholt, E., & Melnyk, B. (2006). *Organizational culture and readiness scale for systems-wide integration of evidence-based practice.* Gilbert, AZ: ARCC, ll.

Fisher, C., Cusack, G., Cox, K., Feigenbaum, K., & Wallen, G. R. (2016). Developing competency to sustain evidence-based practice. *Journal of Nursing Administration, 46*(11), 581–585.

French, B., Thomas, L. H., Baker, P., Burton, C. R., Pennington, L., & Roddam, H. (2009). What can management theories offer evidence-based practice? A comparative analysis of measurement tools for organisational context. *Implementation Science, 4*(28), 1–15. doi:10.1186/1748–5908-4-28

Funk, S. G., Champagne, M. T., Wiese, R. A., & Tornquist, E. M. (1991). BARRIERS: The barriers to research utilization scale. *Applied Nursing Research, 4,* 39–45.

Funk, S. G., Tornquist, E. M., & Champagne, M. T. (1989). A model for improving the dissemination of nursing research. *Western Journal of Nursing Research, 11*(3), 361–367.

Gallagher-Ford, L. (2014a). Implementing and sustaining EBP in real world health settings: Transformational evidence-based leadership: Redesigning traditional roles to promote and sustain a culture of EBP. *Worldviews on Evidence-Based Nursing, 11*(2), 140–142.

Gallagher-Ford, L. (2014b). Implementing and sustaining EBP in real world settings: A leader's role in creating a strong context for EBP. *Worldviews on Evidence-Based Nursing, 11*(1), 72–74.

Gallagher-Ford, L. (2015). Leveraging shared governance councils to advance evidence-based practice: The EBP council journey. *Worldviews on Evidence-Based Nursing, 12*(1), 61–63.

Gawlinski, A., & Rutledge, D. (2008). Selecting a model for evidence-based practice changes: A practical approach. *AACN Advance Critical Care, 19*(3), 291–300.

Gerrish, K., Ashworth, P., Lacey, A., Bailey, J., Cooke, J., Kendall, S., & McNeilly, E. (2007). Factors influencing the development of evidence-based practice: A research tool. *Journal of Advanced Nursing, 57*(3), 328–338.

Gifford, W., Davies, B., Graham, I., Tourangeau, A., Woodend, A., & Lefebre, N. (2013). Developing leadership capacity for guideline use: A pilot cluster randomized control trial. *Worldviews on Evidence-Based Nursing, 10*(1), 51–65

Greenhalgh, T., Robert, G., Macfarlane, E., Bate, P., & Kyriakidou, O. (2004). Diffusion of innovations in service organizations: Systematic review and recommendations. *The Milbank Quarterly, 82*(4), 581–629.

Greiner, A., & Knebel, E. (Eds.). (2003). *Health professions education: A bridge to quality.* Washington, DC: National Academic Press. Retrieved from https://www.ncbi.nlm.nih .gov/books/NBK221528

Hatfield, L. A., Kutney-Lee, A., Hallowell, S. G., Guidice, M. D., Ellis, L. N., Verica, L., & Aiken, L.H. (2016). Fostering clinical nurse research in a hospital context. *Journal of Nursing Administration, 46*(5), 245–249.

Helfrich, C. D., Li, Y. F., Sharp, N. D., & Sales, A. E. (2009). Organizational readiness to change assessment (ORCA): Development of an instrument based on the Promoting Action on Research in Health Services (PARIHS) framework. *Implementation Science, 4*(38), 1–13. doi:10.1186/1748–5908–4-38

Herman, S., Gish, M., & Rosenblum, R. (2015). Effects of nursing position on transformational leadership practices. *Journal of Nursing Administration, 45*(2), 113–119.

Hopewell, S., Clarke, M., Stewart, L., & Tierney, J. (2007). Time to publication for results of clinical trials. *Cochrane Database Systematic Riverview,* Issue 2, MR000011. doi:10.1002/14651858.MR000011.pub2

Innis, J., Dryden-Palmer, K., Perreira, T., & Berta, W. (2015). How do health care organizations take on best practices? A scoping literature review. *International Journal of Evidence-Based Healthcare, 13*(4), 254–72.

Institute for the Advancement of Social Work Research. (2007). *Partnerships to integrate evidence-based mental health practices into social work education.* Washington, DC: National Institute of Mental Health.

Institute of Medicine. (2011). *The future of nursing: Leading change, advancing health.* Washington, DC: National Academies Press. Retrieved from https://www.ncbi.nlm.nih .gov/books/NBK209880

Iowa Model Collaborative. (2017). Iowa model of evidence-based practice: Revision and validation. *Worldviews on Evidence-Based Nursing, 14*(3), 175–182.

Jennings, B. M., Disch J., & Senn, L. (2008). Leadership. In R. Hughes (Ed.), *Patient safety and quality: An evidence-based handbook for nurses* (chap. 20, pp. 551–564). Rockville, MD: Agency for Healthcare Research and Quality.

Johantgen, M., Weiss, M., Lundmark, V., Newhouse, R., Haller, K., Unruh, M., & Shirey, M. (2017). Building research infrastructure in Magnet hospitals. *Journal of Nursing Administration, 47*(4), 198–204.

Kajermo, K. N., Boström, A. M., Thompson, D. S., Hutchinson, A. M., Estabrooks, C. A., & Wallin, L. (2010). The BARRIERS scale—The barriers to research utilization scale: A systematic review. *Implementation Science, 5*(32), 1–22. doi:10.1186/1748–5908-5-32

Kaplan, L., Zeller, E., Damitio, D., Culbert, S., & Bayley, K. B. (2014). Improving the culture of evidence-based practice at a Magnet hospital. *Journal of Nurses in Professional Development, 30*(6), 274–280.

Kelly, K. P., Turner, A., Gabel Speroni, K., McLaughlin, M. K., & Guzzetta, C. E. (2013). National survey of hospital nursing research, Part 2. *Journal of Nursing Administration, 43*(1), 18–23.

Kim, S. C., Brown, C., Ecoff, L., Davidson, J., Gallo, A., Klimpel, K., & Wickline, M. (2013). Regional evidence-based practice fellowship: Impact on evidence-base practice implementation and barriers. *Clinical Nursing Research, 22*(1), 51–69.

Kim, S. C., Stichler, J. F., Ecoff, L., Gallo, A., & Davidson, J. E. (2017). Six-month follow-up of a regional evidence-based practice fellowship program. *Journal of Nursing Administration, 47*(4), 238–243.

Kinney, S., Lima, S., McKeever, S., Twomey, B., & Newall, F. (2012). Employing a clinical governance framework to engage nurses in research. *Journal Nursing Care Quality, 27*(3), 226–231.

Kitson, A., & Harvey, G. (2016). Methods to succeed in effective knowledge translation in clinical practice. *Journal of Nursing Scholarship, 48*(3), 294–302.

Kitson, A., Harvey, G., & McCormack, B. (1998). Enabling the implementation of evidence based practice: A conceptual framework. *Quality in Health Care, 7*(3), 149–158.

Kouzes, J. M., & Posner, B. Z. (n.d.). *The leadership challenge website.* Retrieved from http://www.leadershipchallenge.com/WileyCDA/Section/id-131011.html

Kouzes, J. M., & Posner, B. Z. (2000, June). *Leadership practices inventory: Psychometric properties.* Retrieved from http://media.wiley.com/assets/56/95/lc_jb_psychometric_properti.pdf

Kouzes, J. M., & Posner, B. Z. (2002). *The leadership practices inventory: Theory and evidence behind the five practices of exemplary leaders.* San Francisco, CA: John Wiley & Sons.

Kouzes, J. M., & Posner, B. Z. (2007). *The leadership challenge* (4th ed.). San Francisco, CA: Jossey–Bass.

Lang, E., Wyer, P., & Haynes, R. (2007). Knowledge translation: Closing the evidence-based practice gap. *Annals of Emergency Medicine, 49*(3), 355–363.

Lavin, P. (2013). Boots on the ground: The role of the Magnet project director. *Nurse Manager, 44*(2), 50–52.

League, K., Christenbery, T., Sandlin, V., Arnow, D., Moss, K., & Wells, N. (2012). Increasing nurses' access to evidence through a web-based resource. *Journal of Nursing Administration, 42*(11), 531–535.

Levin, R. F., Fineout-Overholt, E., Melnyk, B. M., Barnes, M., & Vetter, M. J. (2011). Fostering evidence-based practice to improve nurse and cost outcomes in a community health setting. A pilot test of the advancing research and clinical practice through close collaboration model. *Nursing Administration Quarterly, 35*(1), 21–33.

Magers, T. L. (2014). An EBP mentor and unit-based EBP team: A strategy for successful implementation of a practice change to reduce catheter-associated urinary tract infections. *Worldviews on Evidence-Based Nursing, 11*(5), 341–343.

Manchester, J., Gray-Miceli, D., & Metcalf, J. (2014). Facilitating Lewin's change model with collaborative evaluation in promoting evidence based practices of health professionals. *Evaluations & Program Planning, 46*, 1–33.

May, C., Johnson, M., & Finch, T. (2016). Implementation, context and complexity. *Implementation Science, 11*(141), 1–13.

McCormack, B., Kitson, A., Harvey, G., Rycroft-Malone, J., Titchen, A., & Seers, K. (2002). Getting evidence into practice: The meaning of 'context'. *Journal of Advanced Nursing, 38*(1), 94–104.

McCormack, B., McCarthy, G., Wright, J., Slater, P., & Coffey, A. (2009). Development and testing of the Context Assessment Index (CAI). *Worldviews on Evidence-Based Nursing, 6*(1), 27–35.

McEvoy, M., Williams, M., & Olds, T. (2010). Development and psychometric testing of a transprofessional evidence-based practice profile questionnaire. *Medical Teacher, 31*(9), e373–e380.

McHugh, M., Kelly, L., Smith H., Wu, E., Vanka, J., & Aiken, L. (2013). Lower mortality in Magnet hospitals. *Medical Care, 51*(5), 382–388.

McLaughlin K., M., Speroni, K. G., Kelly, K. P., Guzzetta, C. E., & Desale, S. (2013). National survey of hospital nursing research, Part 1. *Journal of Nursing Administration, 43*(1), 10–17.

Melnyk, B. M., & Fineout-Overholt, E. (2002). Putting research into practice, Rochester ARCC. *Reflections on Nursing Leadership, 28*(2), 22–25.

Melnyk, B. M., & Fineout-Overholt, E. (2015). *Evidence-based practice in nursing and healthcare: A guide to best practice.* Philadelphia, PA: Lippincott Williams & Wilkins.

Melnyk, B. M., Fineout-Overholt, E., Gallagher-Ford, L., & Kaplan, L. (2012). The state of evidence-based practice in US nurses. *Journal of Nursing Administration, 42*(9), 410–417.

Melnyk, B. M., Fineout-Overholt, E., Giggleman, M., & Choy, K. (2017). A test of the ARCC model improves implementation of evidence-based practice, healthcare culture, and patient outcomes. *Worldviews on Evidence-Based Nursing, 14*(1), 5–9.

Melnyk, B. M., Fineout-Overholt, E., & Mays, M. (2008). The evidence-based practice beliefs and implementation scales: Psychometric properties of two new instruments. *Worldviews on Evidence-Based Nursing, 5*(4), 208–216.

Melnyk, B. M., Gallagher-Ford, L., Long, L. E., & Fineout-Overholt, E. (2014). The establishment of evidence-based practice competencies for practicing registered nurses and advanced practice nurses in real-world clinical settings: Proficiencies to improve healthcare quality, reliability, patient outcomes, and costs. *Worldviews on Evidence-Based Nursing, 11*(1), 5–15.

Melnyk, B. M., Gallagher-Ford, L., Troseth, M., & Szalacha, L. (2016). A study of chief nurse executives indicates low prioritization of evidence-based practice and shortcomings in hospital performance metrics across the United States. *Worldviews on Evidence-Based Nursing, 13*(1):6–14.

Mick, J. (2017). Call to action How to implement evidence-based nursing practice. *Nursing, 47*(4), 36–43.

Mitchell, S., Fisher, C., Hastings, C., Silverman, L., & Wallen, G. (2010). A thematic analysis of theoretical models for translational science in musing: Mapping the field. *Nursing Outlook, 58*(6), 285–300.

Mohide, E. A., & Coker, E. (2005). Toward clinical scholarship: Promoting evidence-based practice in the clinical setting. *Journal of Professional Nursing, 21*(6), 372–379.

Mollon, D., Fields, W., Gallo, A., Wagner, R., Soucy, J., Gustafson, B., & Kim, S. (2012). Staff practice, attitudes, and knowledge/skills regarding evidence-based practice before and after an educational intervention. *Journal of Continuing Education in Nursing, 43*(1), 411–419.

Moore, L. (2017). Effectiveness of an on-line education module in improving evidence-based practice skills of practicing registered nurses. *Worldviews on Evidence-Based Nursing, 14,* (5), 358–366. doi:10.1111/wvn.12214

Morgeson, F., DeRue, D., & Karam, E. (2010). Leadership in teams: A functional approach to understanding leadership structures and processes. *Journal of Management, 36*(1), 5–39.

Morris, Z., Wooding, S., & Grant, J. (2011). The answer is 17 years, what is the question: Understanding time lags in translational research. *Journal of the Royal Society of Medicine, 104,* 510–520.

Muller, A., McCauley, K., Harrington, P., Jablonski, J., & Strauss, R. (2011). Evidence-based practice implementation strategy. The central role of the clinical nurse specialist. *Nursing Administration Quarterly, 35*(2), 140–151.

Newhouse, R. (2010). Instruments to assess organizational readiness for evidence-based practice. *Journal of Nursing Administration, 40*(10), 404–407.

Newhouse, R., & Johnson, K. (2009). A case study in evaluating infrastructure for EBP and selecting a model. *Journal of Nursing Administration, 39*(10), 409–411.

Newhouse, R., & Spring, B. (2010). Interdisciplinary evidence-based practice: Moving from silos to synergy. *Nursing Outlook, 58*(6), 309–317.

O'Donnell, C. A. (2004). Attitudes and knowledge of primary care professionals towards evidence-based practice: A postal survey. *Journal of Evaluation in Clinical Practice, 10*(2), 197–205.

Olsen, L., Aisner, D., & McGinnis, J. M. (Eds.). (2007). *Roundtable on evidence-based medicine: The learning environment.* Washington, DC: National Academies Press.

Page, A. E. (Ed.). (2004). Committee on the work environment for nurses and patient safety. *Keeping patients safe: Transforming the work environment of nurses.* Washington, DC: National Academic Press. Retrieved from https://www.ncbi.nlm.nih.gov/books/NBK216190

Parkosewich, J. (2013). An infrastructure to advance the scholarly work to staff nurses. *Yale Journal of Biology and Medicine, 86*, 63–77.

Patterson, A. E., Mason, T. M., & Duncan, P. (2017). Enhancing a culture of inquiry. The role of a clinical nurse specialist in supporting the adoption of evidence. *Journal of Nursing Administration, 47*(3), 154–158.

Paul, F., Connor, L., McCabe, M., & Ziniel, S. (2016). Psychometric testing of the Quick-EBP-VIK survey: A survey instrument measuring nurses' values, implementation and knowledge of evidence-based practice. *Journal of Nursing Education and Practice, 6*(5), 118–126

Pfadenhauer, L., Gerhardus, A., Mozygemba, K., Bakke Lysdahl, K., Booth, A., Hofman, B., . . . Rehfuess, E. (2017). Making sense of complexity in context and implementation: The Context and Implementation of Complex Intervention (CICI) framework. *Implementation Science, 12*(21), 1–17.

Phillips, A. C., Lewis, L. K., McEvoy, M. P., Galipeau, J., Glasziou, P., Hammick, M., . . . Williams, M. T. (2014). A systematic review of how studies describe educational interventions for evidence-based practice: Stage 1 of the development of a reporting guideline. *BMC, 14*(152), 1–11. doi:10.1186/1472-6920-14-152

Pierson, M. A., & Schuelke, S. A. (2009). Strengthening the use of evidence-based practice: Development of an independent study packet. *Journal of Continuing Education in Nursing, 40*(4), 171–176.

Pravikoff, D., Tanner, A., & Pierce, S. (2005). Readiness of U.S. nurses for evidence-based practice. *The American Journal of Nursing, 105*(9), 40–51.

Pryse, Y., McDaniel, A., & Schafer, J. (2014). Psychometric analysis of two new scales: The evidence-based practice nursing leadership and work environment scales. *Worldviews on Evidence-Based Nursing, 11*(4), 240–247.

Ramos-Morcillo, A. J., Fernández-Salazar, S., Ruzafa-Martínez, M., & Del-Pino-Casado, R. (2015). Effectiveness of a brief, basic evidence-based practice course for clinical nurses. *Worldviews on Evidence-Based Nursing, 12*(4), 199–207.

Reeves, S., Perrier, L., Goldman, J., Freeth, D., & Zwarenstein, M. (2013). Inrerprofessional educational: Effects on professional practice and health care outcomes (update) (Review). *The Cochrane Collaboration,* (3), CD002213. doi:10.1002/14651858.CD002213.pub3

Rickbeil, P., & Simones, J. (2012). Overcoming barriers to implementing evidence-based practice. A collaboration between academics and practice. *Journal for Nurses in Staff Development, 28*(2), 53–56.

Rogers, E. M. (2003). *Diffusions of innovations* (5th ed.). New York, NY: Free Press.

Rolfe, G., Segrott, J., & Jordan, S. (2008). Tensions and contradictions in nurses' perspectives of evidence-based practice. *Journal of Nursing Management, 16*, 440–451.

Ross, E., Fitzpatrick, J., Click, E., Krouse, H., & Clavelle, J. (2014). Transformational leadership practices of nurse leaders in professional nursing associations. *Journal of Nursing Administration, 44*(4), 201–206.

Rutledge, D. N., & Skelton, K. (2011). Clinical expert facilitators of evidence-based practice: A community hospital program. *Journal for Nurses in Staff Development, 27*(5), 231–235.

Ruzafa-Martinez, M., Lopez-Iborra, L., Moreno-Casbas, T., & Madrigal-Torres, M. (2013). Development and validation of the competence in evidence based practice questionnaire (EBP-COQ) among nursing students. *BMC Medical Education, 13*(19), 1–10. doi:10.1186/1472-6920-13-19

Rycroft-Malone, J. (2004). The PARIHS framework—A framework for guiding the implementation of evidence-based practice. *Journal of Nursing Care Quality, 19*(4), 297–304.

Rycroft-Malone, J., Burton, C., Wilkinson, J., Harvey, G., McCormack, B., Baker, R., . . . Williams L. (2015). Collective action for knowledge mobilization: A realistic evaluation of the collaborations for leadership in applied health research and care. *Health Services and Delivery Research, 3*, 44.

Rycroft-Malone, J., Kitson, A., Harvey, G., Seers, K., Titchen, A., & Estabrooks, C. (2002). Ingredients for change: Revisiting a conceptual framework. *Quality and Safety in Health Care, 11*(2), 174–180.

Rycroft-Malone, J., Seers, K., Chandler, J., Hawke, C., Crichton, N., Allen, C., . . . Strunin, L. (2013). The role of evidence, context, and facilitation in an implementation trial: Implications for the development of the PARiSH framework. *Implementation Science, 8*(28), 1–13.

Rycroft-Malone, J., Seers, K., Titchen, A., Harvey, G., Kitson, A., & McCormack, B. (2004). What counts as evidence in evidence-based practice? *Journal of Advanced Nursing, 47*(1), 81–90.

Rycroft-Malone, J., Wilkinson, J., Burton, C., Andrews, G., Arris, S., Baker, R., . . . Thompson, C. (2011). Implementing health care research through academic and clinical partnerships: A realistic evaluation of Collaborations for Leadership in Applied Health Research and Care (CLAHRC). *Implementation Science, 6*(74), 1–12.

Salbach, N. M., & Jaglal, S. B. (2011). Creation and validation of the evidence-based practice confidence scale for health care professionals. *Journal of Evaluation in Clinical Practice, 17*(4), 794–800.

Sandstrom, B., Borglin, G., Nilsson, R., & Willman, A. (2011). Promoting the implementation of evidence-base practice: A literature review focusing on the role of nursing leadership. *Worldviews on Evidence-based Nursing, 8*(4), 212–223.

Satterfield, J., Spring B., Brownson, R., Mullen, E., Newhouse, R., Wakler B., & Whitlock, E. (2009). Towards a transdisciplinary model of evidence-based practice. *The Milbank Quarterly, 87*(2), 368–390.

Scala, E., Price, C., & Day, J. (2016). An integrative review of engaging clinical nurses in nursing research. *Journal of Nursing Scholarship, 48*(4), 423–430.

Schaffer, M., Sandau, K., & Diedrick, L. (2012). Evidence-based practice models for organizational change: Overview and practical applications. *Journal of advanced Nursing, 69*(5), 1197–1209.

Schmidt, N., & Brown, J. (2007). Use of Innovation-decision process teaching strategy to promote evidence-based practice. *Journal of Professional Nursing, 23*(3), 150–156.

Shaw, T. (2005). Leadership in practice development. In M. Jasper & M. Jumaa (Eds.), *Effective healthcare leadership* (1st ed., pp. 207–221). Oxford, England: Blackwell Publishing.

Shirey, M. (2013). Lewin's theory of planned change as a strategic resource. *Journal of Nursing Administration, 43*(2), 69–71.

Sigma Theta Tau International Clinical Scholarship Task Force. (1999). *Clinical scholarship resource paper.* Retrieved from https://www.nursingsociety.org/docs/default-source/position-papers/clinical_scholarship_paper.pdf?sfvrsn=4

Smith, J. R., & Donze, A. (2010). Assessing environmental readiness: First steps in developing an evidence-based practice implementation culture. *Journal of Perinatal and Neonatal Nursing, 24*(1), 61–71.

Smith, M., Saunders, R., Stuckhardt, L., McGinnis, J. M. (Eds.). (2013). Best care at lower cost: The path to continuously learning health care in America (Chapter 7). Washington, DC: National Academies Press. Retrieved from https://www.ncbi.nlm.nih.gov/books/NBK207234

Spiva, L., Hart, P. L., Patrick, S., Waggoner, J., Jackson, C., & Threatt, J. L. (2017). Effectiveness of an evidence-based practice nurse mentor training program. *Worldviews on Evidence-Based Nursing, 14*(3), 183–191.

Squires, J., Hayduk, L., Hutchinson, A., Mallick, R., Norton, P., Commings, G., & Estabrooks, C. (2015). Reliability and validity of the Alberta Contect Tool (ACT) with professional nurses: Findings from a multi-study analysis. *PLOS ONE, 10*(6), 1–17.

Stavor, D., Zedreck-Gonzaletz, J., & Hoffmann, R. (2017). Improving the use of evidence-based practice and research utilization through the identification of barriers to implementation in a critical access hospital. *Journal of Nursing Administration, 47*(1), 55–61.

Stetler, C. B., & Marram, G. (1976). Evaluating research findings for applicability in practice. *Nursing Outlook, 24*(9), 559–563.

Stetler, C. B., Ritchie, J., Rycroft-Malone, J., & Charns, M. (2014). Leadership for evidence-based practice: Strategic and functional behaviors for institutionalizing EBP. *Worldviews on Evidence-Based Nursing, 11*(4), 219–226.

Stevens, K., & Ovretveit, J. (2013). Improvement research priorities: USA survey and expert consensus. *Nursing Research and Practice, 2013*, Article ID 695729, 1–8. doi:10.1155/2013/695729

The Joint Commission. (2003). *Putting evidence to work: Tools and resources.* Washington, DC: The Joint Commission Resources.

Titler, M. (1997). Research utilization: Necessity or luxury. In J. C. McCloskey & H. Grace (Eds.), *Current issues in nursing* (5th ed. pp. 104–117). St. Louis, MO; Mosby.

Tucker, S. J., Olson, M. E., & Frusti, D. K. (2009). Evidence-based practice self-efficacy scale: Preliminary reliability and validity. *Clinical Nurse Specialist: The Journal for Advanced Nursing Practice, 23*(4), 207–215.

Turkel, M. (2014). Leading from the heart: Caring, love, peace, and values guiding leadership. *Nursing Science Quarterly, 27*(2), 172–177.

Ubbink, D., Guyatt, G., & Vermeulan, H. (2013). Framework of policy recommendations for implementation of EBP: A systematic scoping review. *BMJ Open, 3*, e001881. doi:10.1136/bmjopen-2012-001881

Underhill, M., Roper, K., Diefert, M. L., Boucher, J., & Berry, D. (2015). Evidence-based practice beliefs and implementation before and after an initiative to promote evidence-based nursing in an ambulatory oncology setting. *Worldviews on Evidence-Based Nursing, 12*(2), 70–78.

Upton, D. (1999). Attitudes towards, and knowledge of, clinical effectiveness in nurses, midwives, practice nurses and health visitors. *Journal of Advanced Nursing, 29*(4), 885–893.

Upton, D., Upton, P., & Scurlock-Evans, L. (2014). The reach, transferability and impact of the evidence-based practice questionnaire: A methodological and narrative literature review. *Worldviews on Evidence-Based Nursing, 11*(1), 46–54.

Waite, R., & McKinney, N. (2015). Findings from a study of aspiring nursing student leaders. *Nurse Education Today, 35*(12), 1307–1311

Wallen, G., Mitchell, S., Melnyk, B., Fineout-Overholt, E., Miller-Davis, C., Yates, J., & Hastings, C. (2010). Implementing evidence-based practice: Effectiveness of a structured multifaceted mentorship program. *Journal of Advanced Nursing, 66*(22), 2761–2771.

Warren, J. I., McLaughlin, M., Bardsley, J., Eich, J., Esche, C. A., Kropkowiski, L., & Risch, S. (2016). The strengths and challenges of implementing EBP in health care systems. *Worldviews on Evidence-Based Nursing, 13*(1), 15–24.

Warren, J. I., Montgomery, K. L., & Friedman, E. (2016). Three-year pre-post analysis of EBP integration in a Magnet-designated community hospital. *Worldviews on Evidence-Based Nursing, 13*(1), 50–58.

Waters, D., Rychetnik, L., & Barratt, A. (2009). The Australian experience of nurses' preparedness for evidence-based practice. *The Journal of Nursing Management, 17*(4), 510–518.

Weiner, B. J. (2009). A theory of organizational readiness for change. *Implementation Science, 4*(67), 1–9. doi:10.1186/1748–5908-4-67

Weiner, B. J., Amick, H., & Lee, S. D. (2008). Review: Conceptualization and measurement of organizational readiness for change. *Medical Care Research and Review, 65*(4), 379–436.

Whitmer, K., Auer, C., Beerman, L., & Weishaupt, L. (2011). Launching evidence-based nursing practice. *Journal for Nursing Staff Development, 27*(2), E5–E7.

Wilkes, L., Mannix, J., & Jackson, D. (2013). Practicing nurses perspectives of clinical scholarship: A qualitative study. *BMJ Nursing, 12*(21), 1–7. doi:10.1186/1472-6955-12-21

Wilson, B., Austria, M., Banner, M., & Wilson, A. (2017). Evaluating the implementation of an interdisciplinary evidence-based practice educational program in a large academic medical center. *Journal for Nurses in Professional Development, 33*(4), 162–169.

Wilson, M., Sleutel, M., Newcomb, P., Behan, D., Walsh, J., Wells J., & Baldwin K. (2015). Empowering nurses with evidence-based practice environments: Surveying Magnet pathway to excellence and non-Magnet facilities in one health care system. *Worldviews on Evidence-Based Nursing, 12*(1), 12–21.

Wintersgill, W., & Wheeler, E. C. (2012). Engaging nurses in research utilization. *Journal for Nurses in Staff Development, 28*(5), E1–E5.

Yackel, E. E., Short, N. M., Lewis, P. C., Breckenridge-Sproat, S. T., & Turner, B. S. (2013). Improving the adoption of evidence-based practice among nurses in army outpatient medical treatment facilities. *Military Medicine, 178*(9), 1002–1009.

Yoder, L., Kirkley, D., McFall, D., Kirksey, K., StalBaum, A. L., & Sellers, D. (2014). Staff nurses' use of research to facilitate EBP. *American Journal of Nursing, 114*(9), 26–37.

Yost, J., Ganaan, R., Thompson, D., Aloweni, F., Newman, K., Hazzan, A., & Ciliska D. (2015). The effectiveness of knowledge translation interventions for promoting evidence-informed decision making among nurses in tertiary care: A systematic review and meta-analysis. *Implementation Science, 10*(98), 1–15.

Zwarenstein, M., Goldman, J., & Reeves, S. (2009). Interprofessional collaboration: Effects of practice-based interventions on professional practice and heath care outcomes (Review). *Cochrane Database of Systematic Reviews*, Issue 3, CD000072. doi:10.1002/14651858 .CD000072.pub2

CHAPTER FOURTEEN

Transformation of Healthcare and Health Information Technology

ANNA SCHOENBAUM

This chapter is dedicated to Lena Sorenson who helped develop its original content.

◼ OVERVIEW

As healthcare transitions to a value-based model, health information technology (IT) is becoming more important in transforming the care delivery landscape. Policy mandates and value-based reimbursement are pressuring health organizations to enhance the patient experience, improve the health of populations, and reduce the per capita cost of healthcare (Institute of Health Improvement [IHI], 2017). With this call for transformation, there is increasing need to better engage patients into all aspects of their health and disease management (Institute of Medicine [IOM], 1999, 2001). Subsequently, health IT systems should include business and clinical processes that provide patient-centric care. Today, health IT is embedded in the fabric of an organization and impacts nursing practice. Doctorate of nursing practice (DNP) graduates need to leverage information systems/technology and patient care technology to improve and transform health and healthcare. The primary goal for this chapter is to present an overview of the driving forces in health IT, basic informatics concepts, and health IT strategies focused on the quality of care, population health, and the cost of healthcare.

◼ DRIVING FORCES IN HEALTH IT

In the last five decades, health IT and the field of informatics have changed dramatically due to the advances in technology and changes to healthcare legislation to support a value-based healthcare delivery model. Technology first appeared in the hospitals in the 1960s when hospitals installed mainframes and storage to support basic accounting and data processing systems. Shortly thereafter, the first electronic health record (EHR) system was introduced for tracking basic patient information (Tripathi, 2012). Over the past 50 years, the EHR and other healthcare technology have advanced due to better IT infrastructure, such as hardware, software, network capabilities, and interface standards (i.e., Health Level Seven [HL7] messaging); however, the implementation and adoption of the EHR was slow. In 2009, the American Reinvestment and Recovery Act (ARRA) and the Health Information Technology for Economic and Clinical Health Act (HITECH) provided incentives through the Centers for Medicare and Medicaid Services (CMS) to stimulate the adoption of the EHRs in a meaningful way (Blumenthal & Tavenner, 2010). The "meaningful use" (MU) of a certified EHR includes three components: (a) use in a meaningful way, (b) use for electronic exchange of health information to improve quality of healthcare, and (c) use to submit clinical quality measures (CQM) and other objectives (HITECH, 2009). The MU program implementation involved two groups: eligible hospitals and eligible providers (replaced with eligible clinicians in 2018). MU Stage 1 promotes the use of electronic data capture in a standardized format to track key clinical conditions and for information sharing. Modified Stage 2 expands these functions into advanced clinical processes with more rigorous health information exchange (HIE), clinical decision support (CDS), care coordination, and patient engagement (U.S. Department of Health & Human Services [HHS], 2015). MU Stage 3 focuses on the use of the certified EHR to improve patient quality and safety through the implementation of care coordination tools, further development in exchanging patient information, and public reporting (HHS, 2015). Overall, the "MU" EHR Incentive Program requirements pushed the EHR industry toward better system design and interoperability across systems. As a result, EHR implementations tripled from 2003 to 2014, growing from 31% to 99% (Pedersen, Schneider, & Scheckelhoff, 2017).

While these MU programs dangled incentives for health organizations and providers, MU Stage 3 posed challenges in implementation, which led the American Medical Association to advocate to the CMS to reevaluate the requirements. Subsequently, Congress passed the Medicare Access and CHIP Reauthorization Act (MACRA, 2016) to streamline existing Medicare programs (i.e., MU, Medicare Physician Quality Reporting System, and the Value-Based Modifier Program) into a single program called the Quality Payment Program (QPP) in 2018 for eligible clinicians. The QPP has two paths: (a) the Merit-Based Incentive Payment System (MIPS) and (b) the Advance Alternative Payment Models (APM) to reward the quality of patient care over volume.

Additionally, CMS announced changes to the Hospital Inpatient Prospective Payment System (IPPS) allowing more flexibility in Certified EHR Technology (CEHRT) and MU Stage requirements, and pushed the mandating MU Stage 3 date to 2019 (HHS, 2017). CMS also shortened the Inpatient Quality Reporting (IQR) program's reporting period and reduced the number of electronic CQMs (eCQMs) for both 2017 and 2018 reporting years (HHS, 2017). The MU requirements, along with other federal and state regulations, are ever changing. It is important for nurses to stay abreast of regulatory changes, understand the technical build required, analyze the data, and ensure the data are accurately and timely submitted. With the rapid pace of technological innovation, informatics expertise has become more integral to organizational strategies that address problems, achieve strategic goals, and monitor outcomes.

■ BASIC INFORMATICS CONCEPTS

BIOMEDICAL INFORMATICS

The field of informatics has expanded with the transformation of the healthcare delivery model and the rapid evolution of technology, especially in biomedical research, clinical care, and public health. Biomedical informatics (BMI) is defined as "the interdisciplinary field that studies and pursues the effective uses of biomedical data, information, and knowledge for scientific inquiry, problem solving, and decision making, motivated by efforts to improve human health" (Kulikowski et al., 2012). BMI encompasses the methods, techniques, and theories of academic research to applied research and practice in the field of nursing, medicine, pharmacology, medical imaging, case management, research, and public health sectors. All informatics disciplines can play a critical role in planning, analyzing, designing, implementing, and evaluating technology for their area of specialty. With the increased volume of health data and advances in technology, informatics has expanded to data mining, natural language or text processing, cognitive science, human interface design, decision support, databases, and algorithms for analyzing large amounts of data generated in public health, clinical research, and genomics.

NURSING INFORMATICS

Nursing informatics (NI) is a domain of the health informatics discipline. The definition of NI has evolved since Graves and Corcoran (1989) first defined it as "computer science, information science, and nursing science combined to assist in the management and processing of nursing data, information and knowledge to support the practice of nursing and the delivery of nursing care" (p. 227). In this original definition, the emphasis was on technology. As the definition evolved, it changed to include the central focus on the concepts of data, information, and knowledge incorporating the critical roles and elements of nursing practice (Staggers & Thompson, 2002). The newest definition expands the definition to recognize the role of "wisdom," a fundamental form of knowledge that goes into designing new processes that improve the quality of healthcare (American Nurses Association [ANA], 2014). NI is the "specialty that integrates nursing science with multiple information management and analytical sciences to identify, define, manage, and communicate data, information, knowledge, and wisdom in nursing practice" (ANA, 2014). In the workplace today, every nurse uses some type of informatics skills.

Informatics has evolved with the explosion in technology and the health policies to support the transition to a value-based care delivery model that is patient-centric focused on individual preferences, needs, and values (IOM, 2001). As a result, technology is redesigning the clinical team roles and how care is being delivered. Today, multiple disciplines can be "digitally linked teams" to provide more effective care through EHR, telehealth, and other mechanisms (IOM, 2011). Doctorate-prepared nurses can use information systems/technology to support and improve the quality of healthcare by promoting care coordination, reducing medical errors, improving population health, and reducing healthcare cost.

■ SYSTEM DEVELOPMENT LIFE CYCLE

While not everyone specializes in informatics, there are basic elements of a system development life cycle that can be applied in implementing new functionality, evaluating outcomes, managing and aggregating data, and assessing the efficacy of technology to support patient care. Understanding the basic concepts of the system development life cycle is essential in the field of informatics and provides a vision for the development of ongoing innovation in healthcare delivery (Skiba, Connors, & Jeffries, 2008; Zeng & Bell, 2008). The system development life cycle includes the following components: planning, discovery and analysis, design and usability testing, development, testing, training, implementation, maintenance, and evaluation (Figure 14.1).

Planning is foundational to project success. In the planning phase, it is essential to understand the project scope; key stakeholders; resources needed (i.e., people, technical infrastructure, funding); organizational readiness; the culture and politics; plans for testing, training, and communication; key performance indicators; and tools to be used for the separate phases of the project. The discovery and analysis phase involves understanding current workflow, what problems exist, and the requirements of the users. The design phase transforms user requirements on how to deliver the required functionality based on the capability of the system. The design of the system and workflow is critical to user adoption, hence, the importance of end-user involvement in usability testing. The development phase involves programming and/or configuration changes based on the identified requirements. The testing phase demonstrates expected outcomes,

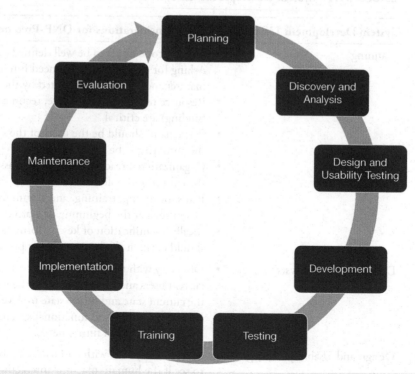

FIGURE 14.1 System development lifecycle.

integrates with other applications, or does not have any downstream implications. The phases of testing include unit, functional, integration, regression, performance, and user acceptance. The length of the testing periods needs to be considered at the beginning of the project. Testing outcomes are documented. Testing issues are addressed following the organizational's IT methods, processes, and procedures for configuration system changes. The training phase is a critical event that contributes to the success of the implementation. Based on the type of implementation and audience, training can be delivered through different mechanisms, such as classroom with instructor-led training, web-based training, or tip sheets. The implementation phase of the project, also considered a "go-live," involves an activation plan with conversion steps from one system to another system, support plan (onsite and/or remote), change management plan, and postsupport plan. Once the implementation is completed, supporting the system is necessary to ensure it is functioning as designed. Any issue should be reported, corrected, and tested following the IT department change management process with proper approval from key stakeholders. After an implementation, modifications to the system may appear as simple system changes but may affect a multitude of other system configurations and many users. The evaluation is also important and often overlooked. The key performance indicators and any metrics used during the project planning should be monitored and analyzed. Throughout the project, a robust communication plan is needed to ensure the right message is delivered to the right audience and delivered in a timely manner. See Table 14.1 for consideration in practice for nurse leaders.

TABLE 14.1 System Development Lifecycle Key Considerations

System Development Lifecycle	Key Considerations for DNP-Prepared Graduates
Planning	• Project scope needs to be well defined and to be realistic. Asking for custom code may need funding, increased maintenance, and not supported by the vendor. • Resource requirements (people, technical infrastructure, funding) are critical. • Participants should be the users of the system and have the authority to be decision makers. • Organizational readiness needs to be assessed, includes the culture and politics. • Plans for testing, training, and communication should be outlined at the beginning of a project. • Ideally, identification of key performance indicators should occur at the beginning of a project.
Discovery and Analysis	• Discovery with the right people is critical. It may include current users and leaders to design the future state. Use the current state and future state to develop a gap analysis. • Identify technical and functional specifications to address current and future needs.
Design and Usability Testing	• Design the system with end users. Usability testing is key to see if the human–machine interaction is optimal.

(continued)

TABLE 14.1 System Development Lifecycle Key Considerations (*continued*)

System Development Lifecycle	Key Considerations for DNP-Prepared Graduates
Development	• Stay involved during the development phase, especially if you are the nurse champion. • Caution—straying away from vendor code may have implications during the implementation and postimplementation. Custom development may lengthen the project timeline, increase cost, require resources to maintain custom code and additional testing, and increase efforts during upgrades.
Testing	• Developing testing scripts with the correct steps is important. Having a peer review of the test script is good practice.
Training	A good training structure, processes, and accountability are needed to improve end-user adoption. Considerations: • Incorporate trainers into the system build, workflow design, and go-live processes to help the trainer better understand the clinician workflows. • Conduct role-based training to demonstrate how various system components and EMR functionality fit into each role's specific workflow. • Enforce utilization of ongoing training checklists to track training progress and ensure end users are appropriately trained around ongoing system updates and compliance requirements. • Coordinate change requests identified by end users during the training phase of the implementation plan.
Implementation	• Implementation plan should include clinical readiness, communication methods and process, elbow support, debriefing meetings, and status reporting. Monitoring of adoption, outcomes, and key performance indicators are a must at go-live.
Maintenance	• Changes to the system should follow the governance process for approval. Communication should occur with changes to the system.
Evaluation	• Monitor effectiveness of implementation. Monitor key performance indicators.

DNP, doctorate of nursing practice; EMR, electronic medical record.

■ HEALTH IT AND TRENDS

There is a demand for technology to enhance the patient experience, to provide quality and safe patient-centered care, to improve the health of populations, and to reduce cost of care across the continuum. These demands have accelerated the need for common technical standards, core structured clinical content, interoperability with other systems, decision support to meet regulatory guidelines, and data analytics capabilities. The proliferation of microprocessors, network capabilities, mobile technology, and artificial intelligence (AI) of computers is also shaping the care delivery model. Furthermore, secure communication and data sharing standards are changing the boundaries of how information is being shared and accessed by providers and patients.

With newer, smarter technologies constantly emerging, nurses must learn to use all information technologies effectively, recognizing the benefits and limitations of the technology and integrating them into their practice (McGonigle, Hunter, Sipes, & Hebda; 2014). Nurses must learn to analyze clinical processes to assess workflow improvements by using technology to solve bottlenecks and to provide better care. With the rapid influx of technology in the healthcare market, nurses need to better understand the health IT trends and how they may impact their practice or organization. The following section highlights the health IT solutions and trends in the transformation of care delivery that focus on enhancing the patient experience and improving the health of populations, which ultimately should lead to a reduction in healthcare cost.

ELECTRONIC HEALTH RECORD

The EHR systems are important clinical tools to enhance the IOM (2001) principles of patient safety, timeliness, and efficiency to deliver patient-centered care in the acute care, ambulatory, and postacute care settings. Today, EHRs are being used almost universally in hospitals and practices. The next leap is to optimize the EHR systems to improve the human–machine interaction, improve workflows, and, most importantly, to improve the quality and safety of the patient. Dartmouth College researchers suggested the elimination of unwarranted variation in their EHR might increase the quality of care and lower cost up to 30% (Bynum, Meara, Chang, & Rhoads, 2016). Streamlining workflows and standardization of contents, such as order sets and clinical paths, will help clinicians adhere to practice and reduce variability.

Considerations for Nurse Leaders

Plan for optimization. Set a target date for the post implementation review (i.e., 90 days, 180 days, or 360 days after an implementation). Prior to optimization changes, review key performance indicators, hold focus groups, and observe users. The American Medical Informatics Association (AMIA) Task Force recommended changes to EHR systems in five areas: (a) simplify and speed documentation, (b) refocus regulation, (c) increase transparency and streamline certification, (d) foster innovation, and (e) support centered care delivery (Payne et al., 2015).

CLINICAL DECISION SUPPORT

Optimization of EHR systems should include CDS tools that are integrated into the clinicians' workflow to provide patient-related information and clinical knowledge for better decision making in caring for the patient. CDS examples include medication alerts (i.e., drug to allergy, drug to drug), documentation reminders, treatment recommendations, and order sets. CDS requests come from organizational leaders and users, but can also be mandated by legislation, such as the MU modified Stage 2 objective to use CDS to improve performance on high-priority conditions (i.e., acute myocardial infarction, stroke, and asthma). Recently, Medicare legislation mandated CDS for advanced diagnostic imaging orders to be in place by January 2020 ("Medicare Program," 2017). As part of the Protecting Access to Medicare Act (PAMA), referring providers are required to consult appropriate use criteria (AUC) prior to ordering advanced diagnostic imaging for Medicare patients (2014). This legislation requires a technical solution to reduce duplicate and/or unnecessary tests and associated costs, which requires a change in workflow for the clinician. For CDS to be applied successfully, it is important to ensure the technical design is intelligent, filtered, and fires at appropriate time to enhance decision making. The ten commandments for effective CDS, published in 2003, are pertinent today. These principles include the following: "speed is everything; anticipate the needs and deliver in real time; fit into the user's workflow; little things can make a big difference; recognize that (clinicians) will strongly resist stopping; changing direction is easier than stopping; simple interventions work best; ask for additional information only when needed; monitor impact, get feedback, and respond; management and maintain knowledge-based systems" (Bates et al., 2003).

Considerations for Nurse Leaders

Implement CDS in the background to monitor the intended effect prior to turning the CDS on to the users. It is also important to monitor the effectiveness of CDS once it is turned on to users.

DATA ANALYTICS

Data analytics is the process of examining data sets to identify and analyze patterns and trends. Nurses can play an instrumental role in ensuring the standardization of data with consistent nomenclatures that reflect the practice of nurses. Data standards are needed to capture, organize, encode, and analyze so that data can be shared between systems. Data standardization is important in designing the EHR. Today, healthcare organizations are using the EHR data to drive clinical, business, and financial improvements. With electronic health data sets so large and complex, a comprehensive approach to data analytics is needed. It is important for healthcare organizations to have robust and scalable data infrastructure, analytical software, and business intelligence tools that help clinicians with using predictive modeling and real-time alerting. If the tools are in place, predictive analysis can drive clinical decisions, such as identifying at-risk patients with real-time clinical data exchange and event notification.

Considerations for Nurse Leaders

Participate in the development of the data quality framework and strategy, which should include a data governance committee to help with data standardization, data validation, and data visualization for completeness—accuracy, timeliness/availability, traceability, use, and monitoring the data.

EVALUATION AND MONITORING OUTCOMES

With the implementation and the optimization of EHR systems actively underway, the next step is to evaluate and monitor outcomes using healthcare IT systems. Is the ogranization improving patient care? Is the ogranization improving the population of health? Is the ogranization reducing healthcare costs? Steps to consider in evaluating outcomes are outlined here (Sengstack & Bodice, 2015, pp. 164–180):

1. Determine what is being evaluated
2. Determine the question being answered
3. Conduct a literature search
4. Determine the data requirements and data sources
5. Determine the study type
6. Determine the data collection method and sample size
7. Collect, analyze, and display data

Considerations for Nurse Leaders

Identify resources needed for data extraction and resources to review/analyze the outcomes in the evaluation process. The time commitment should not be overlooked.

POPULATION HEALTH MANAGEMENT

Population health management (PHM) is an increasingly important strategy as healthcare transitions to the value-based healthcare model. The strategy to manage population health and the technology to aggregate patient data across multiple health information systems is sweeping the industry. Before investing in new population health technology, organizations need to have a clear vision of their PHM strategy and how health technology can be leveraged to support the continuum of care. The five strategic objectives to assist organizations in building technology capabilities for population health measurement activities are as follows (Office of the National Coordinator for Health Information Technology [ONC], 2013):

1. Build collaboration, consensus, and commitments among key stakeholders.
2. Identify and engage data sources and owners to obtain access to required data.
3. Design and implement data access, transmission, and analytics processes.
4. Continuously monitor and improve data quality.
5. Develop and implement reporting on population health measures.

Health IT components to support PHM programs may require infrastructure, connectivity, software, and devices, such as care coordination tools, exchange of health data, analytical tools, and mobile technology.

Considerations for Nurse Leaders

Identify interoperability requirements of an EHR system and other healthcare systems prior to acquisition. Specifically, the evaluation of a PHM system should support the organization's strategic population health vision and requirements, such as interoperability of the system, the tools, dashboards/reports specifically for quality metrics and cost reporting, and workflows. Once a PHM system is selected, it is important to develop a road map by setting priorities.

PHM DATA AND ANALYTICS

The PHM systems vary widely on how data are controlled, analyzed, and visualized. While many EHR vendors have expanded their platform to include population health tools and data analytics tools, new PHM vendors are popping up in the industry. Organizations will have to assess PHM system features, interoperability with data sources, data models, and how to view the data. Data from clinical claims and other data from multiple sources aggregated into a data warehouse with disease registry systems should provide a comprehensive, actionable clinical picture of patients. Key features in a PHM system include the ability to identify gaps in care, alert notification to clinicians and care managers when patients need attention, dashboards to predict and stratify patients, benchmark reports and ability to compare performance, tools to monitor and control costs, and ways to engage patients. Data visualization of metrics is, also, necessary for the organization (i.e., quality measures, utilization metrics, and cost of care).

Considerations for Nurse Leaders

PHM data source requirements should be discussed once the organization has a good understanding of what it is trying to accomplish. Possible outside data sources may include patient health data from any EHR, claims data, patient satisfaction, CMS data, cost data, and medication management (i.e., prescription drugs).

CARE COORDINATION TOOLS

Care coordination is the deliberate organization of managing patient care activities and sharing information to achieve safer and more effective care (Agency for Healthcare Research and Quality [AHRQ], 2017). To manage the health of patients effectively and efficiently, health IT tools are needed to exchange continuity of care documents, facilitate care coordination activities (i.e., care planning; discharge planning), monitor patients, especially in at-risk populations, and send reminders to engage patients, caregivers, and care managers. This may require further development in the EHR to facilitate care coordination workflows in different settings: inpatient, ambulatory, skilled nursing facility, and at home (or just about anywhere in the community). Care coordination tools may include the following: the ability to document and flag care coordination notes, which contain social determinant factors; ability to identify at-risk patients through algorithms and analytic tools; create a longitudinal clinical plan that can be shared; ability to document patients when calling them at home or anywhere; ability to send messages or reminders to patient portals; and ability to send secure texts to communicate among care teams. Further development between health organizations, HIEs, and other agencies will be required to transmit health information electronically.

Considerations for Nurse Leaders

Care coordination workflows are complex, especially if a patient is seen at multiple hospitals. Having access to at-risk patient data, such as care coordination notes from all patient encounters, provides opportunities to understand, monitor, and measure the risk implications of the plan of care for patients.

HEALTH INFORMATION EXCHANGE

HIE allows clinical information to move electronically among disparate health information systems (Mastrian, McGonigle, & Farcus, 2014, pp. 175b–176b). The clinical information provides a longitudinal data record on each patient (i.e., clinical notes, radiology and lab results), which can be automatically shared across healthcare organizations. HIE improves the speed, quality, safety, and cost of patient care (ONC, 2014). HIE can specifically promote care coordination among at-risk patients with complex physical, behavioral, and social needs, especially in the primary care, urgent care, and emergency room setting. The common HIE industry standard methods of data exchange are HL7 interfaces and Consolidated-Clinical Document Architecture (C-CDA). HL7 is a set of standards, formats, and definitions for exchanging clinical and administrative data between software applications (McGonigle, Mastrian, & Nedra, 2012). Common examples of a HL7 interface are demographic data. CDA is an architecture standard based on coding, semantic framework, and markup language to create electronic clinical documents to exchange health information (ONC, 2017). It is the preferred method to aggregate and push out health information in the health industry. An example of C-CDA is care coordination note exchange from hospital to hospital.

Accessing data across systems and organizations continues to be a challenge. Open application programming interface (API) based on HL7 Fast Healthcare Interoperability Resources (FHIR) and blockchain are closing in on the interoperability challenges. FHIR is an application standard of HL7 to assist with data sharing among health IT systems. FHIR may eventually replace the current data exchange technology. Blockchain technology is being considered the next big health technology innovation to improve interoperability and privacy needs in the transaction of patient data without a centralized database or administrator. It enables interoperable distributed systems to send secure transactions that have been approved and verified. Blockchain can facilitate data sharing among a patient and provider or a provider and a payer without a third party.

Considerations for Nurse Leaders

Privacy and security must be at the forefront of healthcare organizations as organizations have more access to data. Policies and processes to support privacy and security are required no matter what technology is used to exchange data.

PATIENT PORTAL, PATIENT HEALTH RECORD, AND MOBILE APPLICATIONS

Health systems are using multiple approaches to engage patients to be actively involved in their healthcare by providing better technology. Patient-centered interactive tools give patients a more meaningful role. Research is beginning to show that many of these innovations improve the quality of health for many patients (Ahern, Woods, Lightowler, Finley, & Houston, 2011; Goldberg et al., 2011; Or & Karsh, 2009; Reed, Graetz, Gordon, & Fung, 2017). Patient portals have become standard tools for many hospitals and practices. They provide a secure web platform on which patients can access their EHR and communicate privately with their providers (Lin, Wittevrongel, Moore, Beaty, & Ross, 2005; Rodriguez, 2010; Sorensen, Shaw, & Casey, 2009). Recently, there has been an increasing emphasis on a consumer-driven system referred to as an electronic personal health record (PHR), which is an electronic health tool used by individual patients to store and share one's health information. There are two kinds of PHRs: stand-alone PHR and tethered/connected PHR (Bobinet & Petito, 2015; ONC, 2013). The stand-alone PHR is usually stored on a patient's computer or on the Internet. The tethered PHR is integrated to a healthcare organization's EHR or to a health plan's information system. The PHR is intended to allow patients to directly manage their care. Having important healthcare information, such as diagnostic test results, lab results, immunization records, and screening due dates, may improve patient engagement by providing the patient the ability to track and manage their health (Jones, Shipman, Plaut, & Selden, 2010). PHRs have functionality to send direct and secure communication between patient and provider, resulting in an improved provider–patient relationship. Additionally, many mobile technologies are providing patients the ability to monitor and enter their own health data and health experiences so it interfaces with Telehealth systems and/or their provider's EHR system. Much of this innovation revolves around mobile phone manufacturers, such as Apple and Samsung. For instance, Apple offers HealthKit for patients to monitor their steps, weight, glucose, and other measurements. These patient-entered data may eventually integrate with the patients' health records for the care teams to actively monitor their patients, which will ultimately enhance a seamless communication and information exchange across the health delivery continuum.

Considerations for Nurse Leaders

MU Stage 3 recommends APIs be available so patients can use any application to retrieve their health information. Organizations will need to prepare for consumer demands to access to their health data.

ARTIFICIAL INTELLIGENCE

AI (also called machine intelligence) is machine logic that can perceive information about its environment and take action to maximize its chance of success at some goal (Miliard, 2017). AI is fast advancing into the healthcare technology platforms that may involve aspects of cognitive computing, machine learning, natural language processing, and neural networks. A well-known AI health vendor is IBM's Watson, which analyzes patient's health information against a wide array of data and evidence-based medicine for informed decision making. Other technology advances include stand-alone Internet-connected devices that can be monitored and/or controlled from different locations, which are being called the Internet of Things (IoT). It is projected that the IoT Healthcare Market Compound Annual Growth Rate will increase by 30.8%, from US $41.22 billion in 2017 to US $158.07 billion in 2022 (Markets and Markets, 2017). IoT digital devices, such as smart wearable devices (i.e., watches), implantables or injectables (i.e., heart monitoring implants), and nonwearables (i.e., weight scales) may eventually be connected to patient health records, thus changing how clinicians monitor patients.

Considerations for Nurse Leaders

Care delivery models, data warehouse platforms, and security infrastructure must be in place prior to adding data from digital devices. Interoperability between digital devices and systems will pose challenges and risks to data security and privacy.

TELEHEALTH

Telehealth solutions are rapidly advancing and changing how care is delivered. Telehealth programs can manage the health of populations and lower healthcare costs by identifying care gaps, monitoring at-risk patients, seeing more patients, and extending services to patients who may not get care otherwise (Bobinet & Petito, 2015; ONC, 2017). At the time of this publication, the Senate Finance Committee approved the Chronic Care Act (S.870), which provides greater flexibility and expansion for telehealth services for Medicare Advantage plans and certain accountable care organizations (i.e., home dialysis and stroke assessments) (AHRQ, 2017).

Considerations for Nurse Leaders

Telehealth and patient portals will change how patients engage with their healthcare providers. Strategic planning needs to look beyond the walls of the hospital and current practices.

PRECISION MEDICINE

Precision medicine is gaining momentum in healthcare. In 2016, the 21st Century Cures Act was passed providing $4.8 billion for precision medicine. Precision medicine improves therapeutic benefits for groups of patients using genomics and molecular profiling (Adams & Petersen, 2016). Nurses are pivotal in identifying personalized healthcare requirements and designing the clinical infrastructure for storing genetic/genomic patient information. Sharing of these profiles and clinical data between clinicians to improve patient outcomes and enhance care experience for patients in diagnosis and treatment plans is a core goal for informatics.

Considerations for Nurse Leaders

A crucial step for precision medicine involves moving to a common database, which makes it easier to manage, aggregate, and secure the data.

■ SUMMARY

Nurses must be central to the implementation of healthcare technology in all healthcare settings, and the goals of new technology directives must be congruent with nursing aims for quality healthcare (Barton, 2011; Jacobsen & Juste, 2010; Murphy, 2009). Nurses have always put the patient at the center of their practice and can identify effective communication across the continuum of care. Specifically, nurses must be knowledgeable about how the design and availability of health information for our communities reflects the unique needs of those patient populations. As the largest group of health providers (55% of all providers), nurses must be aware of regulatory changes and be prepared for the transformation of healthcare delivery through the diffusion of innovative technologies (Booth, 2006; Gassert, 2008; Greenhalgh, Robert, MacFarlane, Bate, & Kyriakidou, 2004; Hersh, 2006; TIGER, 2009). Understanding the ever-changing legislation, the basic concepts of informatics, and latest health IT trends provides nurses the foundation to effectively infuse this knowledge into their practice.

■ REFERENCES

Adams, S. A., & Petersen, C. (2016). Precision medicine: Opportunities, possibilities, and challenges for patients and providers, *Journal of the American Medical Informatics Association, 23*(4), 787–790.v

Agency for Healthcare Research and Quality. (2017). Care coordination. Retrieved from https://www.ahrq.gov/professionals/prevention-chronic-care/improve/coordination/index.html

Ahern, D. K., Woods, S. S., Lightowler, M. C., Finley, S. W., & Houston, T. K. (2011). Promise of and potential for patient-facing technologies to enable meaningful use. *American Journal of Preventive Medicine, 40*(5 Suppl. 2), S162–172.

American Nurses Association. (2014). *Nursing informatics practice scope and standards of practice* (2nd ed.). Washington, DC: Author.

Barton, A. J. (2011). The electronic health record and "meaningful use": Implications for the clinical nurse specialist. *Clinical Nurse Specialist, 25*(1), 8–10.

Bates, D. W., Kuperman, G. J., Wang, S., Gandhi, T., Kittler, A., Volk, L., ... Middleton, B. (2003). Ten commandments for effective clinical decision support: Making the practice of evidence-based medicine a reality. *Journal of the American Medical Informatics Association, 10*(6), 523–530. doi:10.1197/jamia.M1370

Blumenthal, D., & Tavenner, M. (2010). The "meaningful use" regulation for electronic health records. *New England Journal of Medicine, 363*(6), 501–504.

Bobinet, K., & Petito, J. (2015). Designing the consumer-centered telehealth & eVisit experience: Considerations for the future of consumer healthcare. Retrieved from https://www.healthit.gov/sites/default/files/DesigningConsumerCenteredTelehealtheVisit-ONC-WHITEPAPER-2015V2edits.pdf

Booth, R. G. (2006). Educating the future eHealth professional nurse. *International Journal of Nursing Education Scholarship, 3*(1), Article 13.

Bynum, J. P. W., Meara, E., Chang, C., & Rhoads, J. (2016). *Our parents, ourselves: Health care for an aging population.* Retrieved from http://www.dartmouthatlas.org/downloads/reports/Our_Parents_Ourselves_021716.pdf

Gassert, C. A. (2008). Technology and informatics competencies. *Nursing Clinics of North America, 43*(4), 507–21.

Goldberg, L., Lide, B., Lowry, S., Massett, H. A., O'Connell, T., Preece, J., ... Shneiderman, B. (2011). Usability and accessibility in consumer health informatics current trends and future challenges. *American Journal of Preventive Medicine, 40*(5, Suppl. 2), S187–S197.

Graves, J. R., & Corcoran, S. (1989). The study of nursing informatics. *Image, 21*(4), 227–231.

Greenhalgh, T., Robert, G., MacFarlane, F., Bate, P., & Kyriakidou, O. (2004). Diffusion of innovations in service organizations: Systematic review and recommendations. *Millbank Quarterly, 82*(4), 581–629.

Health Information Technology for Economic and Clinical Health Act. (2009). 74, No. 209 Fed. Reg. 56123–56131. Retrieved from https://www.hhs.gov/hipaa/for-professionals/special-topics/hitech-act-enforcement-interim-final-rule/index.html

Hersh, W. (2006). Who are the informaticians? What we know and should know. *Journal of the American Medical Informatics Association, 13*(2), 166–170.

Institute for Healthcare Improvement. (2017). IHI triple aim initiative. Retrieved from http://www.ihi.org/Engage/Initiatives/TripleAim/Pages/default.aspx

Institute of Medicine. (1999). *To err is human: Building a safer health system.* Washington, DC: National Academy of Sciences.

Institute of Medicine. (2001). *Crossing the quality chasm: The IOM health care quality initiative.* Washington, DC: National Academy of Sciences.

Institute of Medicine. (2011). *The future of nursing: Leading change, advancing health.* Washington, DC: National Academies Press.

Jacobsen, T., & Juste, F. (2010). Nursing in the era of "meaningful use". *Nursing Management, 41*(1), 11–13.

Jones, D. A., Shipman, J. P., Plaut, D. A., & Selden, C. R. (2010). Characteristics of personal health records: Findings of the Medical Library Association/National Library of Medicine Joint Electronic Personal Health Record Task Force. *Journal of the Medical Library Association, 98*(3), 243–249.

Kulikowski, C. A., Shortliffe, E. H., Currie, L. M., Elkin, P. L., Lawrence, H. E., Johnson, T., ... Williamson, J. J. (2012). AMIA Board white paper: Definition of biomedical informatics and specification of core competencies for graduate education in the discipline. *Journal of the American Medical Informatics Association, 19*(6), 931–938.

Lin, C. T., Wittevrongel, L., Moore, L., Beaty, B. L., & Ross, S. E. (2005). An Internet-based patient-provider communication system: Randomized controlled trial. *Journal of Medical Internet Research, 7*(4), e47.

Markets and Markets. (2017). *IoT healthcare market by component (medical device, systems & software, service, connectivity technology), application (telemedicine, work flow management, connected imaging, medication management), end user, and region - Global Forecast to 2022*. Retrieved from https://www.marketsandmarkets.com/Market-Reports/iot-healthcare-market-160082804.html

Mastrian, K. G., McGonigle, D., & Farcus, N. (2012). Ethical applications of informatics. In D. McGonigle & K. G. Mastrian (Eds.), *Nursing informatics and the foundation of knowledge* (2nd ed., pp. 69–88). Burlington, MA: Jones & Bartlett.

McGonigle, D., Hunter, K., Sipes, C., & Hedda, T. (2014). Why nurses need to understand nursing informatics. *Association of periOperative Registered Nurses, 100*(3), pp. 324–327.

McGonigle, D., Mastrian, K., & Nedra, F. (2012). Other organizations assisting HIPPA. In D. McGonigle & K.G. Mastrian (Eds.), *Nursing informatics and the foundation of knowledge* (2nd ed., pp. 175b–176b). Burlington, MA: Jones & Bartlett.

Medicare Access and CHIP Reauthorization Act (MACRA) of 2015. 2016. 81 Fed. Reg. § 77008 (to be codified at 42 CFR pts. 414 and 495).

Medicare Program; Revisions to Payment Policies Under the Physician Fee Schedule and Other Revisions to Part B for CY 2018; Medicare Shared Savings Program Requirements; and Medicare Diabetes Prevention Program, 82 Fed. Reg. §219 (final rule Nov. 15, 2017). Retrieved from https://www.gpo.gov/fdsys/pkg/FR-2017-11-15/pdf/2017-23953.pdf

Miliard, M. (2017). With machine learning and AI in healthcare, can you speak the language? *Healthcare IT News*. Retrieved from http://www.healthcareitnews.com/news/machine-learning-and-ai-healthcare-can-you-speak-language

Murphy, J. (2009). Meaningful use for nursing: Six themes regarding the definition of meaningful use. *Journal Healthcare Information Management, 23*(4), 9–11.

Office of the National Coordinator for Health Information Technology. (2013). *Building technology capabilities to aggregate clinical data and enable population health measurement*. Retrieved from https://www.healthit.gov/sites/default/files/onc-beacon-lg6-it-for-pop-hlth-measmt.pdf

Office of the National Coordinator. (2014). Health information exchange. Retrieved from http://www.healthit.gov/HIE

Office of the National Coordinator. (2017). *Health IT Playbook*. Retrieved from https://www.healthit.gov/playbook/introduction

Or, C. K., & Karsh, B. T. (2009). A systematic review of patient acceptance of consumer health information technology. *Journal of the American Medical Informatics Association, 16*(4), 550–560.

Payne, T. H., Corley, S., Cullen, T. A., Gandhi., T. K., Harrington, L., Kuperman, G., ... Zaroukian, M. (2015). Report of the AMIA EHR-2020 Task Force on the status and future direction of EHRs. *Journal of the American Medical Informatics Association, 22*(5), 1102–1110.

Pedersen, C. A., Schneider, P. J., & Scheckelhoff, D. J. (2017). ASHP national survey of pharmacy practice in hospital settings: Prescribing and transcribing—2016. *American Journal of Health-System Pharmacy*. Retrieved from http://www.ajhp.org/content/early/2017/07/21/ajhp170228?sso-checked=true

Protecting Access to Medicare Act of 2014, Pub. L 113-93, 128 Stat. 1040, codified as amended at title U.S.C § 1834(q)(1)(B) (2014). Retrieved from https://www.gpo.gov/fdsys/pkg/FR-2017-11-15/pdf/2017-23953.pdf

Reed, M., Graetz, I., Gordon, N., & Fung, V. (2015). Patient-initiated e-mails to providers: associations with out-of-pocket visit costs, and impact on care-seeking and health. *American Journal Managed Care, 21*, 632–639.

Rodriguez, E. (2010). Using a patient portal for electronic communication with patients with cancer: Implications for nurses. *Oncology Nursing Forum, 37*(6), 667–671.

Sengstack, P., & Boicey, C., (2015). Conducting healthcare IT outcomes and evaluations: Guidelines and resources. *Mastering Informatics: A Healthcare Handbook for Success* (pp. 164–180). Indianapolis, IN: Sigma Theta Tau International.

Skiba, D., Connors, H. R., & Jeffries, P. R. (2008). Information technologies and the transformation of nursing education. *Nursing Outlook, 56*(5), 225–230.

Sorensen, L., Shaw, R., & Casey, E. (2009). Patient portals: Survey of nursing informaticists. *Studies in Health Technology and Informatics, 146*, 160–165.

Staggers, N., & Thompson, C. B. (2002). The evolution of definitions for nursing informatics: A critical analysis and revised definition. *Journal of the American Medical Informatics Association, 9*(3), 255–261.

Technology Initiative Guiding Educational Reform. (2009). *Collaborating to integrate evidence and informatics into nursing practice and education: An executive summary.* Retrieved from http://www.himss.org/collaborating-integrate-evidence-and-informatics-nursing-practice -and-education-executive-summary

Tripathi, M. (2012). EHR evolution: Policy and legislation forces changing the EHR. *Journal of American Health Information Management Association, 83*(10), 24–29.

21st Century Cures Act. (2016). U.S.C. 114–255. Retrieved from https://www.gpo.gov/ fdsys/pkg/PLAW-113publ1/html/PLAW-113publ1.htm

U.S. Department of Health & Human Services. (2015). Electronic health record incentive programs Stage 3 and modifications to meaningful use in 2015 through 2017; final rule, 80 Fed. Reg. § 200 (to be codified at 42 CFR pts. 412 and 495).

U.S. Department of Health & Human Services. (2017). Hospital inpatient prospective payment systems for acute care hospitals and the long-term care hospital prospective payment system and policy changes and fiscal year 2018 rates; quality reporting requirements for specific providers; Medicare and Medicaid electronic health record incentive program requirements for eligible hospitals, critical access hospitals, and eligible professionals, 82 Fed. Reg. § 37990 (Aug. 14, 2017) (to be codified at 42 CFR pts. 405, 412, 413, 414, 416, 486, 488, 489, 495).

Zeng, X., & Bell, P. (2008). Web 2.0: What a health care manager needs to know. *Health Care Manager, 27*(1), 58–70.

CHAPTER FIFTEEN

Outcomes Measurement

LISA COLOMBO

Measurement of outcomes is a broad topic that has different meaning based on the context in which it is considered. Why something is being measured and what measures will inform the processes of care are important considerations in outcomes measurement. Measurement is done for various reasons in healthcare. The driving force for measurement in doctor of nursing practice (DNP) practice is for improvement in the quality of patient care. This chapter reviews the purpose of outcomes measurement as it relates to DNP practice and discusses the use of measurement in improvement of quality of care for patients, safety for healthcare organizations, and to meet requirements from payers and regulators. The interrelationship between each of these perspectives is also discussed.

■ OUTCOMES

Broadly, the term "outcomes" refers to the results of treatment or interventions or a change in health status as a result of care that is provided. They measure healthcare quality and efficacy (Kleinpell & Gawlinski, 2005; Oermann & Floyd, 2002). As the emphasis on patient safety and quality has increased exponentially over the last several years, measurement of outcomes, or results, is essential to demonstrate effectiveness of care. The first step in managing outcomes for patients is measuring them. The measurement of outcomes provides useful information for the design and delivery of care and the continuous improvement in care processes (Hamric, Spross, & Hanson, 2009).

■ PURPOSE OF MEASURMENT

The fundamental question to ask when reviewing outcomes measures is, "Why are we measuring?" The answer to this question will guide the journey to quality improvement. In general, measurement in healthcare is done for three specific purposes: research, improvement, and judgment. In research, measurement of outcomes is used to develop new knowledge. In practice, measurement of outcomes is used to drive improvement in processes, which will lead to improved patient outcomes (Solberg, Mosser, & McDonald, 1997). We also use outcomes measures to make judgments about evidence that results both from research and improvement initiatives. For example, individuals (patients) *judge* the quality of their lives based on their perception of their health. In this example, health perception is an outcome of interest to an individual. A patient's judgment of their health status has more recently been recognized as a "patient-reported outcomes measure" (Griggs, Schneider, Kazis, & Ryan, 2017). This concept becomes important later in this chapter when we discuss outcomes of interest to individuals, where the individual is the patient.

In healthcare, measurements are often used for reporting aggregate results to regulators, legislators, and other parties that *judge* the data against specific standards or rules (Institute of Healthcare Improvement, 2011).

The Essentials of DNP practice (American Association of Colleges of Nursing, 2006) describes the competencies required for DNP-prepared nurses. All of the essentials require skill at the doctoral level in outcomes measurement and the interpretation and use of outcomes measures to demonstrate competency. Essential II, *Organizational and Systems Leadership for Quality Improvement and Systems Thinking*, makes the case that outcomes measurement in practice is paramount to the improvement of quality of patient care and health outcomes.

In short, the overarching purpose for measurement in practice is to understand if improvements in practice lead to improvement in outcomes. Choosing the appropriate measures by which to judge process improvement is also important to the success of the effort.

■ DIFFERENCES BETWEEN MEASUREMENT FOR RESEARCH AND MEASUREMENT FOR IMPROVEMENT

Measurement for research is done to develop new knowledge and identify knowledge that will support improvement in quality of care. Measurement in practice is then used to bring that new knowledge into practice. Both are necessary to improve care; however, the methods of data collection and approaches to measurement vary according to the paradigm (see www.ihi.org/knowledge/Pages/HowtoImprove/ScienceofImprovement EstablishingMeasures.aspx for the comparison).

In research, there is a focus on rigor in research methods to control for biases and to ensure generalizability. In measurement for improvement, the goal is to perform rapid cycle tests of change, identify metrics to judge the effects of change, and incorporate learning from those interpretations into each consecutive improvement cycle to achieve the outcomes suggested by the research. In practice, measurement for improvement is the primary purpose for outcomes measurement.

■ TYPES OF MEASUREMENTS

It is important to understand that there are three types of measures, one of which is outcomes measures (Institute of Healthcare Improvement, 2011). These indicators give signals as to how a system is performing and what results are being achieved. Outcomes measures represent the voice of the customer (Lloyd, 2004). An example of an outcomes measure is the incidence of ventilator-associated pneumonia (VAP) in a population of critical care patients. VAP is the outcome of interest to the patient/customer/population.

Process measures represent the voice of the system (Institute of Healthcare Improvement, 2011). Evidence-based processes of care are processes which, when performed correctly, lead to improved patient outcomes (Chassin, Loeb, Schmaltz, & Wachter, 2010). Process measures help us to evaluate whether or not the system is performing as planned (Institute of Healthcare Improvement, 2011). Using VAP as the example again, measurement of the compliance with evidence-based VAP bundle (i.e., elevation of the head of the bed, daily "sedation vacations," peptic ulcer prophylaxis, deep vein thrombosis prophylaxis, and daily oral care with chlorhexidine) would constitute process measures, which would identify if the established system was working properly. The question to be asked is, "Does the system or processes produce the desired results?" The desired result is reduction in VAP.

In practice, it is important to measure both process and outcomes measures to evaluate the effectiveness of the processes intended to improve care. Measuring one without the other, such as measuring process without respect for outcomes, can lead to conclusions that may not support the improvement of quality of care.

The third type of measure is the balancing measure. This measure looks at a system from a different perspective and is intended to identify if changes made to improve outcomes have resulted in new problems in other parts of the system (Institute of Healthcare Improvement, 2011). For example, evaluation of processes that are put in place to reduce the length of stay for a population of patients should include the balancing measure of readmissions for that same population of patients. It would be important to know if reducing length of stay results in an increase in readmissions.

■ IMPORTANCE OF MEASUREMENT

The fundamental question is, "Why measure?" The answer is simple. Successful measurement is the cornerstone to successful improvement and, in practice, this is where the rubber meets the road. It helps us to determine if changes in practice lead to improvement.

Improvement in quality of care is not just a goal; it is a requirement in today's healthcare environment. In 1998, The Joint Commission (TJC) introduced the ORYX initiative, which was the first national program for hospital quality measurement (Chassin et al., 2010). This initiative required hospitals to collect and transmit data to TJC for a minimum of four core measure sets (TJC, 2017b). Examples of core measure sets are acute myocardial infarction, heart failure, pneumonia, and the surgical care improvement project. For a complete listing of current Centers for Medicare and Medicaid Services (CMS) core measures see Medicare/Quality-Initiatives-Patient-Assessment-Instruments/QualityMeasures/CMS-Measures-Inventory.html. The initial intent was to promote quality improvement efforts in TJC-accredited hospitals. The core measures, essentially, are evidence-based process of care measures, which, when executed correctly, lead to better patient outcomes. In 2004, the CMS aligned their efforts to collect quality data and began financially penalizing hospitals that did not report to CMS the same data that they collected and reported to TJC (Chassin et al., 2010). Today, CMS reimburses hospitals for performance against a broad set of value-based purchasing (VBP) metrics. Payment is based on a combination of adherence to process measures, achievement of outcomes measures, and measurement of the patient's experience of care. Hospitals now have up to 2% of their total Medicare reimbursement at risk for their performance on the established core measure sets. Private insurance carriers have worked together with CMS and state-funded healthcare programs on alignment of core measures, allowing healthcare organizations to focus on the process and outcomes indicators that most significantly impact mortality (CMS, 2017a). Although the topic of VBP is outside the scope of this chapter, it is used as an example of the importance of measurement to payers.

Healthcare economics have also dictated that care should not only be effective but also be *cost-effective*. In 2016, CMS began applying an efficiency measure to its VBP system. In 2017, it added cost-reduction and weighted the efficiency and cost reduction domain at 25% for purposes of determining performance in the VBP system (CMS, 2017b).

The delivery and continuous improvement of high-quality, high-value healthcare requires attention to meaningful outcomes. Organizations that are high performers in the delivery of quality services are consistently asking whether or not specific processes of care add genuine value and if changes to those services represent improvement (Nelson, Batalden, Godfrey, & Lazar, 2011). Measurement answers both those questions and provides meaningful information to inform the improvement process.

■ RELATIONSHIP BETWEEN PROCESS AND OUTCOMES

More than 30 years ago, a physician named Avedis Donabedian proposed a model for assessing healthcare quality based on structures, processes, and outcomes. He suggested that there was a relationship between structure, process, and outcome, and that each is influenced by the other. In effect, structure influences process and process influences outcome (Donabedian, 2005; see sphweb.bumc.bu.edu/otlt/MPH-Modules/HPM/AmericanHealthCare_Quality-Cost-Outcomes/AmericanHealthCare_Quality-Cost-Outcomes_print.html for Donabedian's framework).

Important to note is that judgments on the appropriateness of processes to achieve desired outcomes are based on the premise that the processes are supported by a sound evidence base (Donabedian, 1988). Following Donabedian's model, compliance with processes known to improve quality will lead to desired outcomes.

Therefore, measurement of processes or compliance with processes is a proxy for outcomes. Process measures can be used to assess the ability of a process to impact an outcome, and therefore should be used in conjunction with outcomes measures. The "goodness" of a process is only as good as the outcome that the process produces. Measurement of outcomes is essential to guide improvement. The goal is not measurement; the goal is improvement.

■ THE HEALTHCARE MEASUREMENT CONTINUUM

Measurement in healthcare can be broadly defined as a continuum that ranges from the subjective perceptions of the patient ("I feel good") to the highly objective data that is used to submit insurance claims. Along the continuum are various stakeholders: individuals/patients, providers, payers and regulators, accrediting bodies, and policy makers. Each stakeholder has a different perspective on what constitutes an outcome of interest to him or her. Perspectives and methods of measurement change as the stakeholder changes. Consider heart failure, diabetes mellitus, and nurse staffing as conditions that have outcomes associated with them. Table 15.1 demonstrates how perspectives change as stakeholders change.

As you move vertically down the table, you can see that the outcomes of interest change as the stakeholder changes. It is important to note that with the move toward VBP, alignment of outcomes of interest is beginning to occur. Take the example of nurse staffing. Both providers and payers are aligned in their concern for the

TABLE 15.1 Progression of Perspectives of Interest by Stakeholder

	CHF	DM	Nurse Staffing
Individuals	Quality of life related to activities of daily living	Perceived disease burden in patients with type 2 diabetes	Nurse burnout
Providers	Treatment adherence related to medications, diet, and daily weight	Perceptions of treatment compliance in patients with type 2 diabetes	Quality of care and nurse-sensitive indicator performance (i.e., falls with injury and healthcare-acquired skin breakdown)
Payers	Cost of care, morbidity and mortality, and hospital readmission rate in the congestive heart failure patient population	Preventive care in diabetics: avoidance of hospital admissions	Nurse-sensitive indicators, nurse-driven serious reportable events (i.e., falls with injury, healthcare-acquired skin breakdown)
Regulators/accreditors	Core measure performance	Change in oral agent compliance related to Medicare prescription drug coverage	The Joint Commission staffing effectiveness and standards compliance

CHF, congestive heart failure; DM, diabetes mellitus.

outcomes of nurse-sensitive indicators such as skin breakdown and falls with injury. For providers, hospital-acquired skin breakdown and falls with serious injury can result in nonpayment for services rendered for either of those conditions. Care must still be rendered, but there is no offset for the cost of care in terms of additional reimbursement to treat the undesirable outcome. For payers, these outcomes may signal issues with quality of care, which can drive the level of reimbursement that they will pay for certain services.

Understanding that improvement versus measurement is the goal, selecting indicators for measurement is dependent on knowing the goal of the improvement process. Given that outcomes of interest are different to different stakeholders, consideration must be given to who the stakeholder is in order to measure what matters to each stakeholder.

■ SELECTION OF INDICATORS

If the goal of measuring outcomes is to manage practice that achieves desired results, then outcomes management is accomplished through quality improvement efforts. Central to any quality improvement process is the selection of the correct or appropriate indicators that inform the process under study.

There are many different types of indicators. There are financial indicators, quality indicators, safety indicators, and patient experience indicators, to name a few. Focusing on only one or two types of indicators may give an incomplete picture of the overall success of a given process (Lloyd, 2004). A balanced approach to indicator selection and measurement is required to truly reflect the success of care processes. Donabedian first proposed that indicator selection should be balanced and indicators of structures, processes, and outcomes should be selected and monitored together in order to give a complete picture of the health of a process (Lloyd, 2004). Since then, other organizations have suggested multiple dimensions from which to select indicators for measurement.

In 2001, the Institute of Medicine's report, *Crossing the Quality Chasm*, identified six aims for improvement, which could be used to categorize indicators. The six aims are safety, effectiveness, patient-centeredness, time lines, efficiency, and equity (Institute of Medicine, 2001; Lloyd, 2004).

In November of 2010, TJC proposed an approach to indicator measurement that focuses clearly on maximizing health benefits to patients (Chassin et al., 2010). This initiative refines the approach initially used in the ORYX initiative by identifying four criteria that each measure must meet, the purpose of which is to separate the measures that advance the goal of maximizing health from those that do not. The four criteria are

1. *Research:* Strong scientific evidence base showing that the care process leads to improved outcomes.
2. *Proximity:* The measure accurately captures whether the evidence-based care process has, in fact, been provided.
3. *Accuracy:* The measure addresses a process that has few intervening care processes that must occur before the improved outcome is realized.
4. *Adverse Effects:* Implementing the measure has little or no chance of inducing unintended adverse consequences. (TJC, 2017a)

Core measures meeting these criteria are now considered accountability measures, and those not meeting these criteria are considered nonaccountability measures. Nonaccountability measures are care processes that are considered "good advice" for patient care but not necessarily contributing directly to the outcome of interest (TJC, 2017b). Nonaccountability measures may be useful for quality improvement and/ or organizational learning and explorations and can be part of a holistic performance improvement program (TJC, 2017a). This move by TJC to separate core measures according to these criteria supports the notion that process indicators should be measured in conjunction with outcomes indicators.

Regardless of the types of indicators that are identified to measure, the important idea is to use a balanced approach to indicator selection. Once you have identified the types of indicators appropriate to measure for a given process or outcome, it is then necessary to select specific indicators that reflect the specific aspect of the process. For example, if you are working on fall prevention, specific indicators for the processes of care associated with falls will include number of patient falls, fall rate (in falls per 1,000 patient days), or percent of patients that fall. These are outcome measures; a balanced approach would also include process indicators such as nursing interventions intended to prevent falls (e.g., frequent toileting, call bell within reach, communication to care team members about fall risk). Using Donabedian's model, you could also collect indicators of structure, such as number of nursing and ancillary staff on at the time of the fall. Collecting measures that reflect structure, process, and outcomes simultaneously provides the balanced approach that is necessary to truly inform improvement processes in healthcare.

■ DATA USE

Once you have determined the appropriate indicators to collect to inform care processes, the data need to be available and understandable to healthcare professionals working to improve the delivery of care. Central to this concept is understanding variation in data.

In order to understand variation, one must first understand the concept of variation and also understand how some simple statistical methods and tools can assist in the understanding of variation (Lloyd, 2004). Webster's *New Collegiate Dictionary* (2008) defines variation as "(a) the act, fact, or process of varying; change or deviation in form, condition, appearance, extent, etc. from a former or usual state, or from an assumed standard; (b) the degree or extent of such change." Although the definition of variation seems clear, the interpretation of it may not. A major factor in the accurate interpretation of variation is the manner in which data are displayed.

In healthcare, data are often displayed in aggregate form. Examples of aggregated data include tools like pie charts, bar charts, and tables with summary statistics, to name a few. Clinical dashboards often contain monthly average scores for selected quality indicators. Data displayed in aggregated form can lead only to judgment, and sometimes to inaccurate judgment. It is not useful in determining if improvement processes are achieving goals. Aggregated data doesn't display variation in data and will not help in determining if variation is due to random or natural faults in a system (common cause variation) or due to special circumstances that enter a system for a short period of time and have an effect that cannot be explained by random variation (Lloyd, 2004; Nelson et al., 2011).

Figure 15.1 is a bar graph of average length of stay in an emergency department (ED) for FY11 Quarter 2. This figure illustrates summary data. One possible judgment from this graph is that the length of stay in April was better than that in either May or June. This approach does not provide information about the processes related to length of stay in the ED over time. Table 15.2 provides the raw data that were aggregated to produce the bar graph in Figure 15.1.

If we change the way that the data are displayed, we can see something very differently (see Figures 15.2–15.4).

When you plot the data over time and by month, what conclusions do you now make? If you were using the summary data in Figure 15.1, you may be led to believe that in April emergency department length of stay (ED LOS) was better than in either May or June. When you look at the line charts by month, you can see a very different story. In fact, the median ED LOS was lowest for the month of June. You cannot tell that from the summary data presented in Figure 15.1. In the three graphs that show data in a time series, you can see that there are days when the LOS is very high and those where it is either at or below the goal of 180 minutes. Further analysis would reveal that the days when the LOS is high are weekend days. This data is now useful for performance improvement. It provides clues as to where there are opportunities for improvement in existing processes. When you overlay the results for all 3 months in the quarter, you can see how each month's performance compares to the goal of 180 minutes.

In Figure 15.5, you can easily see that the months of May and June had most of its data points below the goal line. The month of April had none of its data points below the goal line. This information tells you that for most of the days in May and June, the LOS was at or below the goal of 180 minutes. When looking at the days when LOS was higher than desired, you can drill down to the potential causes in

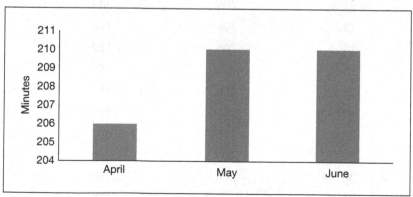

FIGURE 15.1 Bar graph of ED LOS by minutes for 3 months.

ED LOS, emergency department length of stay.

TABLE 15.2 Example of Raw Data for ED by Days for 3 Months

	ED LOS (GOAL: 180)		
Day	April 2011	May 2011	June 2011
1	206	300	150
2	206	160	160
3	206	235	340
4	206	165	340
5	206	160	160
6	206	165	165
7	206	308	150
8	206	300	150
9	206	180	160
10	206	180	340
11	206	180	340
12	206	160	165
13	206	160	160
14	206	310	165
15	206	340	160
16	206	160	170
17	206	165	340
18	206	165	340
19	206	160	160
20	206	160	165
21	206	308	180
22	206	300	180
23	206	170	160
24	206	189	340
25	206	180	340
26	206	165	165
27	206	170	150
28	206	300	165
29	206	310	160
30	206	160	180
31	–	160	–
Average in minutes	206	210.48	210.00

ED LOS, emergency department length of stay.

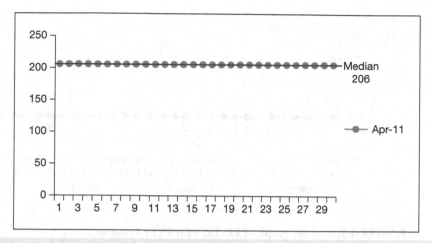

FIGURE 15.2   Run chart of ED LOS, April 2011.

ED LOS, emergency department length of stay.

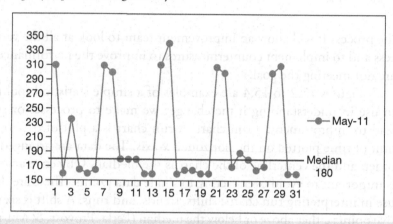

FIGURE 15.3   Run chart of ED LOS, May 2011.

ED LOS, emergency department length of stay.

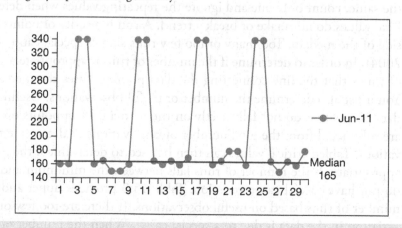

FIGURE 15.4   Run chart of ED LOS, June 2011.

ED LOS, emergency department length of stay.

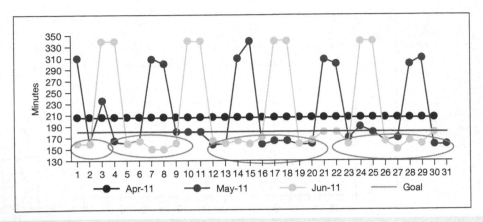

FIGURE 15.5 Line graph of ED LOS for FY11 Quarter 2.

ED LOS, emergency department length of stay.

the process. It will allow an improvement team to look at all the variables in the process and to implement countermeasures to improve the performance on the days that are not meeting the goal.

Figures 15.2 to 15.4 are examples of a simple statistical tool that is important to use in understanding if the changes we make to processes or systems over time lead to improvement: a run chart. A run chart is a plot of data over time with the unit of time plotted on the horizontal *x*-axis. The data are arranged in chronological order, and the centerline of the chart is the median. Objective analysis of run charts is important to avoid overreacting to single data points. There are three basic rules to use in interpreting run charts: shifts, trends, and runs. A shift is six or more consecutive points either above or below the median (Perla, Provost, & Murray, 2011). Points that fall on the median do not count in the shift. A trend is five or more consecutive points all going up or down (Perla et al., 2011). If two or more consecutive values are the same, count only one and ignore the repeating values when determining a shift. Like values do not make or break a trend. A run is a series of points in a row on one side of the median. Too many or too few runs signals special cause variation (Lloyd, 2004). In order to determine if the number of runs is appropriate, count the number of times that the line connecting the data points crosses the median and add one. You must also determine the number of useful observations. Useful observations are data points that do not fall exactly on the median. Data points on the median line are subtracted from the total number of observations to determine the useful observations. Tabled critical values can then be used to determine if the number of runs is appropriate. If the number of runs falls between the minimum and maximum, you do not have special cause variation. Table 15.3 provides upper and lower limits for number of runs based on useful observations. If there are too few or too many runs, variation in the data is due to a special cause. When the number of runs falls below the upper and lower limits, variation is from common cause or random variation in processes (Lloyd, 2004).

TABLE 15.3 Test for Too Many or Too Few Runs on a Run Chart

Total Number of Data Points That Do Not Fall on the Median	Lower Limit for the Number of Runs	Upper Limit for the Number of Runs
10	3	9
11	3	10
12	3	11
13	4	11
14	4	12
15	5	12
16	5	13
17	5	13
18	6	14
19	6	15
20	6	16
21	7	16
22	7	17
23	7	17
24	8	18
25	8	18
26	9	19
27	10	19
28	10	20
29	10	20
30	11	21
31	11	22
32	11	23
33	12	23
34	12	24
35	12	24
36	13	25
37	13	25
38	14	26
39	14	26
40	15	27

Source: Adapted from Perla, R. J., Provost, L. P., & Murray, S. K. (2011). The run chart: A simple analytical tool for learning from variation in healthcare processes. *BMJ Quality & Safety, 20,* 46–51.

There are other useful tools and techniques to guide the use of data. The control chart offers another method to display data over time. The major difference between a run chart and a control chart is that the centerline is the mean (vs. median) and there are both upper and lower control limits in the control chart. The control limits define the boundaries of variation around the mean (Lloyd, 2004). Points between the boundaries represent normal variation around a mean and points outside the limits signals a special cause (Lloyd, 2004). The method to construct a control chart is beyond the scope of this chapter. Further information can be obtained in classical statistics textbooks.

■ MEASUREMENT FOR IMPROVEMENT: WHERE THE RUBBER MEETS THE ROAD

We learned earlier in this chapter that the driving force for measurement in practice is to inform improvement processes. It is important to understand if changes we make to processes result in actual improvements. The Institute for Healthcare Improvement (IHI) provides a framework for this.

The IHI's Model for Improvement (see www.ihi.org/knowledge/Pages/HowtoImprove/default.aspx) outlines a structure for testing change ideas that are expected to result in improvements. The model starts with three questions that help to focus the improvement project: "What are we trying to accomplish?" or "What is the aim of the work?"; "How will we know that a change is an improvement?" or "What are the measures for the project?"; and "What changes can we make that will result in an improvement?" or "What are the changes that will be implemented and tested?" The second part of the model provides the structure for executing small tests of change using the plan–do–study–act, or PDSA, method, pioneered by Walter Shewhart and promoted by W. E. Deming (Nelson et al., 2011). The planning phase is where the objective and specific changes to be tested are outlined. It details all of the steps necessary to carry out the test, including roles, functions, education needed, how data will be collected, and how long the test will last. In the "do" phase, execution of the test is carried out, and the "study" phase is used to analyze the data collected during the "do" phase. When conclusions from the data are drawn, the act phase occurs and modifications to the plan are made if expected results are not achieved. If desired results were achieved, plan for dissemination can then be made.

It is extremely important to select a balanced set of measures to inform improvement processes. A scorecard that incorporates process, outcome, and balancing measures will provide a comprehensive set of data to inform the effectiveness of the improvement effort (Institute of Healthcare Improvement, 2011).

There are some pitfalls to measurement for improvement that need to be considered and avoided. Aside from the principles discussed, it is important to ensure that working definitions for your outcomes are established and understood by all who are involved in the improvement process. For example, how do you define a patient fall? The Agency for Healthcare Research and Quality (AHRQ) defines a fall as:

> an unplanned descent to the floor with or without injury to the patient. Include falls when a patient lands on a surface where you wouldn't expect to find a patient. All unassisted and assisted falls are to be included whether they result from physiological reasons (fainting) or environmental reasons (slippery floor). (AHRQ, 2013)

Without clarification of working definitions there is potential for multiple interpretation of a fall, such as exclusion of assisted falls and falls which result in patients landing on surfaces other than a floor. Lack of clarity on this definition will result in inaccurate outcomes measures. Clearly articulating working definitions and educating all improvement team members to those definitions is essential in achieving desired results.

Another, and perhaps equally important consideration is that clarifying the single data source (source of truth) for all data collection elements is essential. Not doing so could lead to data being gathered in multiple manners and from different sources, which will invalidate the findings of the improvement work. In today's healthcare environment, electronic health records are required and should be relied on to the greatest extent possible since discrete data can be extracted relatively easily and can be formatted for ease of use in improvement work.

The final consideration, and perhaps the most frequent error, in measurement for improvement is the failure to collect baseline data prior to the implementation of any countermeasures or interventions. If you don't know where you started, it is impossible to know if what you have done resulted in improvement.

Regardless of the framework used for improvement, measurement and analysis of data in a systematic way should be what drives improvement. It is important for DNP-prepared nurses to be competent in the techniques and tools used to evaluate the performance of processes and to then translate that knowledge to inform improvements in care.

■ SUMMARY

This chapter discusses various concepts in outcomes measurement. It is important to understand the purpose of measurement in order to select appropriate measures. Measurement for research differs from measurement for judgment or improvement. We use measurement in research as the platform for evidence-based practice. In practice, measurement is used primarily to drive improvement. Translating research into practice requires the use of basic performance improvement frameworks and concepts. Identifying best practices through research and comparing the outcomes of research to those in practice will help to identify areas in need of improvement. Use of an improvement framework, such as the IHI's Model for Improvement, provides structure for improvement work. Selecting balanced metrics to reflect the effectiveness of the improvement effort raises the probability of success. Knowledge of some basic statistical tools and analysis, as well as an understanding of the common pitfalls of measurement, is an important competency for the DNP-prepared nurse to have in order to lead improvement efforts in practice.

It is important to remember that the goal is not measurement; rather, the goal is improvement. Measurement provides information to inform processes of care that will result in better outcomes for patients in both quality and safety arenas.

■ REFERENCES

Agency for Healthcare Research and Quality. (2013). Preventing falls in hospitals. Retrieved from http://www.ahrq.gov/professionals/systems/hospital/fallpxtoolkit/fallpxtk5.html

American Association of Colleges of Nursing. (2006). *The essentials of doctoral education for advanced practice nursing.* Retrieved from http://www.aacnnursing.org/Portals/42/Publications/DNPEssentials.pdf

Centers for Medicare & Medicaid Services. (2017a, July). Core measures. Retrieved from https://www.cms.gov/Medicare/Quality-Initiatives-Patient-Assessment-Instruments/QualityMeasures/Core-Measures.html

Centers for Medicare & Medicaid Services. (2017b, September). *Hospital value-based purchasing.* Retrieved from https://www.cms.gov/Outreach-and-Education/Medicare-Learning-Network-MLN/MLNProducts/downloads/Hospital_VBPurchasing_Fact_Sheet_ICN907664.pdf

Chassin, M. R., Loeb, J. M., Schmaltz, S. P., & Wachter, R. M. (2010). Accountability measures: Using measurement to promote quality improvement. *New England Journal of Medicine, 363*(7), 683–688.

Donabedian, A. (1988). The quality of care: How can it be assessed? *The Journal of the American Medical Association, 260*(12), 1743–1748.

Donabedian, A. (2005). Evaluating the quality of medical care. *The Milbank Quarterly, 83*(4), 691–729.

Griggs, C. L., Schneider, J. C., Kazis, L. E., & Ryan, C. M. (2017). Patient-reported outcomes measurement. *Annals of Surgery, 265*(6), 1066–1067.

Hamric, A. B., Spross, J. A., & Hanson, C. M. (Eds.). (2009). *Advanced practice nursing: An integrative approach* (4th ed.). St. Louis, MO: Saunders Elsevier.

Institute of Healthcare Improvement. (2011). Science of improvement: Establishing measures. Retrieved from http://www.ihi.org/knowledge/Pages/HowtoImprove/ScienceofImprovementEstablishingMeasures.aspx

Institute of Medicine. (2001). *Crossing the quality chasm: A new health system for the 21st century.* Washington, DC: National Academies Press.

Kleinpell, R., & Gawlinski, A. (2005). Assessing outcomes in advanced practice nursing practice: The use of quality indicators and evidence-based practice. *AACN Clinical Issues, 16*(1), 43–57.

Lloyd, R. (2004). *Quality health care: A guide to developing and using indicators.* Sudbury, MA: Jones & Bartlett.

Nelson, E. C., Batalden, P. B., Godfrey, M. M., & Lazar, J. S. (Eds.). (2011). *Value by design: Developing clinical microsystems to achieve organizational excellence* (1st ed.). San Francisco, CA: Jossey-Bass.

Oermann, M. H. W., & Floyd, J. A. (2002). Outcomes research: An essential component of the advanced practice nurse role. *Clinical Nurse Specialist, 16*(3), 140–144.

Perla, R. J., Provost, L. P., & Murray, S. K. (2011). The run chart: A simple analytical tool for learning from variation in healthcare processes. *BMJ Quality & Safety, 20*, 46–51.

Solberg, L. I., Mosser, G., & McDonald, S. (1997). The three faces of performance measurement: Improvement, accountability, and research. *Joint Commission Journal on Quality Improvement, 23*(3), 135–147.

The Joint Commission. (2017a). Facts about accountability measures. Retrieved from https://www.jointcommission.org/facts_about_accountability_measures

The Joint Commission. (2017b). Facts about ORYX® for hospitals (National hospital quality measures). Retrieved from http://www.jointcommission.org/facts_about_oryx_for_hospitals

Variation. (2008). In *Webster's New World College Dictionary* (4th ed.). Boston, MA: Houghton Mifflin Harcourt.

Introduction: Policy, Politics, and the DNP

STEPHANIE W. AHMED

America's present need is not heroics but healing; not nostrums but normalcy; not revolution but restoration.
                                                            —Warren G. Harding

The American healthcare landscape is undergoing rapid change. Within our society, there are economic and social implications of policy decisions that can influence the health of the nation—they present to us as opportunities to create a *healthier future for all*. With respect to national debates around access to healthcare coverage and payment reform, we are being asked not only to consider health as a value but further challenged to create equitable access and improve the outcomes. While a strong recognition exists for how biology, genetics, or even how individual behaviors might influence health, we must broaden traditional conversations, considering the social, economic, and environmental factors that influence the health of individuals—social determinants of health (Healthy People 2020, 2017).

DNPs, through their diverse roles, must not only be conversant relative to practice-specific issues, they must also be positioned to make an impact through participation in policy development and the larger legislative process. In this section, Ober and Wilkie create a foundational understanding of health policy for the DNP, with content that supports the practice of effective advocacy. Sroczynski, Cadmus, and Polansky transport us to the intersection of health policy and cross-sector partnerships, where they highlight how nurses are engaging community partners, seeking to create health as a shared value and fostering collaboration that promises to create healthier, more equitable communities. Further, given nursing's social contract with society, we are reminded by Davis, Corless, and Nicholas that such efforts should not be limited to home, effective DNPs must be able to translate the policy and advocacy skill-set to the global arena, seeking to impact larger public health agendas.

◼ REFERENCE

Healthy People 2020. (2017, September 8). *Determinants of health*. Retrieved from https://www
.healthypeople.gov/2020/about/foundation-health-measures/Determinants-of-Health

Effective Policy and Advocacy for Nurses Engaged in Advanced Practice

STACEY OBER AND SARAH WILKIE

Healthcare reform initiatives that address payment and delivery transformation have created a new landscape within the U.S. healthcare system. Nurses are being asked to assume new and enhanced roles in the delivery of care. After all, nursing has consistently been reported to be the most trusted of occupations (Norman, 2016). However, barriers to realization of these opportunities persist. For instance, optimization of the nursing workforce to the full extent of education and training is impeded by antiquated laws and regulations.

Successful changes that ultimately benefit patients can be achieved through effective policy and advocacy, however. Accordingly, nurses are in a unique position to influence policy makers because they comprise a sizeable and trusted voice. Taking advantage of the profession's inherent credibility depends upon being motivated, organized, and policy-savvy. The proximity of nurses to their patients makes them a knowledgeable resource for policy makers. Further, the profession's social justice underpinnings establish a clear duty to patients who can provide nurses with strong motivation to act. This chapter is designed to review fundamentals of public policy development so nurses engaged in advanced nursing practice can appreciate how to best advocate beyond the patient's bedside into the greater healthcare reform environment in ways that positively impact delivery systems and patients within the United States.

■ THE PUBLIC SECTOR

Before discussing the importance of health policy and its impact on the profession of nursing and the patients they serve, it is essential to understand the basics of public policy in the United States. Unlike most countries around the globe, as

Massachusetts founding father John Adams famously opined, "We are a government of laws, not men" (John Adams Quotes, n.d.). As citizens of a nation governed by law, it is essential to understand how laws are made and how democracy works.

In adopting the U.S. Constitution, the founding fathers wrote the principles for the branches of government and established public policy domains. There were decisions about what subject matters required uniformity across these newly independent but joined states, and what decisions would be better left to the discretion of each sovereign state entity. Nursing practice lacks uniformity today because of this concept of state sovereignty. Areas of federal jurisdiction are limited, clearly spelled out in the Constitution, and include matters of national importance such as interstate commerce, taxation, and the military. The thirteen colonies that first formed our union made clear that each would still enjoy the freedom to legislate and regulate everything not detailed in the Constitution as a federal matter of importance, from real and personal property to matters of public health, safety, and welfare. State legislatures take the separation of power seriously and may at times push back against federal influence over their public policy decision making. Legislative bodies, Congress or state lawmakers, make the laws. Under the Constitution and its doctrine of separation of powers, it is the executive branch with its responsible agencies, the president, or a state's governor that is responsible for implementing and enforcing the laws through rules and regulations.

The third branch of government is the judicial system. Under the Constitution, the executive branch is solely charged with carrying out and enforcing the law. At times, the executive branch may be viewed as overreaching its authority while implementing the laws adopted by the legislative branch. The line of demarcation between federal and state lawmaking authority or "jurisdiction," and the extent and reach of each, may at times become obscured. Moreover, efforts expended by Congress at the federal level are frequently designed to expand federal influence and control over the states by either granting or cutting federal funding in exchange for state adoption of specific policies. Typically, where there is a lack of clarity, the judicial branch provides guidance by issuing court decisions or advisory rulings after reviewing the law and set of facts presented. Such court decisions, known as "case law," provide necessary policy guidance at times. These principles and dynamics most certainly all play out during health policy formation as well. One of the most significant examples is the U.S. Supreme Court's decision in National Federation of Independent Business v. Sebelius, 567 U.S. 1 (2012), 183 L. Ed. 2d 450, 132 S.Ct. 2566. In this case, the U.S. Supreme Court stated that the Patient Protection and Affordable Care Act (ACA) was not an unconstitutional exercise of power by the U.S. Congress, which required nonexempt individuals to obtain health insurance or be penalized under Congress's constitutional federal authority to tax and spend. The policy debate around how much Congress believes it ought to tax individuals and spend on healthcare coverage is an ongoing policy conversation in Washington, DC, but confirmation that Congress does have the constitutional authority to do it was settled by the Supreme Court of the United States in 2012.

POWERS TO REGULATE NURSING RESERVED FOR THE STATES

Laws and regulations applying to healthcare and nursing practice are proposed, debated, and signed at both the state and federal levels of government. At the turn of the 20th century, state legislatures began adopting laws overseeing the health professions in the interest of the public's health, safety, and general welfare. Shortly thereafter, due to the nature of the work of healthcare providers and their potential to do the public harm, state laws established professional licenses to authorize a scope of activities, or "practice," for specific professions. This is referred to as the state's legal scope of practice. Boards of registration issuing licenses are the state agencies within the executive branch with responsibility for overseeing the profession consistent with state law and ensuring that rules and regulations align with professional organizations' safe standards of practice. While a health professional today may be educated and trained consistent with uniform national educational standards, a state's restrictive legal scope of practice and implementing regulations may either expressly prohibit specific practice activities or fail to include certain activities by licensees. As advances in healthcare technology are made, antiquated laws and regulations pose real challenges for the health professions because changes to their legal scope of practice often do not keep pace with evolving national standards of professional practice.

The U.S. Constitution provides the legal backdrop for why state legislators continue to be encumbered with decision making regarding the health professions' legal scope of practice. A natural consequence of this jurisdictional framework enjoyed by the individual states is the potential for wide variation in state laws affecting access to care, services covered by health plans, and employment laws, for example. In the case of healthcare, this may mean that patients receive a very different type of care when crossing state lines. Therefore, many professional nurse organizations adopt a state-by-state approach when working to reform state licensure restrictions, among other policy issues that fall within the state's jurisdiction.

The AANP and State-Level Issues: Among AANP's policy agenda items, there are a number of priorities which must be addressed at the state level because they fall under state jurisdiction, such as modernizing state licensure laws, streamlining care delivery with nurse practitioner (NP) signature recognition, and building flexible and sustainable reimbursement and care delivery models (American Association of Nurse Practitioners, 2018).

When the federal government directs federal resources for state programming, they can have substantial influence over policy details traditionally left for the states to determine. There is no finer example than the specific and ever-changing rules promulgated by the Centers for Medicare and Medicaid Services (CMS). In 1965, Congress enacted laws establishing the Medicare and Medicaid programs and defined the eligibility requirements to become a beneficiary of the programs' health coverage (Rettig, 2011). Federal law requires an individual be 65 years or older in order to qualify for Medicare coverage and proof of disability or low income is required to qualify for Medicaid coverage (Rettig, 2011). The U.S. federal government finances the Medicare program independently, while it shares the cost

NCSBN's Consensus Model: Oftentimes, state legislators voice feeling ill-equipped to determine legal scope of practice for professions. As a result, the participation of nurses in policy regarding their scope of practice is critical in informing legislators with the specifics that likely fall outside of the legislator's expertise. To establish uniformity across the states on how to best regulate nurses and protect the public, the National Council of State Boards of Nursing (NCSBN) developed the Advanced Practice Registered Nurse (APRN) Consensus Model Legislation for adoption by individual state legislatures (APRN Consensus Work Group & The National Council of State Boards of Nursing APRN Advisory Committee, 2008). The model relies on accreditation processes for education and certification of APRNs. Also developed was the Nurse Licensure Compact aligning consistency in nursing preparation and practice. The goal was not to usurp state lawmakers' authority to legislate in this area, but to create consistency in regulating nurses along the lines of uniform education, training, and expected patterns of practice behavior. The NCSBN's expertise in drafting model licensure language has been a benefit to lawmakers in providing policy guidance based upon extensive research. Great progress has been made at the state level in the adoption of Nurse Licensure Compact's legal language which permits a nurse licensed in a Compact state to care for patients not only in that specific state but also in all other states that have legislatively adopted Compact licensure language. In this sense, Compact licensure, which offers consistency in practice standards and promotes fluidity in movement across state lines, can be likened to licensure to operate a motor vehicle. Motorists licensed in one state may lawfully drive in another, and this makes sense. So too does this type of uniformity make sense for nursing practice. Nationally, more work remains to be done to create uniformity; for example, adopting NCSBN's model legislative text licensing APRNs would authorize full practice authority across all participating states.

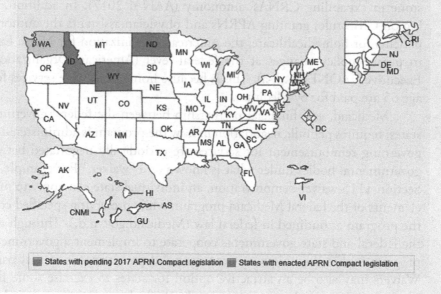

Source: National Council of State Boards of Nursing. (2017). Advanced Practice Nurse Compact [Map]. Retrieved from https://www.ncsbn.org/aprn-compact.htm

of Medicaid in partnership with the individual states. This financial arrangement, debated by Congress and spelled out in federal law, directly influences the structure of how these two programs work. For example, the ability to dialyze an end-stage renal disease (ESRD) patient and prevent imminent death was new technology back in the 1960s. Advocates dialyzed a patient during a Congressional hearing in the presence of members of Congress and, as a result, ESRD is the only chronic disease condition included in the eligibility requirements for Medicare. If an individual is diagnosed with ESRD it results in Medicare payment for health services regardless of age (Rettig, 2011). The aforementioned is a powerful example of the impact advocates had on an entire patient population by participating in the lawmaking process.

A necessary component of CMS programs' administration is the payment structure, which CMS dictates through federal regulations promulgated by the executive branch to specify the terms and amount of payment. According to Medicare regulations, all participating hospitals and providers must demonstrate certain conditions of participation to receive reimbursement in exchange for services delivered to the beneficiaries of this public, government-sponsored program. National accreditation is routinely required as a condition of payment for healthcare facilities. Another example of such a condition is provider type of licensure. In the case of APRNs, CMS early on did not recognize APRNs in their program's payment structures. In fact, advocacy efforts led by the American Association of Nurse Anesthetists (AANA) informed the Omnibus Budget Reconciliation Act of 1986 adopted by Congress, which included a direct reimbursement provision for certified registered nurse anesthetists (CRNAs) (American Association of Nurse Anesthetists [AANA], 2017). This provision made CRNAs the first nursing specialty to gain the right to bill Medicare directly for services and receive reimbursement, which symbolized a significant milestone in expanding CRNAs' autonomy (AANA, 2017). In addition, when working on CMS rules granting APRNs and physician assistants the authority to certify patients for home healthcare, the American Organization for Nurse Executives had to pursue policy changes at the federal level (American Organization for Nurse Executives [AONE], n.d.-a). This is because home healthcare services for those over age 65 are paid for by Medicare.

Medicaid, as a financial partnership between the federal government and the states, requires periodic negotiation in how the program is administered. Regulations governing reimbursement for services are periodically negotiated between the two governmental bodies under what is known as a "waiver." For example, through the Section 1115 waiver demonstration, an individual state can apply to modify certain elements of the federal Medicaid program, while preserving specified core tenants of the program as outlined in federal law (Medicaid.gov, n.d.). Through these waivers, the federal and state governments cooperate to implement a government-sponsored program within the unique environment and patient needs of that particular state. Waivers may also be an attractive option for states to exercise some flexibility and experimentation in the manner through which they administer their Medicaid program, while still maintaining the overarching federal objectives of the program as Congress intended.

ADVOCATING FOR A DEVELOPING NURSE WORKFORCE AT THE FEDERAL LEVEL

Another area the federal government commonly exercises its influence with the states is through nursing workforce development. Nursing education is key to maintaining the high standard of excellence that nurses have established, expanding nurses' role in filling gaps in the healthcare system, and recruiting faculty to prepare the next generation of nurses. Workforce development was first supported by the federal government in 1964 through the passage of the Nurse Training Act, Title VIII of the Public Health Service Act (PHSA) (Reyes-Akinbileje, 2005). At the time of passage, there was recognition by studies conducted by the Surgeon General that there was a nursing shortage, expected to grow, if left unaddressed (Reyes-Akinbileje, 2005). Through Title VIII, federal money was allocated to support nursing education. Over time, the Act was reauthorized and expanded to include sponsorship for student loan programs and construction grants for nursing schools (Reyes-Akinbileje, 2005). However, the role of the federal government in financially continuing to support the nursing workforce was unclear and there were competing priorities for the federal funds devoted to nurse workforce development. Congress did not unanimously agree on how the federal government should support the nursing workforce and even debated the magnitude of the nursing shortage itself (Reyes-Akinbileje, 2005). The Institute of Medicine (IOM) was commissioned by Congress to evaluate the state of nursing in the United States and to make recommendations to Congress for further funding. In 1979, the IOM determined that while there was still a nursing shortage, generalist education alone would suffice in supporting development of the nursing workforce. As a result, many provisions of Title VIII were repealed in the 1980s (Reyes-Akinbileje, 2005). Over the past several decades, the role of the federal government remains uncertain, as those funding levels, known as "appropriations", continue to change despite widespread belief of an impending nursing shortage that will result from aging baby boomers, retiring caregivers, and growing career options for women. As a result, professional nurse organizations today must continue to annually advocate in Washington, DC, for additional workforce development resources. Along with other professional nursing organizations, the American Organization of Nurse Executives continues to make nursing workforce development a policy priority and annually advocates for educational funding in the federal budget to specifically prepare nurses to practice in underserved areas, support loan forgiveness programs, and create opportunities for nursing faculty (AONE, n.d.-a).

Because healthcare services are inextricably entwined with public safety, it is one of the most highly regulated industries in the United States. Reimbursement for health services is contingent upon adherence to many federal agency rules. In addition, healthcare facilities must also comply with their state licensure rules and other state operating requirements designed to ensure public safety. Professional organizations frequently provide their members with educational resources and assistance in monitoring the ongoing changes to these public rules in order to ensure continued compliance.

■ THE PRIVATE SECTOR

In addition to public laws and regulations that guide a healthcare professional's practice, private entities such as healthcare systems, provider groups, and health plans all have the authority and responsibility to adopt their own policies and procedures. Private entities are free to enter into business relationships, contracts, and financial risk arrangements that reflect their business operations. These terms of agreement between private entities may also significantly influence the daily practice of an advanced practice nurse.

Many hospitals were initially established as nonprofit corporations and categorized as charitable organizations formed in the interest of the public good. With exemptions from some tax requirements and limitations on exposure to liability, charitable organizations may have responsibilities to the communities they serve as defined in state law as community benefits. Healthcare organizations today may also be for-profit corporations owned by investors, a multihospital system, or other parent corporation. Whether for profit or nonprofit, healthcare entities have a private governance structure that is responsible for operations, ensuring compliance with all laws, regulations, and rules, and also for adopting policies and formulating rules. It is important to understand that public laws, regulations, and rules create a floor, or a minimum set of expectations. The private healthcare entity, however, can create a ceiling of additional expectations for themselves, as long as they do not break the law or violate an individual's constitutional rights when doing so.

For instance, selection and review of the performance of medical staff is an important function of the hospital governance structure. Likewise, a hospital bylaw or physician group practice's policy may provide a job description for an APRN employee that is more restricted than what the state's legal scope of practice authorizes the APRN to do. When an APRN accepts a job, at minimum, restrictions on practice are set according to law. However, nothing in the law requires that a private entity compensate the APRN to provide all of those services for which they are actually authorized by state law to perform. Furthermore, if state law does not require physician supervision of the APRN, an employing private physician or hospital bylaw may still require supervision, if they choose. On the contrary, a hospital bylaw or group practice cannot provide a job description that is outside the legal scope or broader than what the state nurse practice act authorizes that APRN to do. Thus, if state law requires physician supervision of APRN practice, the legal requirement cannot just be ignored by consenting professionals without risk of serious disciplinary consequences detailed in the licensing bodies' disciplinary regulations.

Policies or requirements may also be established by private stakeholders through private contractual agreements. Before state law expressly prohibited it, health plans in Massachusetts healthcare provider network contracts routinely included a refusal to contract with any provider that already had an affiliation with another health plan. In this instance, if a patient wanted to see a specific provider, they would be forced to select the health plan whose network included that provider. The Massachusetts legislature concluded that these types of business practices were anti-competitive and not in the public's best interests. Similarly, the state was experiencing a serious primary care physician shortage. While Massachusetts state law permitted nurse practitioners (NPs) to serve as primary care providers (PCPs), some health plans were declining to contract with NPs as PCPs on their provider networks. The members of the Massachusetts Coalition of Nurse Practitioners collectively advocated that a health plan's refusal to contract with a provider based upon the provider's type of licensure be made unlawful too. A major healthcare reform proposal subsequently passed with this legal prohibition included (See Mass Gen Laws c. 176D § 3(4)).

When evaluating whether a private stakeholder's business practices or policies violate the law, an examination should be made of both the statutory language in the law itself and the accompanying regulations interpreting it. The law as adopted by Congress or the state legislature takes precedence over any regulation if there is inconsistency or confusion. Because regulations are adopted by the executive branch, they are subject to political influence when either the U.S. president or governor of the state changes and regulations are subsequently amended. Sometimes a review of an old regulation that presents barriers to nursing practice may be found to be inconsistent with what the law actually states and what was originally intended by the legislative branch.

Obviously, it can be very useful to have a lawyer on the advocacy team to provide legal research and analysis. Advocates must be aware, however, that a federal or state law is only as effective as the ability to enforce it. If there is no incentive to comply with a law, individual private entities may choose to ignore it and perhaps risk the financial or punitive consequences. Therefore, when engaging in effective advocacy to change the law, it is important to ensure there are provisions included to ensure compliance. These enforcement tools may take the form of fines, lawsuit, and loss of licensure or even incarceration. In some instances, there may be financial incentives identified to encourage certain business practices, such as public recognition as a certified patient-centered medical home (PCMH) or the opportunity to even contract with the federal or state government for the provision of services. The Medicare Shared Savings Accountable Care Organization (ACO), an alternative payment model developed by CMS, is one example of financial incentives used to shape private business practices because implementing such a program reforms the way healthcare is paid for, which ultimately changes how services will be delivered in practice. As the largest payer of healthcare services, Medicare has enormous influence over how healthcare is delivered and paid for in our country. Once Medicare began allowing APRNs to directly bill for their services, for instance, the private health plans followed suit and changed their private policies to reflect the new Medicare rules.

Private healthcare entities must establish policies and adopt rules to guide their professional practice and business operations, which directly impacts the day-to-day work of nurses. Establishing policy by adopting white papers, guidelines, and professional standards are areas where national organizations are important policy contributors. The professional organization may convene subject matter experts and form committees or taskforces to conduct literature reviews and inform others on best practices. The current National Academy of Medicine, formerly the IOM, is a nonprofit, nongovernmental organization that provides guidance on issues relating to science, medicine, and health. It aims to provide unbiased, objective, evidence-based authoritative information on how to improve our nation's health, upon the request of Congress or governmental agencies (The National Academies of Sciences, Engineering, and Medicine, 2017). In relation to the nursing profession, the IOM issued a landmark report in 2010, *The Future of Nursing: Leading Change, Advancing Health* (IOM, 2011b). The IOM's guidance is held in high regard and has provided direction for practitioners, researchers, and policy makers. Report recommendations for scope of practice, education, and the elimination of barriers to APRN practice are among the current policy priorities of most specialty nurse organizations and affected stakeholders such as AARP.

Central to specialty nurse organizations' advocacy efforts are their work to educate stakeholders, from both private industry and federal and state government, on the use of APRNs to ameliorate issues facing the U.S. healthcare system. Organizations achieve this by producing and distributing fact sheets or hosting briefings. In recognition that members are often responsible for educating the public and policy makers on their role and what they do, the American College of Nurse-Midwives (ACNM) equips members with a comprehensive library of position statements on topics ranging from breastfeeding to climate change, which can supplement educational pursuits (F. Purcell, personal communication, June 26, 2017). Specialty nurse organizations are wonderful places to commence research when seeking to learn more about a particular topic or when developing private institutional policies and procedures for the practice setting.

> **Guidance on Policy Is Fluid and Dynamic:** Nurse researchers and members of the American College of Nurse-Midwives (ACNM), found that the impact of climate change falls disproportionately on women and children and brought this research to the ACNM, which led to the first ACNM-developed position statement on climate change (F. Purcell, Personal communication, June 26, 2017).

Those issues which are most fervently pursued by members or represent the current subject of debate among lawmakers can often become the nurse organization's policy priorities. For example, national APRN associations may issue guidance on issues such as health reform, nursing ethics, staffing, nursing workforce development, and numerous other topics. Policy priorities are fluid and appropriately change as the healthcare payment and delivery landscape also changes. Professional organizations and their members must be nimble in order to tailor their organization's advocacy focus on those issues most relevant at any given point in time.

■ WHERE CAN ADVOCACY FOR ADVANCED PRACTICE NURSING HAVE INFLUENCE?

The nature of healthcare is a matter of life and death. It's no wonder the industry is the most highly regulated in our country, with healthcare practitioners poking and prodding, testing, and prescribing to help extend lives (Livni, 2016). Therefore, there are numerous opportunities where monitoring and participating in the process of policy change can occur. An advanced practice nurse may consider engaging as an individual, or through a collective body, such as a professional organization. Establishing and executing specific policy agendas is one of the most time-consuming and critical services provided by professional nurse organizations on behalf of members. All actively practicing nurses should be invested in this process and at minimum maintain membership for this reason. In addition to receiving updates from the professional nurse organization about the ever-changing healthcare policy environment, there are many sources of reliable and timely information available that individual nurses may subscribe to for free online. The Campaign for Action, supported by the Robert Wood Johnson Foundation and AARP, is working to implement the recommendations from the IOM's *The Future of Nursing* report and distributes a newsletter with updates and advocacy tools. At the state level, the campaign has created active regional action coalitions (RACs) to collaborate and work toward policy updates. The Robert Wood Johnson Foundation has also dedicated resources to a Center for Health Policy at the University of New Mexico to conduct research and policy analyses that address the many social, political, and economic factors that contribute to the inequities observed in health and healthcare in our society. Politico .com, a global news and information online resource, issues daily emails on the topic of health policy and eHealth summarizing federal health initiatives being examined. The Kaiser Family Foundation also distributes a daily health news briefing. Among the first female philanthropists to establish a foundation, Mrs. Stephen V. Harkness, created the Commonwealth Fund. With a mission to promote a high-performing healthcare system, it, too, serves as a source of independent research and provides email alerts on policy topics nurses are likely to care most about. Similar state-based news outlets exist that also summarize valuable information regarding what policy is being considered by whom on the state level and when.

Whether an advanced practice nurse chooses to act as an individual or a collective, there are some key considerations to make before taking action. Federal and state lawmakers develop laws in accordance with their subject matter jurisdiction. Researching lawmakers' expertise and which bills they have previously supported can be an indicator as to which lawmakers will be most likely to support and lead around a particular policy problem or bill. It is also important to identify the appropriate level of government in order to be effective. Any proposed legislation is either federal, being debated by Congress in Washington, DC, or a state proposal being considered by the respective state's legislature. Due to the separation of state and federal subject matter jurisdictions, members of Congress do not take action on state legislation and state lawmakers do not take action on pending federal legislation. The ability to recognize the delineation between federal and state jurisdiction, and advocating at the appropriate level, is a key competency for an effective nurse advocate (J. Webb, personal communication, July 15, 2017). It is easy to determine where pending legislation is being proposed by either obtaining a copy of federal legislative text from the Library of Congress website or searching the state's legislative website for free. The Library of Congress can be accessed at www.congress.gov/quick-search/legislation.

Influencing which legislative proposals are adopted requires influencing those who get elected to make those decisions. Nursing associations typically establish political action committees (PACs) to financially support those candidates for elected office who research demonstrates either act in direct support or are philosophically in alignment with the association's policy agenda. Though money and politics may feel contrary to a nurse's character, there are strict campaign contribution reporting requirements for PACs and political candidates to ensure transparency and weed out corruption.

ACTING AS AN INDIVIDUAL

An individual citizen's voice can be heard in a number of ways. The first is simply to vote in national and local elections. By researching candidates' positions on issues related to healthcare and nursing, a vote can be cast for a candidate with favorable opinions on the policy issues related to the nursing profession. Once in office, representatives can be contacted in person, by phone, email, or letter. Contributing money to a federal or state nursing association PAC is another area where you can have influence by strengthening the PAC's financial resources. PACs may endorse an executive branch candidate for president or governor and ultimately that official will have decision making power over how federal or state laws will be interpreted and implemented via regulations and executive orders.

Individuals have numerous ways to act independently, but may also work together with other like-minded individuals as a collective, pooling resources. It is vital for individuals to raise their voice, but to be heard with many others is very valuable in advocacy efforts (F. Purcell, personal communication, June 26, 2017). Strength in numbers usually translates to more attentive lawmakers.

ACTING AS A COLLECTIVE

Setting the Policy Agenda at the ANA: The policy agenda is developed and updated regularly, based on policy positions and advocacy for a host of issues that align with ANA's mission to improve health for all (P. Cipriano, personal communication, June 26, 2017). Ideas for the agenda, prioritized based on opportunity, importance, and urgency, may come from scanning the environment or surveying members and ANA state constituents. The agenda includes positions pro or con on pending legislation, Supreme Court decisions, or issues ANA wants to advance (P. Cipriano, personal communication, June 26, 2017).

Joining a professional organization is an effective way to coalesce professionals around advocacy activities related to their livelihood. Further, the professional organizations' staff provides valuable expertise. Leaders within organizations are responsible for setting the policy direction for work being performed by the association. This is a key area for advanced practice nurses to actively shape public policy in a number of ways. Internally, the organization may have subject matter committees or taskforces where members or the organization's staff perform literature reviews, discuss findings, and then draft fact sheets, guidelines, or position papers. These authoritative sources may be referenced by health systems, practicing licensees, or the organization's own board of directors in establishing business practices, procedures, public positions, and official testimony. Specifically, specialty nurse organizations' legislative committee participation requires the analysis of how proposed legislation or regulation would impact the ability to access patients, provide quality services, and get appropriately compensated. On behalf of the individual organization, legislative committees typically devise and implement a strategic plan to promote a policy solution to any issue sought to be addressed by a proposed policy change that impacts its interests. These members serve a vital role as the culture and subject matter experts for the advocacy team of lawyers and lobbyists hired to represent the organization in the halls of government. Organizations will often survey their members or solicit feedback from state chapters when defining their policy agenda each year. In addition to the president, member leaders may also represent an organization externally as an appointee to a policy-making committee, advisory council, or taskforce established by a governmental body or elected official. There are also numerous opportunities to volunteer in grassroots efforts or in other volunteer positions.

Participation in a professional organization has a multiplicative effect on advocacy due to the practice of working in coalitions. One professional organization may partner with another to advance policy for shared interests. Working together with other groups can amplify the voice for policy change, but may be challenging at times to find and maintain alignment of mutual goals. The National Council of State Boards of Nursing (NCSBN) assists groups looking to collaborate by providing a consensus-building guide, which can be found in the Resources and Getting Started section of this chapter.

A professional organization may also hold conferences or other events to educate and engage members. The American Nurses Association's (ANA) annual Membership Assembly brings together representatives from its state constituents to conduct the business and set policy for the organization. The meeting, held in Washington, DC, includes "Hill Day," an opportunity to visit members of Congress and speak with them about issues important to nursing. AONE, AANA, American Association of Nurse Practitioners (AANP), ACNM, and NCSBN similarly host annual meetings for members. Additionally, nursing service organizations (NSOs) may also provide networking or mentorship opportunities that can enhance the experience of an advanced practice nurse.

Informing the Agenda as a Member: Within a professional organization, members may be able to directly influence that organization's policy agenda. For example, members of ACNM may participate in committees, including Government Affairs, at both national and state levels with participation at either the national or state chapters, which includes opportunities to communicate issues to the Board or to other organizations in the field (F. Purcell, personal communication, June 26, 2017).

Lastly, with professional organization participation, members are representatives of the profession. Educating the public, in addition to policy makers, is a duty that comes with membership; in fact, in the absence of such education, lack of awareness poses a great barrier to policy change (P. Cipriano, personal communication,

June 26, 2017). Such education may include explaining the work of nurses, or perhaps describing what defines and differentiates the APRN-recognized titles and their respective training. It may include the analysis of clinical outcome data and disseminating an alternative delivery model of care that results in savings to public and private payers. The informational tools, such as fact sheets and white papers, developed by the professional organizations can also serve as a resource that members can distribute. It is important to also educate the public, because as constituents of their respective elected officials, their opinions will strongly influence policy makers.

■ WHY MUST YOU ENGAGE?

After years of rigorous clinical training, nurses are prepared to deliver a high level of care to patients. While their clinical training is comprehensive and focused on excellence, the healthcare system today demands that nurse leaders acquire new competencies, including the ability to analyze policy and understand implications for the profession and therefore patient care. Though nursing academic programs do not commit extensive time and energy toward understanding the fundamentals of advancing health policy within the curriculum, there are, however, numerous reasons why nurses must be active participants in advocating for policies impacting a multitude of healthcare delivery issues such as health disparities, cultural sensitivity, ethics, access to quality care, healthcare finances, and social justice in the delivery of care and the integrity of the profession itself. Among the most salient reasons to engage are the nurse's duty to patients, a business case for nursing, and a rapidly transforming payment and delivery system.

DUTY TO PATIENTS

CRNAs and Pain Management: CRNAs have addressed their duty to patients by advocating to increase their role in pain management (B. Schoneboom, personal communication, June 8, 2017). The National Academy of Medicine estimates that about 100 million Americans face chronic pain (IOM, 2011a). Annually, CRNAs deliver about 43 million anesthetics each year, and so are uniquely positioned to provide relief to patients in chronic pain (AANA, n.d.-b). In support, AANA provides members with clinical, educational resources on pain management, in addition to continually advocating to Congress for increased utilization of CRNAs in chronic pain management (B. Schoneboom, personal communication, June 8, 2017).

Nurses stereotypically have an intrinsic social justice core and a desire to care for patients has influenced their chosen profession. The profession enjoys a social and ethical contract with society (Fowler, 2015). This duty to patients extends outside of the traditional clinical healthcare system into the political world of health policy. When it comes to advocacy, nurses speak on behalf of their patients (C. Cooke, personal communication, June 13, 2017). Motivation to engage in policy making can be a natural fit for nurses because the consequence of public policy adoption has a direct impact on patients and the fabric of our social safety net. For example, Medicaid is one of the largest programs supporting the old, poor, and sick in the United States. Changes to the program, such as budget cuts, time and again result in real challenges for patients to appropriately access the right care in the right setting at the right time. The powerful practice experiences of the nurse are stories that illuminate the impact of such policy changes on the patient and further have the potential to positively influence those forming policy decisions. Research supports that patients are proponents of expanded roles for advanced practice nurses. One such study, surveying consumers on primary care utilization, found that although the majority of patients had a physician as their primary care provider, consumers were open to the option to see an NP instead of waiting to see a physician (Dill, Pankow, Erikson, & Shipman, 2013). In this example, antiquated laws may prevent NPs from practicing to the full extent of their education and training, which directly impacts access to comprehensive healthcare. By not engaging in the policy-making process, nurses disadvantage those patients seeking access to quality care and further risk not being able to practice to the full extent of their education and training.

A BUSINESS CASE FOR EXPANDED ROLES FOR ADVANCED PRACTICE NURSES

Healthcare expenditures are a large and growing proportion of total U.S. expenditures (Peterson-Kaiser, n.d). As a result, policies related to the cost-effectiveness of healthcare delivery are critical. According to *The Future of Nursing* report's argument, evidence suggests that nursing care may attribute to cost savings, though calls for additional research (IOM, 2011b). Research can provide policy makers with evidence and the business case for expanding APRN roles. For example, a study on the cost-effectiveness of anesthesia providers found that CRNAs working as the sole

All healthcare providers are needed and all can contribute to continually improving outcomes (M. Cahill, NCSBN, personal communication, August 11, 2017): APRNs have practiced and prescribed without the required oversight of another profession for more than 25 years in several states. The quality outcomes of that care is no different than in restricted states, and in many cases, full practice states rank among the highest for overall state health (M. Cahill, NCSBN, personal communication, August 11, 2017). Across states with barriers to APRN full practice, legislation is introduced aimed at reducing those barriers and is opposed strenuously by organized medical groups, which the Federal Trade Commission suggests may be about competition and the ability of APRNs to provide the same quality of care more efficiently; however, the very states that have such barriers have shortages of physicians, and that higher demand for their services could increase physician payments (M. Cahill, NCSBN, personal communication, August 11, 2017). Despite the perception that physician salaries suffer in states with full practice authority for APRNs, at least one study has concluded that physician income is not negatively impacted (Pittman & Williams, 2012). APRNs don't practice medicine but do provide health services competently.

anesthesia provider for patients are the most cost-effective delivery option (Hogan, Seifert, Moore, & Simonson, 2010). Further, this study demonstrated that the costs to train a CRNA were less than that of other anesthesia providers (Hogan et al., 2010). In their advocacy efforts, the AANA can leverage this study to demonstrate that anesthesia delivery by CRNAs is not only safe and high quality but also fiscally responsible. Nurse researchers play a key role in advocating a business case that promotes nursing by producing and publishing research examining the cost implications of policy issues under debate.

HEALTHCARE DELIVERY TRANSFORMATION

National expenditures for healthcare spending have grown to an unsustainable level over the past several decades; in 2015, the United States spent $32 billion on healthcare (Peterson-Kaiser, n.d.). The government, through Medicare and Medicaid, and private health plans are attempting to reduce national spending on healthcare by reforming the way that services are reimbursed. Healthcare is increasingly being paid for by demonstrating quality, rather than quantity/volume of services performed, as has been done historically. Providers are measured by select quality metrics, graded according to prespecified benchmarks, and paid accordingly. These payment schemes grade providers and pit healthcare delivery institutions against each other in order to incent continual improvement. However, the data of those providers who deliver healthcare, but do not bill in an identifiable way for their services are excluded. This occurs because old fee-for-service claims data is what is currently available, and therefore used to calculate alternative payment methodologies. Assessment of quality performance is conducted through the National Provider Identifier (NPI) number and attributed to the provider submitting the claims rather than who rendered the care. For example, if a supervising physician submits claims for services rendered by an NP, the quality metrics, which would be most accurately attributed to the NP, are instead attributed to a billing physician's NPI #. While healthcare payment policies promise to shift the incentives to wellness and prevention of illness rather than treating chronic illness, a perhaps unintended consequence of billing under the NPI # is that the data may not accurately represent the care delivered by advanced practice nurses and limit the intended transparency, accountability, and recognition of clinical outcomes-based reimbursement structures. Submitting independent or identifiable claims for services rendered by APRNs is a public and private policy matter critical to their ability to quantify how their practices can positively impact delivery models of care in a value-based healthcare business climate. AANP has supported legislation in Congress which would authorize NPs to certify patients for home care services, and given the past history of the Congressional Budget Office (CBO) scoring, there is a possibility that Congress may view this policy change as resulting in more home care services and more costs to the delivery system (C. Cooke, AANP, personal communication, June 13, 2017). Clearly, the CBO is missing the point that without this change, patients may deteriorate in the home and eventually present to the hospital much

Medicare Reimbursement Under the Quality Payment Program: Nurse executives are increasingly being tasked with protecting and advancing the role of nursing through advocacy (J. Webb, personal communication, June 15, 2017). In 2015, Medicare reformed the way that physicians, advance practice nurses, and physician assistants are reimbursed through the Medicare Access and CHIP Reauthorization Act of 2015 (MACRA) and establishment of the Quality Payment Program (AONE, n.d.-c). As a result, AONE is committed to educating their nurse executive members on key provisions where they must comply and advocating with CMS to ensure that annual updates to the program appropriately measure and reimburse advance practice nurses appropriately (AONE, n.d.-c).

sicker for a lengthy and costlier hospital stay. Opportunity cost refers to the financial impact of making one choice or decision over the cost of making another alternative one. When educating decision makers about policy proposals, nurse leaders can have significant impact by quantifying the "opportunity cost" to the delivery system if their proposed policy changes, such as allowing NPs to certify patients for home care services, are not adopted.

An aging population and the transition of services out of the inpatient setting present additional opportunities to adapt the role that advanced practice nurses have typically held in the United States. For example, a systematic review of the effectiveness of advanced practice nurses in long-term care demonstrated favorable outcomes to patients receiving care from clinical nurse specialists and NPs, including fewer preventable hospitalizations, lower rates of urinary incontinence, fewer pressure ulcers and reports of aggressive behavior and loss of affect, and improved morale of nursing home residents among patients receiving care from NPs (Donald et al., 2013).

The training of advanced practice nurses prepares them to assume new roles within the structure of a changing healthcare system; advocating for policies which support these roles assures improved care for patients and professional satisfaction.

CURRENT GAPS AND FUTURE UNCERTAINTY

In the words of Abraham Lincoln, "The best way to predict your future is to create it." Simply put, there are ways in which the healthcare system in its current form disadvantages patients by impeding the development and practice of advanced practice nurses. The future in healthcare does not guarantee inclusion without advanced practice nurses' participation in collectively advocating for change. In business and politics, you get what you promote, not what you deserve. This sentiment is perhaps not a comfortable concept for a compassionate profession such as nursing, but it is important to understand and accept nonetheless.

Several current issues present opportunities for nurse leaders to impact policy change and provide clear examples of why the professions' voice has an important role to play. For example, the National Institutes of Health (NIH) is a federal research center which funds clinical research. Within NIH, the National Institute of Nursing Research (NINR) holds responsibility for nursing research and research training. In the Fiscal Year 2017, the NINR reported appropriations of approximately $147 million, much of which is distributed through research awards (NINR, 2016). This budget, however, must continually increase to appropriately match the growing magnitude of nurses practicing in the United States. The Bureau of Labor Statistics estimated that there were approximately 2.7 million jobs in the United States for registered nurses alone, and that job outlook was growing much faster than the average rate of job growth (Bureau of Labor Statistics & U.S. Department of Labor, 2016). Further, *The Future of Nursing Report* calls for a substantial increase in the proportion of nurses with a baccalaureate degree and for the number of nurses with a doctorate degree to double by 2020 (IOM, 2011b). If the profession is going to successfully incorporate evidence-based research into clinical practice during this movement toward value-based payment for health services, nurse researchers need adequate resources to study, publish, and share their results. Decision makers, both public and private, will need this knowledge to be shared with them in a clear manner that details the cost implications, including the opportunity costs, of not delivering care differently.

Further, the IOM and other stakeholders have recommended the use of advanced practice nurses to fill current gaps in the healthcare system that leave patients without appropriate care because barriers exist to fully implement these changes. Although establishing residencies for newly graduated APRNs is one IOM recommendation many agree has real value, the funding is missing. Unlike the medical residency program funded by additional Medicare payments for those institutions that accept and mentor new physicians, there is no comparable funding formula for institutions to provide the same support to new APRNs. Until a similar payment stream is secured, chief nursing officers within institutions may have great difficulty establishing such residency programs. For lawmakers, whether federal or state, what is included in the budget blueprint, debated and adopted annually, best reflects the values, and therefore the program funding priorities, of those holding elected office. The budget process is a key policy-making opportunity that should not be missed.

Another glaring gap in advancing the nursing profession through policy is simply that nurses are not provided with sophisticated policy and advocacy training. Nursing program curriculum is comprehensive in clinical training, seeking to prepare students to pass the NCLEX exam upon graduation. Some professional organizations believe the absence of policy fundamentals on the NCLEX itself may therefore be a serious omission, one that perpetuates a perspective that keeping abreast of policy changes and participation in the process is best left to those in the chief executive's suite who better understand the business of healthcare. The aforementioned thinking is not only erroneous, but further fails to express the voice of the professional discipline, which is the authority trusted by patients to ensure the quality and safety of care received.

■ HOW TO BE EFFECTIVE

The ability to positively affect public policy is a skill set that requires timing, accuracy, strategy, and policy-savviness. Nurses hold accurate information in high regard, given the emphasis on clinical excellence during their education and training. Before any patient intervention, nurses are taught to make certain they know what they are doing and why they are doing it. In the world of developing public policy, however, politics reigns. Together with the merit of a policy, the process of adopting policy is managed by a variety of individuals with any number of motives. The unpredictable nature that is politics can have a chilling effect on the desire of nurses to participate in the democratic process. There are, however, absolute patterns of behavior among elected officials. Nurse leaders armed with this know-how can have a collective impact moving forward their agenda on behalf of patients and the profession. The process of how a bill becomes a law and the nuances of congressional or state legislatures' rules can easily be learned from your professional nurse organizations or a review of government websites. Learning how to effectively influence policy making requires learning about a policy maker's personal values and experiences so you can communicate a message that resonates with them after determining strategic action based upon whether you are supporting or opposing a specific policy change.

CRAFTING YOUR ARGUMENT

When a policy problem is raised that may influence the profession, there is traditionally an opportunity to weigh in with support, opposition, or another policy solution. Efforts to support or oppose pending policy proposals are equally important as they both hold potential to directly affect your livelihood, and ultimately patient care. Elected officials will be faced with numerous perspectives that are both different and competing, and will want to understand the perspective of constituents.

To be effective, one must be clear. When promoting adoption, outline the merits of the proposal by first identifying the issue or problem in need of resolution. Second, reference the current federal or state statute or regulation, or recent court decision interpreting the law, that is causing the problem. Always apply the current policy to a real-life set of circumstances to demonstrate how the policy is problematic to clinical practice or for patients. Assist the policy maker in understanding how the proposed change would solve this problem. Finally, anticipate which stakeholder(s) might be opposed to the policy change and outline for the policy maker a response to the opposition's anticipated arguments. Most policy makers are going to research all sides of an issue before making their own decision. This information can be communicated in face-to-face meetings, through briefings, or fact sheets. Following this framework will guide effective communication to convey the merit of a proposal. Professional organizations provide resources to assist members in learning how to craft a strong argument, such as the toolkits provided by the AANP referenced in the Resources and Getting Started section of this chapter.

Stakeholders opposed to a policy change may communicate any number of questions to prevent a policy maker from taking forward action on a measure. The first concern is, most frequently, financial. Lawmakers will be concerned about how much the measure is going to cost the government (federal or state) or who else will be responsible for paying. Advocates and special interest groups must be prepared to provide support for their political priorities by offering an analysis of the financial impact. Legislative bodies will also seek their own objective analysis. Congress relies upon the CBO to provide an impartial fiscal analysis of all proposed legislation. Similarly, state legislatures rely upon a "ways and means" committee. If the measure costs nothing, it is budget neutral and has an easier path to passage. Beware if the opposition is proposing changes to a policy proposal that would result in costs! This could result in implementation expenses that policy makers are not willing to assume and therefore stall passage. At every step of the policy-making process, it is extremely important to follow the money. It will point to natural opponents and may identify a barrier to successful passage. By drafting a policy measure that is either budget neutral or generates the revenue to cover the cost of implementation, policy makers are more likely to consider adoption.

Opponents to a policy proposal may produce data to convey there is no issue or problem that needs to be solved. To thwart state legislation from granting full practice authority to APRNs, medical organizations may present data to suggest there is no shortage of physician providers, and therefore no patient need to enact the legislative proposal. Producing evidence-based research, surveys, or polling data can be a powerful contributor to the debate. Stakeholders that want to maintain the status quo or perceive changed policies as a financial risk to their bottom line may employ any number of delay strategies. By leveraging the evidence-based research, either primary or secondary research, advocates can successfully craft an argument to support a position or dispute the opposition.

Another barrier to successful policy adoption occurs when an issue is currently before the courts for interpretation. Legislators are loath to change the law if the judicial branch of government has a court case under its review. It is common for legislators to wait until the court renders a final decision to see if the law needs clarification or is not working as intended. The aforementioned represents the constitutional principle of separation of power among the executive, legislative, and judicial branches of government. Alternatively, opponents may point to federal law and complain to policy makers that the issue is not appropriate for state lawmakers to decide. With federal policy, opponents could argue to members of Congress that the subject is one for the states to decide and not within the federal government's jurisdiction. An example of this dynamic is the ongoing tension around financing the Medicaid program. How much should the federal government contribute financially to the coverage for beneficiaries versus the states in their partnership to provide for the disabled and low-income citizens who are in need of a safety net remains an ongoing debate.

COMMUNICATION STRATEGY AND WORKING WITH POLICY MAKERS

Anyone with advocacy experience knows that elected officials do not weigh merit alone when adopting a public position on policy proposals. Therefore, it's essential to review political concepts that can guide a clear communication strategy. Whether advocating for support or opposition to pending policy proposals, it is imperative to research the background of the policy maker. One of the most significant mistakes an advocate could make is approaching an elected official with the goal of convincing them to see things "their way." Legislators bring a host of professional and life experiences to the job. Exercise caution not to stereotype along partisan lines of Democrat or Republican. Conduct background research to obtain an understanding of who the policy maker is and what their philosophical leanings might be. Assessing a policy maker is no different than first assessing a patient before taking any action. To be effective, communication must correspond accordingly. Remember that a policy maker who does not support a specific cause of interest could still be a real asset on a future initiative (J. Webb, personal communication, June 15, 2017). Politics is about relationships, which is another area where nurses are skilled experts.

Elected officials also respond to internal and external political pressures. Re-election is on the forefront of their minds, so a policy maker's priorities are also highly reliant upon and representative of what is important to their constituents. Political campaigns for elected office can be very expensive, so policy makers must engage in significant fundraising in order to win re-election and keep the job. This element of our democracy, although essential, can seem distasteful. However, the overwhelming majority of candidates do comply with campaign finance rules, and effective organizations routinely make financial contributions to candidates for office. In addition, avoiding conflict among constituents is ideal for elected officials because it insulates them from angry voters and decreases any risk to their re-election. Oftentimes, policy makers wait for stakeholders to arrive at a compromise instead of immediately choosing a political side of an issue. When credible stakeholders on the same side of an issue come together to form a coalition, the sheer numbers of advocates can sway a policy makers' position. A coalition may represent different perspectives too, which helps the policy maker understand the measure's full impact and importance. The advocacy in support of full practice authority for APRNs by AARP is a wonderful example of how consumers joining a nursing legislative effort has resulted in gains for the profession despite organized medicine's opposition. If parties for and against are unable to reach a compromise on their own, policy makers may broker a compromise they determine to be fair.

Much like the leadership hierarchy that exists within healthcare systems and other provider organizations, the legislative branches operate under the leadership of elected officials who have been chosen by their legislative colleagues to organize the rules and procedures by which decisions are to be made by the chamber. The two-party system of our democracy results in the members of either the Democratic or Republican Party making up the majority, and the others serving as the minority party within the chamber. The majority party has control over prioritizing what legislation will be debated and when. The head of the majority party at the start of each legislative session appoints members of their own party to chair bipartisan committees charged with analyzing legislative proposals and making recommendations. Successfully negotiating a compromise between stakeholders at odds over pending legislation may take pressure off leadership and fellow policy makers from their constituents and can result in positive recognition among legislative colleagues or even promotions to more powerful posts within their chamber of government. Policy makers in leadership positions, such as committee chairs, are frequently called upon to serve in this negotiator role and may take the political heat for everyone by advocating one position over another. The public position by a committee chair can be a signal by the leadership to the members of a policy-making body on how it prefers the members to vote on an issue. Never underestimate the power of recognition. If a specialty nurse organization has the support of an elected official serving in a leadership position, it should be shared broadly with other policy makers. Such information can influence the decision of rank and file members to get onboard or publicly risk being on the wrong or "losing" side of an issue. Recognition can also help build support among and win favor with policy makers. If an elected official takes a favorable action on a matter of interest or perhaps assists in thwarting a measure that is harmful, the savvy advanced practice nurse should make certain that their professional colleagues have been made aware of it. Give credit where credit is due. This promotes the establishment of lasting credible political relationships.

Experiences communicating with elected officials can be frustrating at times. This can be a real hurdle to promoting activism. Rest assured that words do matter in the political world. One must listen attentively to what is actually being said, something nurses are proficient at as well. The trick is figuring out what motivates the elected official. Is it good public policy? Is it getting along with legislative colleagues? Is it getting elected to a more powerful position? Once this knowledge is obtained, it can be used to an advantage to help shape the argument and to articulate how a specific policy aligns with their motivations. If an elected official has aspirations for higher office, for example, sharing polling data on how the public feels about an issue would be of keen interest to them.

To avoid conflict among their constituent voters, politicians can become expert at communicating a message in such a way that is ambiguous, while it is often perceived as essentially what the listener wanted to hear. This communication style can contribute to a negative perception of elected officials, but may only be a matter of not listening closely enough to what is being said.

> **Chair:** Thank you for coming in today to speak with me and my staff. You have been a long-time supporter of me and I really want to learn more about the legislation you are working on.
>
> **Advocate:** Yes, I'm grateful to have the opportunity to review our legislation and explain why it is important to my professional association and the patients we serve. The bill and an explanatory fact sheet are reviewed in the meeting.
>
> **Chair:** Great, thank you for the information. You know I support you. Thank you again for coming in.

Remember, words matter and such conversations require attentive listening skills. Holding policy makers accountable also requires clear communication on what you are asking them to do and why they should do it. In this scenario, the advocate departed from the office believing the chair supported the bill. However, examination of the chair's language suggests the policy maker has reserved the future right to vote either way on the bill. Any public position taken by this policy maker later could reflect how party leadership wants to move on the matter despite this constituent meeting. Without a specific "ask" for support, an opportunity to effectively influence policy outcomes is missed. If the chair's support for the bill was secured during the meeting, the chair might have felt pressed to then advocate on the bill's behalf with leadership, rather than wait for a directive from above. After this meeting, this advocate can only say that the chair supports the advocate's association, but has no idea where the chair stands on the actual legislation.

■ RESOURCES AND GETTING STARTED

Desire is the only prerequisite to becoming an effective advocate (J. Webb, personal communication, June 15, 2017). When the desire and willingness to engage is present, the remaining necessary fundamentals can easily be taught; so find a mentor. There are numerous resources to educate and guide a nurse advocate that can assist both beginners and more seasoned, policy-savvy DNP graduates. When searching for places to learn more about how to participate in policy making, the following resources are good places to start.

Professional nursing organizations provide opportunities for nurses to learn about current policies affecting their profession. These organizations also direct nurses to opportunities to engage in advocacy, by either supplying toolkits or through membership benefits. Following are a number of nursing professional organizations and a sampling of their policy priorities and resources:

AMERICAN ASSOCIATION OF NURSE PRACTITIONERS

- *Policy Priorities:* Improve healthcare by removing barriers to NP practice and patient care. Modernizing NP licensure; streamlining care delivery, such as certification to document a Medicare beneficiaries' eligibility for home health services, authorization to perform admitting exams, and assessments for Medicare beneficiaries in Skilled Nursing Facilities; direct and sustainable reimbursement for NP services, including NP participation in insurance exchanges and other new payment models as full participants; patient-centric health reform in support of advancement of NP roles; funding for Nurse Education Programs.
- *Tools and Resources:* AANP provides toolkits on pursing policy at federal or state policy levels, including talking points, issue briefs, data, and tips on finding your senator and representative (AANP, n.d.-a; n.d.-b).

AMERICAN ORGANIZATION OF NURSE EXECUTIVES

- *Policy Priorities:* Funding for Nursing Workforce Education, proliferation of nursing research and outcomes, support of nurse reimbursement for Medicare services through the Quality Payment Program (J. Webb, personal communication, June 15, 2017).
- *Tools and Resources*: Educational guides on the legislative process, tips for how to communicate with legislators, and a glossary of legislative terms and other resources are made available by the American Organization of Nurse Executives (AONE, n.d.-b).

AMERICAN NURSES ASSOCIATION

- *Policy Priorities*: Healthcare reform ensuring access to affordable insurance and care for all, scope of practice with full practice authority for APRNs; nurse staffing; funding for workforce development (P. Cipriano, personal communication, June 26, 2017).
- *Tools and Resources*: ANA provides educational tools on conducting a political environmental scan, a guide for interpreting proposed regulations, talking points, and a Coalition Building Guide (ANA, n.d.).

AMERICAN ASSOCIATION OF NURSE ANESTHETISTS

- *Policy Priorities*: Ensuring Access to Anesthesia in Rural communities; promotion of pain management services delivered by CRNAs; expanded roles for CRNAs within alternative payment models (B. Schoneboom, personal communication, June 8, 2017).
- *Tools and Resources*: Members may access guides detailing State Legislative and Regulatory Requirement summaries, Opt-Outs and Federal Supervision Requirement, and talking points on CRNA practice (AANA, n.d.-a).

AMERICAN COLLEGE OF NURSE-MIDWIVES

- *Policy Priorities:* Expanded roles for Nurse-Midwives through full practice authority, hospital credentialing, and reimbursement; state licensure of birth centers and home births; state recognition of the Certified Midwife and Certified Professional Midwife Credential (F. Purcell, personal communication, June 26, 2017).
- *Tools and Resources:* ACNM equips members with guidance documents, fact sheets, and a Legislative Tracking tool (ACNM, n.d.).

NATIONAL COUNCIL OF STATE BOARDS OF NURSING

- *Policy Priorities:* State-to-state uniformity in APRN regulation; improved collection and analysis of nursing workforce data; inclusion of nurse regulators in Health Policy discussions; educating others about Nursing regulation (M. Cahill & N. Livanos, personal communication, June 27, 2017)
- *Tools and Resources:* The NCSBN supplies a guides for working in coalitions to create consensus called the APRN Consensus Model Toolkit (NCSBN, n.d.).

State agencies and nonprofits can also be helpful resources for an effective advocate:

- GovTrack is a search engine that can be used to identify and track bills currently in the House and Senate (www.govtrack.us).
- Free access to federal legislative text is available through the Library of Congress (www.congress.gov/quick-search/legislation).
- The Centers for Disease Control and Prevention (CDC) created an analytical framework for assessing problems facing the healthcare system and policy solutions that educates readers to identify a problem, formulate a policy solution, and analyze proposed policies (www.cdc.gov/policy/analysis/process/analysis.html).
- The CDC also provides the "Core Economic and Budgetary Indicators" framework and criteria for making a business case for a healthcare problem, such as reporting the cost savings or costs averted (www.cdc.gov/policy/analysis/docs/oadp_fact-sheet_economicindicators.pdf).
- A beginner's guide to learning about the federal budget can be found through the National Priorities Project (www.nationalpriorities.org/about/mission).

There are also numerous ways to advocate on behalf of the nursing profession to members of Congress:

- To find a representative use the U.S. House of Representatives website's "Find Your Representative" search engine (www.house.gov/representatives/find).
- To contact a representative by phone, use the U.S. Capitol Switchboard at 202-224-3121.
- To contact a member of Congress by mail, use this address format:

For Senators
The Honorable (Full Name)
[Room #] [Building Name] Senate Office Building
United States Senate
Washington, DC 20510

For Representatives
The Honorable (Full Name)
[Room #] [Building Name] House Office Building
United States House of Representatives
Washington, DC 20515

■ CALL TO ACTION

Today represents a critical time for the nursing profession. Nurses engaged in advanced practice are situated at the nexus of a rapidly evolving healthcare system with shifting payments based on quality and value of care and the endurance of antiquated laws and regulations governing nursing practice. Joyce Clifford, RN, PhD, the former Chief Nursing Officer of the Beth Israel Hospital in Boston, Massachusetts, is remembered for her leadership and mentoring of future nurse leaders. She thought that education, practice, and policy should happen along a continuum, and influencing one requires making a correction to the other (J. Clifford, personal communication to S. Ahmed). Similarly, advocacy is a life-long expectation for the nurse engaged in advanced practice (P. Cipriano, personal communication, June 26, 2017). Health policy must keep pace with the evolution of standards of nursing practice and adapt to fit the changing landscape of the U.S. healthcare system. No stakeholder is better suited to advocate for the nursing profession, and the patients they serve, than those nurses engaged in advanced nursing practice.

■ REFERENCES

American Association of Nurse Anesthetists. (n.d.-a). State government affairs. Retrieved from https://www.aana.com/advocacy/state-government-affairs

American Association of Nurse Anesthetists. (n.d.-b). *Support the role of CRNAs in pain care and patient safety*. Retrieved from http://www.future-of-anesthesia-care-today.com/pdfs/mya2017-04-%201pager-chronic-pain.pdf

American Association of Nurse Anesthetists. (2017). Certified registered nurse anethe-tists fact sheet. Retrieved from https://www.aana.com/membership/become-a-crna/crna-fact-sheet

American Association of Nurse Practitioners. (n.d.-a). Federal policy toolkit. Retrieved from https://www.aanp.org/legislation-regulation/policy-toolkit

American Association of Nurse Practitioners. (n.d.-b). State policy toolkit. Retrieved July from https://www.aanp.org/legislation-regulation/state-policy-toolkit

American Association of Nurse Practitioners. (2018). *AANP's 2017 state policy priorities*. Retrieved from https://www.aanp.org/images/documents/state-leg-reg/State%20Policy%20Priorities.pdf

American College of Nurse-Midwives. (n.d.). State resource center. Retrieved from http://www.midwife.org/State-Resource-Center

American Nurses Association. (n.d.). Policy & advocacy. Retrieved from http://www.nursing world.org/MainMenuCategories/Policy-Advocacy

American Organization for Nurse Executives. (n.d.-a). Key issues : Sustain and grow funding for nursing. Retrieved from http://advocacy.aone.org/key-issue/sustain-and-grow-funding-nursing

American Organization for Nurse Executives. (n.d.-b). Legislative basics. Retrieved from http://advocacy.aone.org/legislative-basics

American Organization for Nurse Executives. (n.d.-c). MACRA-quality payment program. Retrieved from http://advocacy.aone.org/key-issue/macra-quality-payment-program

APRN Consensus Work Group & the National Council of State Boards of Nursing APRN Advisory Committee. (2008). *Consensus model for APRN regulation: Licensure, accreditation, certification & education* (APRN Joint Dialogue Group Report).

Chicago, IL: National Council of State Boards of Nursing. Retrieved from https://www .ncsbn.org/Consensus_Model_for_APRN_Regulation_July_2008.pdf

Bureau of Labor Statistics and U.S. Department of Labor. (2016). *Occupational outlook handbook, 2016-17 Edition.* Retrieved from https://www.bls.gov/ooh/healthcare/ registered-nurses.htm

Dill, M. J., Pankow, S., Erikson, C., & Shipman, S. (2013). Survey shows consumers open to a greater role for physician assistants and nurse practitioners. *Health Affairs, 32*(6), 1135–1142. doi:10.1377/hlthaff.2012.1150

Donald, F., Martin-Misener, R., Carter, N., Donald, E. E., Kaasalainen, S., Wickson-Griffiths, A., . . . DiCenso, A. (2013). A systematic review of the effectiveness of advanced practice nurses in long-term care. *Journal of Advanced Nursing, 69*(10), 2148–2161. doi:10.1111/ jan.12140

Fowler, M. (2015). *Guide to nursing's social policy statement: Understanding the profession from social contract to social covenant.* Silver Spring, MD: American Nurses Association.

GovTrack. (n.d.). Home. Retrieved from https://www.govtrack.us/

Hogan, P. F., Seifert, R. F., Moore, C. S., & Simonson, B. E. (2010). Cost effectiveness analysis of anesthesia providers. *Nursing Economics, 28*(3), 159.

Institute of Medicine. (2011a). *Relieving pain in America: A blueprint for transforming prevention care, education, and research.* Washington, DC: The National Academies Press.

Institute of Medicine. (2011b). *The future of nursing: Leading change, advancing health.* Washington, DC: National Academies Press.

John Adams Quotes. (n.d.). *John Adams Historical Society.* Retrieved from http://www .john-adams-heritage.com/quotes

Livni, E. (2016). Regulation nation: What industries are most carefully overseen? [Blog post] Retrieved from http://blogs.findlaw.com/free_enterprise/2016/02/regulation-nation -what-industries-are-most-carefully-overseen.html

Medicaid.gov. (n.d.). About section 1115 demonstrations. Retrieved from https://www .medicaid.gov/medicaid/section-1115-demo/about-1115/index.html

National Council of State Boards of Nursing. (n.d.). APRN consensus model toolkit. Retrieved from https://www.ncsbn.org/739.htm

National Institute of Nursing Research. (2016). *The NINR strategic plan: Advancing science, improving lives.* Bethesda, MD: Author.

Norman, J. (2016, December 19). Americans rate healthcare providers high on honesty ethics. *Gallup.* Retrieved from http://www.gallup.com/poll/200057/americans-rate -healthcare-providers-high-honesty-ethics.aspx?g_source=Social%20Issues&g_ medium=lead&g_campaign=tiles

Peterson-Kaiser. (n.d.). *Health spending explorer.* Retrieved from http://www.healthsystem tracker.org/interactive/?display=U.S.%2520%2524%2520Billions&service=Hospita ls%252CPhysicians%2520%2526%2520Clinics%252CPrescription%2520Drug& source=Total%2520National%2520Health%2520Expenditures&tab=0

Pittman, P., & Williams, B. (2012). Physicians wages in states with expanded APRN scope of practice. *Nursing Research and Practice, 2012,* 1–5. doi:10.1155/2012/671974

Rettig, R. A. (2011). Special treatment? The story of medicare's ESRD entitlement. *New England Journal of Medicine, 364*(7), 596–598. doi:10.1056/NEJMp1014193

Reyes-Akinbileje, B. (2005). *Nursing workforce programs in title VIII of the public health service act* (CRS Report to Congress). Washington, DC: Congressional Research Service, The Library of Congress. Retrieved from http://congressionalresearch.com/RL32805/document. php?study=Nursing+Workforce+Programs+in+Title+VIII+of+the+Public+Health+Service+Act

The National Academies of Sciences, Engineering, and Medicine. (2017). *Frequently asked questions*. Retrieved from http://www.nationalacademies.org/about/faq/index.html

CHAPTER SEVENTEEN

Advancing Systems Thinking and Cross-Sector Collaboration to Create a Culture of Health

MAUREEN SROCZYNSKI, EDNA CADMUS, AND PATRICIA POLANSKY

The ferocious and unnamed storm that hit the Gulf of Maine in October of 1991 was immortalized as the "perfect storm" because of the way in which a combination of forces converged, amplified one another, and fed each other in a cycle of increasing potency. These factors were a unique combination of meteorological events that caused major changes in the ocean environment and threatened the northeast fishing industry (National Climatic Data Center, 1991). Similarly, another "perfect storm" is in the making in the American healthcare sector and this storm threatens to create a public health crisis. The combination of forces swirling within the healthcare sector include the need for increased access, changes in reimbursement, the increasingly complex and technology-driven environments, and a heightening focus on quality and safety (Thompson, 2008).

In 2008, the Robert Wood Johnson Foundation (RWJF) partnered with the Institute of Medicine (IOM) to develop an initiative on the future of nursing. The collective work of these two prestigious organizations served as a foundation to the IOM report *The Future of Nursing: Leading Change, Advancing Health*. This report details the convergence of forces contributing to the decline in quality, increase in fragmentation, and rise in costs of healthcare (IOM, 2011), thus recognizing that quality patient care can only be achieved through a total transformation of the healthcare system. Offering an action-oriented blueprint for the future of nursing and improvement of healthcare, the report further highlights that such change would only be achievable by advancing the role of nurses in today's healthcare system.

The report concludes that no one entity alone can effectively address all of these forces and makes recommendations for nursing to develop strategic alliances with policy makers, regulators, government leaders, philanthropic groups, and consumer organizations to advance the transformation that is needed within the healthcare system (IOM, 2011).

Following the release of the IOM (2011) report, the RWJF partnered with AARP and the AARP Foundation to form the Center to Champion Nursing in America and the Campaign for Action (CFA) (2017). The purpose of this collaboration is to ensure that all Americans have access to high-quality, patient-centered care in which nurses contribute as essential partners in a system-wide transformation. The CFA, comprised of action coalitions in every state, focuses on developing strategies to implement the IOM recommendations. The CFA targets six main areas or "pillars" for action: (a) advancing education transformation, (b) removing barriers to practice and care, (c) leveraging nursing leadership, (d) promoting diversity, (e) fostering interprofessional collaboration, and (f) bolstering workforce data (National Academies of Sciences, Engineering, and Medicine [The Academies], 2016). The Academies assessed the progress of the CFA and concluded that its work would be better advanced by building a "broader coalition to increase awareness of the nurses' ability to play a full role in health professions education, collaboration, and leadership" (2016, p. 4). This report again stressed the changing climate of healthcare policy and practice and the need for nurses to lead and partner in teams that provide services and develop healthcare policy across the continuum of care (The Academies, 2016).

■ A CULTURE OF HEALTH

In 2014, the RWJF worked to expand its vison of enabling our diverse society to lead healthier lives for generations to come (Lavizzo-Mourey, 2014). In partnership with the RAND Corporation, the RWJF focused on building a national movement to accelerate an integrated course of action among individuals, organizations, and communities across the country to achieve a Culture of Health (COH). In this process, a framework for a COH was defined as linking healthcare, family, and community life to cultivate a shared vision, increase awareness among all Americans, and discover and invest in solutions. This COH framework is built on the beliefs that good health can flourish across geographic, demographic, and social sectors with all individuals and families having the means and opportunities to lead the healthiest lives possible, regardless of where they live, how much money they make, or where they come from (Lavizzo-Mourey, 2014).

In collaboration with RWJF, the Future of Nursing CFA developed key messages to identify the important role of nurses in developing a COH which includes the following:

- Everyone deserves to live the healthiest life possible: This message focused on the fact that improving health for everyone is one of the most pervasive challenges of our time and requires the shift toward building a COH.
- Nurses are essential to building a COH: Because of their ever-present role in our communities, nurses play a vital role in realizing this vision.

- Nurse are transforming health and healthcare: The CFA is equipping and empowering nurses to build a COH by building on the recommendations of *The Future of Nursing* report.
- Nurses cannot do this alone: The CFA focuses on identifying and working with other stakeholders to collaborate across sectors of healthcare to create a COH.

THE COH ACTION FRAMEWORK

The RWJF COH framework identifies four areas where action is needed to build a COH (Figure 17.1) These action areas include (a) making health a shared value, (b) fostering cross-sector collaboration to improve well-being, (c) creating healthier, more equitable communities, and (d) strengthening the integration of health services and systems with an outcome of population health and well-being surrounded by health equity (Plough, 2015). The action areas and drivers define the structure of the framework and identify the priorities while the measures are adaptable to keep pace with changing conditions (Plough, 2015). Each action area has a set of drivers and measures to promote cross-sector collaboration and provide a structure to align its own work (Weil, 2016). Table 17.1 highlights the action areas and their drivers and measures. The Action Framework is a long-term initiative that requires the input of

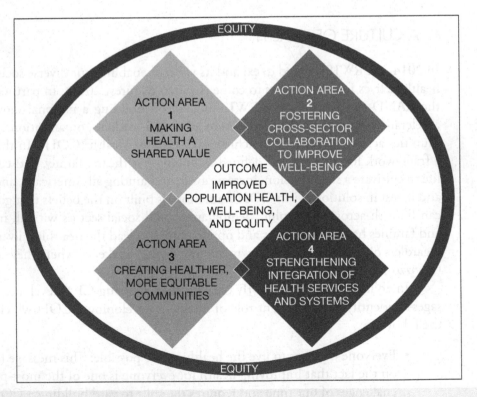

FIGURE 17.1 COH framework.

COH, Culture of Health.

TABLE 17.1 Culture of Health Framework: Action Areas, Drivers, and Measures

1. Making Health a Shared Value	
Drivers	**Measures**
Mindset and expectations	• Value of health interdependence • Value of well-being • Public discussion on health promotion and well-being
Sense of community	• Sense of community • Social support
Civic engagement	• Voter participation • Volunteer engagement

2. Fostering Cross-Sector Collaboration to Improve Well-Being	
Drivers	**Measures**
Number and quality of partnerships	• Local health department collaboration • Opportunities to improve health for youth at schools • Business support for workplace health promotion and Culture of Health
Investment in cross-sector collaboration	• U.S. corporate giving • Federal allocations for health investments related to nutrition and indoor and outdoor physical activity
Policies that support collaboration	• Community relations and policing • Youth exposure to advertising for healthy and unhealthy food and beverage products • Climate adaptation and mitigation • Health in all policies (support for working families)

3. Creating Healthier, More Equitable Communities	
Built environment/physical conditions	• Housing affordability • Access to healthy foods • Youth safety
Social and economic environment	• Residential segregation or evenness of racial/ethnic distribution across communities • Early childhood education • Public libraries
Policy and governance	• Complete streets policies • Air quality

4. Strengthening Integration of Health Services and Systems	
Access	• Access to public health • Access to stable health insurance • Access to mental health services • Routine dental care

(continued)

TABLE 17.1 Culture of Health Framework: Action Areas, Drivers, and Measures (*continued*)

4. Strengthening Integration of Health Services and Systems (*continued*)	
Consumer experience and quality	• Consumer experience—CAHPS • Population covered by an ACO
Balance and integration	• Electronic medical record linkages • Hospital partnerships • Practice laws for nurse practitioners • Social spending relative to health expenditure
5. Outcome-Improved Population Health, Well-Being, and Equity	
Enhanced individual and community well-being	• Well-being rating in areas of health, life satisfaction, and work/life balance • Caregiving burden
Managed chronic disease and reduced toxic stress	• ACEs • Disability associated with chronic conditions
Reduced healthcare costs	• Family healthcare cost • Potentially preventable hospitalization rates • Annual end of life expenditures

ACEs, adverse child experiences; ACO, accountable care organization; CAHPS, Consumer Assessment of Healthcare Providers and Systems.

Source: Plough, A., & Chandra, A. (2015). *From vision to action: A framework and measures to mobilize a culture of health—Executive summary.* Princeton, NJ: Robert Wood Johnson Foundation. Retrieved from https://www .cultureofhealth.org/content/dam/COH/RWJ000_COH-Update_CoH_Report_1b.pdf. Copyright 2015. Robert Wood Johnson Foundation. Used with permission from the Robert Wood Johnson Foundation.

many stakeholders across the country and provides an opportunity for nurses to be full partners and leaders of this effort to create equity in health across the country.

BUILDING ON THE IOM TO CREATE A COH

In alignment with the IOM (2011) conclusion that no one entity can address all the forces facing healthcare, RWJF notes that the creation of nationwide COH will take time, determination, and the input of many (Plough, 2015). The past president of RWJF noted that "building a COH in America is much like assembling a quilt" which requires many hands working together (Lavizzo-Mourey, 2016, p.1). All the elements of the Framework for Action are interconnected and build on the RWJF mission to improve health and healthcare. In alignment with this framework, the CFA is now focusing on building on the work being done by state action coalitions to advance the IOM (2011). As part of this process, CFA circulated a set of Campaign Imperatives (CFA, 2013) to encourage action coalitions to move beyond nursing and involve diverse stakeholders who are critical to the success of the campaign. Through a process of examination and questioning, Action coalitions were encouraged to review their current activities established to advance IOM recommendations and identify potential linkages to the COH framework (CFA, 2016). The following possible linkages were identified:

- Promoting diversity activities can be linked to the action area of making health a shared value, with the drivers of mind-set and expectations, sense of community, and civic engagement
- Removing barriers to practice and care can be linked to strengthening integration of health services and systems, with the drivers of access, consumer experience and balance, and integration
- Leveraging nursing leadership activities can be linked to creating healthier more equitable communities, with the drivers of policy and governance
- Advancing nursing education can be linked to fostering cross-sector collaboration, with the drivers of number and quality of partnerships, investment in cross-sector collaboration, and policies that support collaboration

Each of the recommendations made in the IOM report to advance nursing can be directly linked to the COH framework. The CFA has helped the nursing community form strong relationships with groups within nursing and other stakeholders outside of nursing, including consumer groups, businesses, educators, and policy makers at both the local and national levels. Nurses are the linchpin of the movement to improve America's health by leading the way in working across sectors and disciplines to provide individuals and populations with the best opportunities to be healthy (CFA, 2015).

LINKING POPULATION HEALTH, POPULATION MANAGEMENT, AND A CULTURE OF HEALTH

In examining the RWJF COH framework, it becomes clear that it encompasses both population health and population health management. Defining population health and how to measure population outcomes is very complex, and different terminology has been used by different groups. Population health was first defined as "the health outcomes of a group of individuals, including the distribution of such outcomes with the group" (Kindig & Stoddart, 2003, p. 381). The National Quality Forum (2016) furthered this definition to include disparities in the population. Population health not only focuses on medical care but also includes the social determinants such as education, transportation, and housing, to name a few. Therefore, population health also includes improving health equity among different groups.

Kindig and Stoddart also distinguished a difference between population health and public health in that they saw population health as broader in scope (Harris, Puskarz, & Golab, 2016; Kindig & Stoddart, 2003). In this context, public health can be considered a tool to ensure health safety and welfare of the public. Population health further needs to be differentiated from disease management as it also focuses on disease prevention and optimization of health along the continuum.

The Triple Aim was introduced in 2008 to improve population health (Berwick, Nolan, & Whittington, 2008). The three aims include improving the patient experience of care, per capita cost, and the health of the population by ensuring a value-based system. A key element of the Triple Aim is to define the population. A population can be defined as a geopolitical area which has boundaries, such as nations, states, communities, or zip codes, and is labeled often as total population. Subpopulations can be defined by income, race/ethnicity, disease, specific healthcare system, or employees. Subpopulations can be any group with shared characteristics.

Another area of potential confusion relates specifically to the definitions of population health and population management which are often used interchangeably but have different meanings. Population management is focused on payment for and delivery of healthcare services for a population to improve population health and quality of care (Loehrer, Lewis, & Bogan, 2016; Steenkamer, Hanneke, Heijink, Baan, & Struijs, 2017). Population management includes key outcome measures that are used to determine the effectiveness of interventions.

CONCEPTUAL MODEL OF NURSING AND POPULATION HEALTH

Fawcett and Ellenbecker (2015) created a proposed conceptual model of nursing and population health (CMNPH) to describe the role that nurses play in population health. This model identifies the social determinants of population health outcomes to include upstream factors (such as socioeconomic and physical environment), population factors (such as genetics, behavioral, physiologic, resilience, and health state), and healthcare system factors (such as providers, organizations and institutions, payers, and policies). These upstream factors help nurses define nursing activities that are population based. This conceptual model provides a context or space for nursing in collaboration with other sector partners to identify interventions. It also provides a model for conducting research to determine the effectiveness of varied interventions with populations. Nurses need to be clear that they must engage in these dimensions to help improve the health of the populations we serve that go beyond the walls of hospitals and into the communities to improve health.

CONVERGENCE OF THE CULTURE OF HEALTH FRAMEWORK AND THE SOCIAL DETERMINANTS OF HEALTH

The outcome of the COH framework is defined as improved population health, well-being, and equity. This outcome requires moving beyond the clinical setting to include social inputs such as housing, education, and employment. These social inputs can include upstream societal factors of personal resources, education, income, and the social environments in which people live, work, study, and engage in recreational activities. Downstream determinants include access to medical care and environmental factors and health behaviors. Intrinsic biological attributes of age, sex, and genes are also determinants of health (Woolf & Braveman, 2011). The COH framework encompasses these environmental and socioeconomic factors in the action areas and drivers. Although most caregivers, academics, and policy makers understand the health impact of the social determinants, the public and some policy makers do not always recognize the link between social policy and health policy (Woolf & Braveman, 2011). The social determinants of health are given very little attention in our current systems of healthcare and social welfare despite the disproportionate role they play in determining life outcomes. The basic reason for the neglect is that the system is primarily set up to treat acute, biomedical problems. Another major cause of the neglect of social determinants of health is the fragmentation within the healthcare system, as well as lack of coordination between healthcare and social welfare systems. The general public is also unaware of the ways in which addressing social determinants might improve health outcomes. A recent survey supported by RWJF concluded that public health advocates and healthcare practitioners should not assume that the importance of personal health in day-to-day life necessarily translates into support for a government role in population health or the public health agenda to address the social determinants of health (Bye, Ghirardelli, & Fontes, 2016). However, the amount of attention being given to the social determinants is growing as national policy imperatives, the need to control healthcare costs, and the larger question of justice in our society are becoming renewed concerns (Benedict-Nelson, 2016). While the United States is a leader in developing innovative technologies, pharmaceutical products, and healthcare treatments, our country also has the highest healthcare costs per capita of any country (Kane, 2012).

While many professionals in healthcare and human services are aware of ways in which the social determinants shape the lives of people they care for, the best way to act on this understanding is often uncertain (Benedict-Nelson, 2016). Substantial work remains to be done if we hope to translate our understanding into practical, specific protocols for care on the individual or community level. Health is often presented as a goal instead of the anchor of community well-being and a fuel for national prosperity (Plough & Chandra, 2015). Despite several promising efforts to coordinate action between healthcare and social welfare systems, our country must embrace a more integrated, comprehensive approach to health as defined in the RWJF COH framework with improved well-being and equity as the center of the target.

NEW POLICY INITIATIVES, EDUCATION FRAMEWORKS, AND MODELS OF CARE

A deeper understanding of the social determinants could also lead to more comprehensive models of health, human welfare, and social justice with tools and perspectives beyond those provided by public health or economic models. The process may require us to rethink our fundamental assumptions and lead to some immediate changes in everyday decision making. To fully address the social determinants in a comprehensive way, all healthcare professionals will need to acquire new skills in using data in decision making, design and innovation, strategic communication, and leadership within systems. The measures within the RWJF COH framework use a variety of data sources to engage different sectors and reflect the complexity of decision making and multipronged ways in which communities get things done (Plough & Chandra, 2015). The annual *County Health Rankings* (University of Wisconsin Population Health Institute, 2017) provide a revealing snapshot of how health is influenced by where we live, learn, work, and play. The rankings also provide a starting point to help communities identify and implement solutions that make it easier for people to be healthy in their neighborhoods, schools, and workplaces. These key factors affecting community and population health outcomes are clearly evident in the RWJF COH framework.

EDUCATIONAL FRAMEWORKS

In order to adequately address social determinants of health, the most important change needed in both professional education and practice is early training and education in interprofessional collaboration and working as part of patient-centered teams that are comprehensive, coordinated, and patient- and family-centered. To develop true competencies in working with teams, professionals need more than a mere familiarity with other disciplines. They need formative, integrative experiences providing actual care alongside other professionals with a focus on the social determinants of health. Such a program of professional education could be grounded in the development of relationships with professional colleagues as well as patients and include empathic listening and respect for the cultural and disciplinary perspectives of others.

The 2004 American Association of Colleges of Nursing (AACN, p.2) statement on the scope of advanced nursing practice defines it as "any form of nursing intervention that influences healthcare outcomes for individuals or populations, including the direct care of individual patients, management of care for individuals and populations, administration of nursing and healthcare organizations, and the development and implementation of health policy." AACN also noted the benefits of practice-focused doctoral programs as the development of advanced competencies for increasingly complex practice, faculty, and leadership roles. *The Essentials of Doctoral Education for Advanced Nursing Practice* outline the curricular elements and foundational outcome competencies that are core to all advance practice roles. *The Essentials* also define that DNP programs prepare graduates to be accountable for quality health; the safety of populations with whom they work; and sensitivity to diverse organizational cultures, populations, and providers (AACN, 2006). Each of these educational outcomes align with the formative and integrative competencies and sensitivity to diverse organizational cultures and populations.

In 2015, the Academies convened a workshop titled "Envisioning the Future of Health Professional Education" (Cuff, 2016). The workshop aimed to (a) explore the shifts in health, policy, and healthcare that could have an impact on health professions education and workforce learning; (b) identify learning platforms that could improve effective knowledge transfer with improved quality and efficiency; and (c) discuss opportunities for building a workforce that understands the role of culture and health literacy in approaches to health and disease. Among the recommendations at the conclusion of the workshop were the need to:

- Focus on competency-based curricula
- Promote interprofessional and transprofessional education
- Adapt to address local community challenges
- Link together networks, alliances, and consortia extending beyond the traditional discovery-care-education continuum and strengthened through external community collaboration

These approaches in relational competence, accountability for quality health-care, and community collaborations could be the scaffolding on which all efforts to address the social determinants of health could be constructed.

INNOVATION CARE MODELS

The Center for Medicare and Medicaid Services (2016) is now providing financial and technical support for State Innovation Models (SIM). This initiative is focused on the development of state-led, multipayer health payment and service models that will improvise health system performance, increase quality of care, and decrease costs for Medicare, Medicaid, and Children's Health (Children's Health Insurance Program [CHIP]). In round one of SIM nearly $300 million was awarded to 25 states to design or test innovative models. In round two the SIM initiative is providing $660 million to 32 awardees. The state models range from community-based transition programs; federally qualified health center (FQHC) advanced primary care practice; frontier community health integration projects; next generation accountable care organization (ACO) models; and strong start for mothers and newborns initiatives. These models, as part of the CMS innovation center, aim to achieve better care for patients and better health for our communities while lowering costs. The Prevention Institute (2013) has developed a model, the community-centered health home, that demonstrates the need for integration between public health and clinical services and further serves as a design for future SIM grants. In 2017, the Academies released a report, *Communities in Action-Pathways to Health Equity*, which provides examples of nine community-driven, multisectorial models that show promise for promoting health equity. Each of these models include and focus on creating shared value and building trust in community, leadership development, fostering creativity, and leveraging community resources.

In 2017, the RAND Corporation examined three nurse-designed care models that have been recognized by the American Academy of Nursing as Edge Runners (Martsolf, Mason, Sloan, Sullivan, & Vilarruel, 2017). These programs include

(a) centering pregnancy, (2) insights into children's temperament, and (c) family practice and counseling network. Each of these programs demonstrates a holistic approach to care or addresses an unmet need of a population. In addition, each of these innovative projects contributes to the COH in the action area of strengthening integration of health services and also demonstrates the leadership role nursing can take in COH-related initiatives. These innovative models for innovation in care and building healthier communities directly align with both the social determinants of health and the RWJF COH framework and highlight the continuing need for cross-sector collaboration to achieve these goals.

SYSTEMS THINKING TO CREATE A COH

Systems thinking means careful consideration of possible consequences of policies and actions, generating scenarios through group working and joint thinking, and taking into account the interactions between health system elements and the context of care (Atun, 2012). Systems thinking provides a methodology to decode the complexity of health systems and design and evaluate interventions that maximize health and health equity (World Health Organization [WHO], 2009). The World Health Organization (WHO) has identified steps to systems thinking in healthcare that includes (a) convening of stakeholders, (b) collective brain storming, (c) conceptualizing effects to map how the intervention will affect health and the health systems, (d) adapting and redesigning to optimize synergies and minimize any negative effects, and (e) designing an evaluation to determine indicators, methods, design, plan and timeline, budget, and source funding. Systems thinking fosters direct links to policy making, better ownership of processes and outcomes, and wider participation. The WHO report examines dynamics and challenges of systems thinking in healthcare with a focus on aligning policies, priorities, and managing and coordinating partnerships and expectations among stakeholders. Both RWJF and the CFA have adopted this approach to garner trust, galvanize support, and inspire others toward meaningful action. The RWJF COH recognizes that we must move toward a comprehensive approach to health that involves policy makers, providers, communities, individuals, and other stakeholders to address the range of complex social factors. The factors that influence the ways in which health systems achieve these goals include the "capacity of both individuals and institutions within the health system; continuity of stewardship; the ability to seize opportunities; and the economic set up" (Atun, 2012, p. iv4).

OPPORTUNITIES FOR DNP-PREPARED NURSES

DNP-prepared nurses are in a unique position to assist professionals working in the healthcare systems, policy makers, and other stakeholders to understand and incorporate the social determinants and COH practices and policies. DNP nursing practice and education includes an organizational and systems leadership component that emphasizes practice, ongoing improvement of health outcomes, and ensuring patient safety (AACN, 2006). From a systems thinking perspective, DNP-prepared practitioners should be able to assess organizations, identify systems issues, and facilitate organization-wide changes in care models and practice delivery. By utilizing political skills, systems thinking, and the business and financial acumen needed to analyze practice quality and costs, DNP-prepared practitioners are well prepared to develop the cross-sector collaboration that is key to the success and advancement of a COH.

■ COLLECTIVE ACTION AND CROSS-SECTOR COLLABORATION

Creating social change in building a COH requires a shifting of mindset from working as individual groups in isolation to working in a collective approach to address complex issues that impact health and healthcare. Health and healthcare are influenced by social concerns. It needs to be recognized that no one organization is responsible for any social problem; therefore, why should an individual organization try to resolve it on its own (Kania & Kramer, 2011). To create large-scale change, cross-sector partners are needed to come together for a common agenda. So, what is collective impact? Collective impact is a community coalition of multisector participants that works to change highly complex systems (Hanleybrown, Kania, & Kramer, 2012; Kania & Kramer, 2011; Preskill, Parkhurst, & Juster, n.d.).

To use this type of approach, organisations must first recognize a sense of urgency. As we look today at the current health and healthcare of populations in the United States, a need exists for us to come together to improve health and healthcare by recognizing that the social determinants impact behaviors toward health. Cost and quality have not been linked to better health outcomes in the United States. The 35 member countries of the Organisation for Economic Co-operation and Development (OECD) monitor events and project short- and medium-term economic development. They compare health indicators by country to help problem-solve and develop policy. For example, in 2015 the United States spent 16.9% of the gross domestic product on healthcare yet infant mortality rates continue to be on the high end of those reported by the OECD countries. The OECD defines *infant mortality rate* as the number of deaths of children younger than 1 year of age expressed per 1,000 live births. Additionally, the United States is not performing well in preventing avoidable hospital admissions for people with chronic conditions, which has a major impact on costs (OECD, 2015, 2016). Therefore, cross-sector partners are needed to help guide the discussion and the collective actions needed to move the needle on health and social outcomes. Leadership is needed to coordinate these organizations toward a common agenda to improve health and healthcare.

There are five conditions that need to be met in order to create and sustain collective impact. These conditions include (a) a common agenda, (b) shared measurement system, (c) mutually reinforcing activities, (d) continuous communication, and a backbone support organization (Kania & Kramer, 2011). A *common agenda* requires a shared vision, a common definition of the problem to be solved, and collective action. Organizations need to recognize that the areas they choose to focus on will either improve populations or individuals depending on their approach. The five-tier health impact pyramid developed by the public health community identifies strategies that improve populations versus individuals. Those strategies that improve populations (from least effective to most effective) are (a) counseling and education, (b) clinical interventions, (c) long-lasting protective interventions, (d) changing the context to make individuals default to healthy decisions, and (e) addressing socioeconomic factors. This public health framework may help guide the coalition toward a common agenda as it relates to population health (Frieden, 2010). A *shared measurement system* is more complex and needs to be considered, but it must be recognized that it cannot hinder the work of the organizations. Cabaj (2014) describes an adaptive approach where planning is dynamic, learning is by doing, and the ability to change course based on data are important. Shared measurement cannot be a substitute for strategic and systemic thinking and key action. There are anticipated and unanticipated outcomes which should be captured during this process. *Mutually reinforcing activities* requires coordination of each organization's contribution to the social problem being addressed by each sector toward a common goal. This does require each organization to take action in the same manner in order to contribute to action on the overall social issue and accelerate corrective progress. *Continuous communication* requires a structure of regular meetings, both structured board meetings as well as one-on-one meetings, to build trust among organizations. This effort takes both time and resources to be effective. Many times these organizations are not-for-profit organizations, governmental, or business associations that are stretched in their work; therefore, the right balance of meetings and connections needs to be considered in the planning phase and beyond. Finally, a *backbone organization* is important to coordinate these efforts. This requires leadership skills to ensure that all ideas are heard and that consensus is reached on the direction of the team (Kania & Kramer, 2011). Backbone organizations serve to ensure there is agreement on the common agenda topic and accountability of the team. They also help prioritize and align activities and goals.

WHAT ARE THE BENEFITS OF COLLECTIVE IMPACT?

Using collective impact as a strategy brings with it benefits to organizations and to the consumer. Initially, as organizations begin to share what their organization is focused on, it quickly becomes evident that there is redundancy of efforts toward a similar problem or social concern. Many times, the organizations are not aware of the other organizations' work. This dialogue creates an opportunity to focus collectively, share resources, and have a larger impact within the communities. When cross-sector groups come together with a common agenda, an expansion of new solutions to old problems is frequently the outcome. Initially, each organization is viewing the problem or social concern through its own lens, which can be limiting. Bringing together multiple lenses creates a kaleidoscope of views that intersect and create new solutions. This is an important strategy to move the needle on change.

In this time of resource and funding scarcity, greater opportunities can be leveraged by a collective group. Funders are more likely to finance those projects that have greater impact. Groups can take on larger projects as each group can take a part of the whole overall cost as well as benefits.

Sustainability is always a key concern of any group. As projects take off, how an organization can sustain the program is often considered challenging. With this approach, more options can be identified and each organization may be able to contribute to the continued success of the initiative. The aforementioned can also help address scalability and focus on long-term systemic change.

WHAT ARE THE PHASES OF COLLECTIVE IMPACT?

There are four phases in the development of collective impact: (1) generating ideas and dialogue, (2) initiating action, (3) organizing for impact, and (4) sustaining action and impact (Foundation Strategy Group [FSG], 2013). These four phases should be evaluated for success based on (a) governance and infrastructure, (b) strategic planning, (c) community involvement, and (d) evaluation and improvement. Key questions for each phase and component assist to identify what phase of collective impact the organizations are in. These questions include: What works well? What is challenging? and What is missing? Getting from phase 1 to phase 4 often requires several years, and in fact, some initiatives may never get to the final phase due to changes in leadership, organizational commitment, and resources. Each phase has a different evaluation approach based on maturity level of the group and the initiative selected. (FSG, 2013; Preskill, Parkhurst, & Juster, n.d).

ALIGNING ACTIVITIES OF CROSS-SECTOR COLLABORATION

In the developmental stage, for better understanding, an inventory of what initiatives organizations are working on may be useful. This inventory can help identify common issues being addressed or gaps. Comparing these initiatives to data that is available from programs such as the County Health Rankings, Livability Index, and Healthy People 2020 can further inform the discussion. The activities selected by the group should be considered using a systems-level approach. Using this approach will help move to new solutions. Building leadership in both the backbone organization and the organizations engaged can help build adaptability and the willingness of the groups to take a new approach to old problems.

Individual organizations should share their projects, which can help shape the discussion and be used to springboard a common agenda. Assessing available data and the level of potential impact the initiative may have on moving the needle to improve population health is an important factor to consider as time and resources will need to be expended. In identifying initiatives, it is important to be clear on the problem and how each constituent in the group defines it and the data to support the concern. There are some key principles that should be considered, including being intentional in the design of the initiative to include equity as a key thread throughout the initiative.

Not every initiative will require the same players, therefore it is important to ensure that the right stakeholders are at the table or are included, such as community members and other key organizations that are concerned about the same issues. Having the communities engaged helps to determine if the problem is one that they see as important in the complexity of improving health and healthcare. These members should help set the agenda. The backbone organization should also consider how many activities the group can take on so as not to overextend or stress the organization.

EXEMPLAR

The New Jersey Action Coalition (NJAC) is used as one example of how action coalitions can impact health and healthcare. Focused on aligning for sustainability, the NJAC has formed a partnership with the New Jersey Collaborating Center for Nursing (NJCCN), which is the nursing workforce center for the state. Both groups have common agendas that can build on each other's work.

The NJAC serves as the backbone organization for building a COH, by unleashing the talents of New Jersey nurses to work with cross-sector organizations in a more organized fashion. The mission of NJCCN is working to ensure that NJ has future-oriented nurses who can help evolve the healthcare system. Through data analysis, the workforce center can target needs through supply and demand data and help facilitate programing.

As a backbone organization, the NJAC created an advisory board structure to align forces for a healthier New Jersey. The cross-sector leaders include AARP, New Jersey Healthcare Quality Institute, New Jersey Department of Health, New Jersey Prevention Network, New Jersey Hospital Association, YMCA, library association, and Rutgers Health. Collectively, these organizations form a board which has come together to identify how nurses can engage in their work and to understand how each group can leverage the work of others with a common goal. In addition to meeting quarterly, the NJAC team meets with each organization to better understand their work, and to identify projects where nurses can bring value by adding leadership and bandwidth to their initiatives.

Nurses have been selected as coaches and aligned to the 21 counties in the state. This helps provide a structure in the recruitment of nurses for community projects. Professional nursing organizations are also engaged by helping to recruit nurses in their region. Nurses can engage in short-term projects or engage in committees and task forces based on their availability and the choice of when and where. To facilitate this communication, a website has been developed that identifies the projects that nurses can engage in. This website allows nurses to offer their services and for the coach to match them to the needs in the community.

An example of projects that benefit communities and where nurses can engage is the work of AARP in translating the livability index into action in communities through offerings such as health education workshops, targeting outreach to caregivers, working on public spaces for walking, and partnering with schools to help those older adults that may be isolated in their homes. Using the talents of nurses goes beyond specific health-related initiatives to integrating the issues that are reflective of the social determinants of health.

Before a common measurement can be created, the areas each group is focused on must be mapped and then analyzed with respect to how they relate to each other to determine common measures. This takes time not only in identifying metrics but also in working with organizations to identify priorities and common goals. This commonality will come through continuous communication and the building successes over time.

■ LIVING THE FUTURE

In *The Art of Innovation* (2001), Thomas Kelley notes that knowing what's next is not a matter of guesswork. It is like putting together a puzzle. He notes that the cyberspace novelist William Gibson gave us the good news by noting that "the future has already arrived, it is just not widely distributed" (Kelley 2001, p. 277). Innovation tends to take root when there are deeply engrained rituals. To move to the future, you need to listen to your own sages. Both the IOM report (2011) and the RWJF COH framework provide all healthcare practitioners with a roadmap and guideposts for the future. We just need to join forces, build momentum, and transform what it means to be a healthy nation.

Culture of Health-Related Resources[a]	
Campaign for Action	https://campaignforaction.org
Communities in Action-Pathways to Health Equity	www.nap.edu/catalog/24624/communities-in-action-pathways-to-health-equity
Community-Centered Health Homes	www.preventioninstitute.org/publications/community-centered-health-homes-bridging-the-gap-between-health-services-and-community-prevention
County Health Rankings	www.countyhealthrankings
Healthy People 2020	www.healthypeople.gov
Interprofessional Education and Collaboration Competencies	www.aacn.nche.edu/educationresources/IPECReport.pdf
Livability Index	https://livabilityindex.aarp.org
Collective Impact Forum	https://collectiveimpactforum.org or http://www.fsg.org/blog/navigating-collective-impact
Prevention Institute	www.preventioninstitute.org
Robert Wood Johnson Foundation	www.rwjf.org
The Future of Health Professions Education	www.nap.edu/catalog/21796/envisioning-the-future-of-health-professional-education-workshop-summary
Winnable Battles	www.cdc.gov/winnablebattles

[a] The authors have assembled this list of resources related to a Culture of Health.

■ REFERENCES

American Association of Colleges of Nursing. (2004). AACN position statement on the practice doctorate in nursing. Retrieved from http://www.aacnnursing.org/Portals/42/News/Position-Statements/DNP.pdf

American Association of Colleges of Nursing. (2006). *The essentials of doctoral education for advanced nursing practice.* Retrieved from http://www.aacnnursing.org/Portals/42/Publications/DNPEssentials.pdf

Atun, R. (2012). Health systems, systems thinking and innovation. *Health Policy and Planning, 27*(Suppl. 4), iv4–iv8.

Benedict-Nelson, A. (2016). *Health plus social—An inquiry into the social determinants of health* (Spring). Los Angeles: University of Southern California School of Social Work–GreenHouse. Retreived from http://ghouse.org/category/andrew-benedict-nelson

Berwick, D., Nolan, T., & Whittington, J. (2008). The triple aim: Care cost and quality. *Health Affairs, 27*(3), 759–769.

Bye, L., Ghirardelli, A., & Fontes, A. (2016). Promoting health equity and population health: How American views differ. *Health Affairs, 35*(110), 1982–1990.

Campaign for Action. (2013). *Campaign* imperatives. Retrieved from https://campaignforaction.org/resource/campaign-imperatives

Campaign for Action. (2015). Campaign leaders discuss culture of health and the next five years. Retrieved from https://campaignforaction.org/campaign-leaders-discuss-culture-health-next-five-years

Campaign for Action. (2016, April 5). Building a culture of health, state by state. Action Coalition web conference. Retrieved from https://campaignforaction.org/resource/building-culture-health-state-state

Campaign for Action. (2017). Our story. Retrieved from http://campaignforaction.org/about/our-story

Cabaj, M. (2014). Evaluating collective impact: Five simple rules. *The Philanthropist, 26*(1), 109–124.

Centers for Medicare & Medicaid Services. (2016). *State innovation models initiative: General information.* Retrieved from https://www.cms.gov/Medicare/Medicare.html

Cuff, P. (2016). *Envisioning the future of health professional education: Workshop summary.* Washington, DC: National Academies of Sciences, Engineering, and Medicine.

Fawcett, J., & Ellenbecker, C. (2015). A proposed conceptual model of nursing and population health. *Nursing Outlook, 63,* 288–298.

Foundation Strategy Group. (2013). Collective impact forum. Retrieved from http://www.fsg.org/blog/navigating-collective-impact

Frieden, T. R. (2010). A framework for public health action: The health impact pyramid. *American Journal Public Health, 100,* 590–595.

Hanleybrown, F., Kania, J., & Kramer, M. (2012). Channeling change: Making collective impact work. *Stanford Social Innovation Review,* 1–8. Retrieved from http://www.fsg.org/publications/channeling-change

Harris, D., Puskarz, K., & Golab, C. (2016). Population health: Curriculum framework for an emerging discipline. *Population Health Management, 19*(1), 39–45.

Institute of Medicine. (2011). *The future of nursing: Leading change, advancing health.* Washington, DC: National Academies Press.

Kane, J. (2012). Health costs: How the U.S. compares with other countries. *PBS News Hour.* Retrieved from https://www.pbs.org/newshour/health/health-costs-how-the-us-compares-with-other-countries

Kania, J., & Kramer, M. (2011, Winter). Collective impact. *Stanford Social Innovation Review*. Retrieved from https://ssir.org/articles/entry/collective_impact

Kelley, T., & Littman, J. (2001). *The art of innovation*. New York, N Y: Doubleday.

Kindig, D., & Stoddart, G. (2003). What is population health? *American Journal Public Health*, *83*(3), 380–383.

Lavizzo-Mourey, R. (2014). *Building a culture of health—2014 president's message*. Robert Wood Johnson Foundation. Retrieved from https://www.rwjf.org/en/library/annual -reports/presidents-message-2014.html

Lavizzo-Mourey, R. (2016). *Joining forces to build momentum—2016-president's message*. Robert Wood Johnson Foundation. Retrieved from https://www.rwjf.org/en/library/ annual-reports/presidents-message-2016.html

Loehrer, S., Lewis, N., & Bogan, M. (2016). Improving the health of populations. *Health Executive, 31*(2), 82–83.

Martsolf, G., Mason, D. J., Sloan, J., Sullivan, C. G., & Villarruel, A. M. (2017). Nurse- designed care models: What can they tell us about advancing a culture of health? Santa Monica, CA: RAND Corporation. Retrieved from https://www.rand.org/pubs/research_ briefs/RB9959.html

National Academies of Sciences, Engineering, and Medicine. (2016). *Assessing progress on the institute of medicine report: The future of nursing*. Washington, DC: National Academies Press.

National Academies of Sciences, Engineering, and Medicine. (2017). *Communities in action- pathways to health equity*. Washington, DC: National Academies Press.

National Climatic Data Center. (2000). The perfect storm. Retrieved from http://www .noaanews.noaa.gov/stories/s451.htm

National Quality Forum. (2016, August) *Improving population health by working with communi- ties: Action guide 3.0*. Retrieved from http://www.qualityforum.org/Publications/2016/08/ Improving_Population_Health_by_Working_with_Communities__Action_Guide_ 3_0.aspx

Organisation for Economic Co-operation and Development. (2015). Health at a glance 2015. Retrieved from http://www.oecd.org/newsroom/healthcare-improving-too -slowly-to-meet-rising-strain-of-chronic-diseases.htm

Organisation for Economic Co-operation and Development. (2016). Health statistics. Retrieved from http://www.oecd.org/els/health-systems/health-statistics.htm

Plough, A. (2015). Measuring what matters: Introducing a new action framework. *Culture of Health blog*. Princeton, NJ: Robert Wood Johnson Foundation. Retrieved from https:// www.rwjf.org/en/culture-of-health/2015/11/measuring_what_matte.html

Plough, A., & Chandra, A. (2015). *From vision to action: A framework and measures to mobilize a culture of health—Executive summary*. Princeton, NJ: Robert Wood Johnson Foundation. Retrieved from https://www.cultureofhealth.org/content/dam/COH/ RWJ000_COH-Update_CoH_Report_1b.pdf

Preskill, H., Parkhurst, M., & Juster, J. (n.d). Guide to evaluating collective impact. Retrieved from http://www.fsg.org/publications/guide-evaluating-collective-impact

Prevention Institute. (2013). *Opportunities for advancing community prevention in the state innovation models*. Retrieved from https://www.preventioninstitute.org/sites/default/ files/editor_uploads/images/stories/Documents/CMMI_SIM_Initiative_Memo_ February_2013.pdf

Steenkamer, B., Hanneke, D., Heijink, R., Baan, C., & Struijs, J. (2017). Defining population health management: A scoping review of the literature. *Population Health Management*, *20*(1), 74–85.

Thompson, P. (2008). Key challenges facing American nurse leaders. *Journal of Nursing Management*, *16*, 912–914.

University of Wisconsin Population Health Institute. (2017). *County health rankings: Key findings report*. Retrieved from www.countyhealthrankings.org

Weil, A. R. (2016). Defining and measuring a culture of health. *Health Affairs*, *35*(11), doi:10.1377/hlthaff,2016.13558

Woolf, S., & Braveman, P. (2011). Where health disparities begin: The role of social and economic determinants and why current policies may make matters worse. *Health Affairs*, *30*(10), 1852–1859. doi:10.3377htlhaff.2011.06

World Health Organization. (Ed.) (2009). *Systems thinking for health systems strengthening*. Geneva, Switzerland: Editor. Retrieved from ww.who.int/alliance-hpsr/resources/9789241563895/en

CHAPTER EIGHTEEN

The Critical Need for Global Nursing Leadership

SHEILA M. DAVIS, INGE CORLESS, AND
PATRICE NICHOLAS

Global: of, relating to, or involving the entire earth; worldwide.
—*American Heritage Dictionary* (2016)

There are numerous challenges in global health. These challenges are perpetuated as global leaders fail to recognize the critical role that nurses play in this area. Nurse leaders must, therefore, fill the global health leadership void and those with a doctor of nursing practice (DNP) can be part of meeting this challenge. In this chapter, we examine the world population workforce challenges and impact on global nursing practice, the Sustainable Development Goals (SDGs), and what is meant by global health leadership.

■ GLOBAL HEALTH

Global health is becoming much more integrated into national and public health discussions across various disciplines. Both nursing and medical schools have content related to global health as part of their curricula, and many students entering the health professions do so with an early commitment aimed at participation in global health activities. Many students are drawn to healthcare delivery in resource-limited settings, and although discussions of global health are often limited to "other" places, it is critical that a more inclusive view of global health be incorporated. While the term "resource-limited" is often reserved for discussions regarding the developing world, it is also an accurate description of many parts of the United States, and therefore it is vital that we incorporate U.S. resource-limited settings in global endeavors.

The United States is considered a "developed" or "resource-rich" country, yet stark health disparities exist and resources are not equally shared among various demographic groups. The United States ranked 169th out of 225 countries in infant mortality in 2016, estimated at a rate of 5.80 deaths per 1000 live births (Central Intelligence Agency, 2017), a measure often used to evaluate the quality of healthcare for a nation (MacDorman et al., 2005). Despite having the highest health expenditure per person in the world, measures of health indicate that the United States lags in the health of some segments of our population. There are many potential explanations for this discrepancy between poor health outcomes and higher expenditure per person in the global and public health arena, but they are beyond the scope of this chapter. However, such startling statistics help focus on the importance of bidirectional global exchange and how "resource-rich" states fail to deliver care to many populations. Lessons learned from other areas of the world can and should be applied to many healthcare delivery models domestically.

Insisting on a more inclusive view of global health serves many critical functions. This shared accountability acknowledges the interconnectedness of our world. Booming industry, social conditions, and modernity have garnered increased international mobility for both people and pathogens. Transmission of infectious diseases across continents is now a reality, while the devastating effects of noncommunicable diseases are also felt through our mutual interconnectedness. No nation can effectively remove itself from this responsibility of addressing global health, nor is it in their best interest.

■ WORLD POPULATION AND GLOBAL WORKFORCE

According to the United Nations Department of Economics and Social Affairs/ Population Division, as published in "World Population Prospects: The 2017 Revision," the percentages of population from 0 to 14 years vary from 16% for Europe to 41% for Africa (p. 10). Likewise, these percentages vary for those 15 to 24 years from 11% in Europe to 19% in Africa. Such statistics have profound implications for the needs of the population, including maternity care, healthcare of infants and children, and education. This vulnerable population cannot survive without adequate food and care. There are other implications as well, including the need for an economy that can support a bolus of 60% of the population that will come into the workforce over the coming decades.

While the statistics in other regions are not as stark, Latin America and the Caribbean have 25% of their population in the 0 to 14 age group and 17% in the 15 to 24 age group, and Asia is similar with 24% in the 0 to 14 age group and 16% in the 15 to 24 age group. This bolus of young people will not only need food and healthcare but education and jobs. And, depending on the economy and the need for workers of various skill levels, the numbers of potential workers may exceed the need with out-migration as a result. The most educated will secure further education and livelihoods in more economically diversified regions and will relocate to those regions where the supply of workers is inadequate. Those individuals who remain in areas of low employment face a challenging future. For those with less or no education, the implications are dire unless there is a spate of agricultural and mining jobs. Without such opportunities, the potential for armed conflict and work as mercenaries for hire increases.

Why, you may wonder, is so much attention being given to the issue of population dynamics? It is because this is the context in which global health nursing practice will transpire, and is doing so already. Regions with a high proportion of individuals 60 years of age and older will have different types of needs for their population than one with a different population composition. With a population 65 years and older, accessible housing, transport, and healthcare are a few areas of the economy that government will need to consider for this segment of the population. Clearly, these considerations will benefit other segments of the population as well. Those countries with a high proportion of the population 60 years and older will potentially also have a need for in-migration of workers, some of whom will emanate from countries with different languages and cultural traditions. This too will have an impact on global nursing practice and the need for healthcare workers, particularly nurses.

The World Health Organization's (WHO, 2016b) "Global Strategy on Human Resources for Health: Workforce 2030" has developed a number of "milestones" to be accomplished by 2020 and 2030. Particularly relevant to the need for global health nursing leadership are the following milestones, the first for 2020 and the second one mentioned for 2030.

- All countries are making progress on health workforce registries to track health workforce stock, education, distribution, flows, demand, capacity, and remuneration (Annex 3)
- All countries are making progress towards halving inequalities in access to a health worker (Annex 3)

In addition to other societal forces, the production of healthcare workers, namely education and labor market dynamics, is influenced by various policies (Sousa, Scheffler, Nyoni, & Boerma, 2013). The production of healthcare workers is affected by the infrastructure, including the physical infrastructure; the availability, enrollment, and selection of students; and the quality and availability of faculty members. The labor market is influenced by policies that address migration, both in-migration and out-migration, as well as currently unemployed healthcare workers. Maldistribution of healthcare workers can also be affected by policies that reward workers for service in underserved areas. Inefficiencies can be reduced by attention to skill mix and productivity/performance (Sousa et al., 2013).

The availability of potential students for education as healthcare workers is directly affected by the opportunity of children for primary and secondary education. Cultural practices that restrict the opportunities for education and travel, and the presence of male determination of female rights and options, are all impediments to the development of an adequate healthcare workforce (WHO, 2016, p. 24). It is to the benefit of society that countries consider investment "in the education and training, recruitment, deployment and retention of health workers to meet national and subnational needs through domestically trained health workers" (WHO, 2016, p. 25). Such investment will assure the supply of culturally congruent healthcare workers who speak the language of their patients and have an understanding of the culture of those whom they serve.

Data on the current practicing healthcare professional workforce and its distribution are essential for sound policy making. Including either those who have completed the programs or whose names are listed and are so-called ghost workers because they are present in name only confuses the reality of currently working healthcare professionals.

The WHO (2016b) data on health professionals groups nurses and midwives together (p. 41). In Table A1.1 in WHO (2016b), data in the millions is depicted for 2013 and 2030 by WHO regions (WHO, 2016b). Africa has the lowest number of nurses/midwives with 1 million, followed by the Eastern Mediterranean (1.3 million), Southeast Asia (2.9 million), the Western Pacific (4.6 million), the Americas (4.7 million), and Europe (6.2 million). By 2030, each of these regions will have increased their numbers of healthcare workers, with the greatest increase in the Americas (8.2 million projected), followed by the Western Pacific (7.0 million projected). Europe will retain its primacy in the sheer numbers of nurses and midwives with 8.5 million workers predicted for 2030.

WHO (2016b) projects that the needs-based shortage will worsen, particularly for Africa (p. 44). From a different perspective, the demand for health workers, including nurses/midwives, physicians, and other health workers, for 2013 and 2030 is lowest in Africa (1.1; 2.4 million), followed by the Eastern Mediterranean (3.1; 6.2 million); Southeast Asia (6.0; 12.2 million); the Americas (8.8; 15.3 million); Europe (14.2; 18.2 million); and the Western Pacific (15.1; 25.9 million). The demand calculations were based on projections of supply, population aged 65+, per capita out of pocket healthcare expenditures, and per capita gross domestic product (GDP) (p. 45). This basis for the demand calculation favors those countries with a greater percentage of population 65 years and older, those with a greater supply of healthcare workers, and countries with a higher GDP.

More specific data on each country indicates the skilled professional density per 10,000 population as 2.8 for both Ethiopia and Liberia, 1.6 for Niger, 3.4 for Sierre Leone, 1.1 for Somalia, and 3.6 for Tonga (World Health Statistics, 2017, Annex B). The skilled professional density refers to physicians, psychiatrists, and surgeons. It is noted that such data for nurses and midwives are challenging to measure and compare across countries but should be included (World Health Statistics Monitoring Health for the SDGs, 2017, p. 10). The bottom line is that they are not included. In addition, there is no data available for multiple countries concerning physicians, psychiatrists, and surgeons for provider density (WHO, 2017).

These data underscore the imbalance in the distribution of healthcare professionals. The question remains as to how this situation can be remedied so that the healthcare providers are available where there is a need for healthcare rather than be clustered where there are medical and social amenities. Wilson and colleagues (2010) found that physicians most likely to practice in rural areas are those who originate from these areas. These authors also examined the use of incentives to bring physicians to rural areas, such as scholarships, and found them helpful.

For nurses in South Africa, satisfaction with supervision was key to job satisfaction (Delobelle et al., 2011). Improved work conditions and financial compensation were also issues that needed to be addressed if nurses were to remain in rural areas. When age, education, years in nursing, and tenure in the unit were controlled in the equation, job satisfaction was key to significantly explaining turnover intent ($p ≤ .001$; p. 371). Obviously, keeping nurses who are already practicing in rural areas is paramount and attention to such findings will be key to retaining these professionals. How else can the misdistribution of nurses be addressed?

The WHO (2016a, 2016c) has published a report on approaches to strengthening the nursing and midwifery workforce in 2016–2020. WHO's third theme in the report states "Working together to maximize the capacities and potentials of nurses and midwives through intra- and interprofessional collaborative partnerships, education, and continuing professional development" (p. 21). The collaborative partnerships include the community, teamwork with health professionals, and intersectoral partnerships.

Four themes are proposed with suggested interventions for countries, regions, and with partners over the years 2016, 2017, 2018, 2019, and 2020, with indicators identified for each year for the evaluation of success in achievement. The themes are as follows:

1. Ensuring an educated, competent, and motivated nursing and midwifery workforce within effective and responsive health systems at all levels and in different settings (pp. 28–29)
2. Optimizing policy development, effective leadership, management, and governance (pp. 30–31)
3. Working together to maximize the capacities and potentials of nurses and midwives through intra- and interprofessional collaborative partnerships, education, and continuing professional development (p. 32)
4. Mobilizing political will to invest in building effective evidence-based nursing and midwifery workforce development (pp. 33–34)

The 64th World Health Assembly in Agenda item 13.4 on May 24, 2001 made six requests of the director-general, four of which directly involved the participation of nurses (WHO, 2016a). This participation included:

- The appointment of professional nurses and midwives to specialist posts in the Secretariat both at headquarters and in regions
- To engage actively the knowledge and expertise of the Global Advisory Group on Nursing and Midwifery in key policies and programmes that pertain to health systems, the social determinants of health, human resources for health and the Millennium Development Goals
- To provide support to Member States in optimizing the contributions of nursing and midwifery to implementing national health policies and achieving internationally agreed health-related development goals, including those contained in the Millennium Declaration
- To encourage the involvement of nurses and midwives in the integrated planning of human resources for health, particularly with respect to strategies for maintaining adequate numbers of competent nurses and midwives (p. 39)

These recommendations incorporate nurses in their implementation, which is a good step. The problem is that they don't resolve the immediate problem of inadequate healthcare resources. How is this to be achieved? One approach is substitution, which has been categorized by Dovlo (2004) as "indirect substitution," or the delegation of some tasks; "direct substitution," or the delegation of most tasks by creating a new cadre of professional; "intra-cadre skills assignment," which involves the delegation of some tasks to those in the same profession who have less training; "delegation of nonprofessional tasks," or the shifting of nonprofessional tasks; and "informal substitution," whereby tasks are assumed by lower cadres of workers in the absence of the appropriate professional (p. 5). The advantages of substitutes are that they are usually local and more likely to be retained and will accept postings to rural areas; the costs, that is salaries, are lower for such workers as is the initial training; the focus of the training is likely to be practical and fewer tests may be ordered; and the workers are more likely to be integrated into the communities (p. 10). Some of the potential disadvantages include the possibility of lower quality care, poor supervision, and that the lower initial costs for salaries over time will be met with demands for compensation similar to that of professionals (p. 10).

Substitution as previously indicated has usually meant the assumption of activities by a lesser trained group of individuals. Another option is that of nurses in nations with a more plentiful supply of nursing professionals working in the areas of other countries where the supply is more limited and augmenting the work of local professionals. Such experiences improve the practice of the incoming and the local nurses as they exchange ideas and approaches.

The concept of bidirectionality allows nurses in more healthcare limited areas to gain experience in a more technically advanced facility either in their home country or out of country. The draw of out-of-country experiences is that the site is usually more technically sophisticated and allows the nurse to obtain new areas of expertise. Families and countries profit from the out-migration as the nurses and others usually send remittances back to their families.

Nurses seeking international experiences and having a commitment to sharing their expertise in other countries will find they too have much to learn by such experiences. The development of partnerships between the nurses from the host and donor countries will bring education and expertise to both. With bidirectionality that is equivalent in numbers, both individuals and home and receiving countries could profit. That profit could extend to the donor countries' rural areas and their immigrant and rural communities. Clearly, nurses with experience in the home countries of some of the immigrants to their country will be in a better position to provide care once they return. Local health becomes global with the mobility of individuals for shorter or longer time. With the potential of migration based on the needs of the host country as well as the donor country, global healthcare becomes local and local care becomes global.

These dynamics have implications for the preparation of future nurses. To be effective in a world of increasing mobility, understanding the implications of diversity and cultural humility are improved by experiences in other countries where the nurse is the stranger with limited knowledge of the language and customs. Such experiences will assist the nurse in being more sensitive to diverse customs and ways of being in the world. Coincidentally this will make the nurse a more sensitive and better healthcare practitioner in his or her home country. Given the potential need for workers in parts of Europe and in other geographic areas where the population is aging, the in-migration of workers from donor countries will require healthcare by nurses knowledgeable about the home countries of the migrants. This is best achieved by nurses from the host country gaining experience in the donor country of the migrants. Such exchanges can be a win-win situation for both countries and individual nurses. Nurses must be the ones to provide the leadership for such developments, working together internationally to improve healthcare for all.

■ UN MILLENNIUM DEVELOPMENT GOALS

In September 2000, a vision for the future of the world was established with the millennium development goals (MDGs). The eight goals addressed were eradicating extreme poverty and hunger, achieving universal primary education, promoting gender equality and empowering women, reducing child mortality, improving maternal health, combating HIV/AIDS, malaria, and other diseases, ensuring environmental sustainability, and a global partnership for development (United Nations [UN], 2011).

The target year for achieving these improvements in health was 2015. The World Health Organization identifies the gaps in achieving the goals as gaps in social justice, responsibility, implementation, and knowledge (WHO, 2006). There are no quick or easy "fixes" for the gaps identified by WHO. Viewing global health as a shared responsibility continues to be difficult in settings of financial stressors and the changing dynamic of the economic and political strife in many countries in the world. Implementation of effective health programs that have measurable outcomes to assess overall impact on the individual and community level remain less of a priority for funders. The silo approach to global health, for example, funding HIV/AIDS programs to prevent transmission of the virus from mother to child and ignoring critical issues such as other methods of HIV transmission or concurrent medical challenges such as TB, have proven to be expensive, duplicative, and often disruptive to the public sector of healthcare. Many donor initiatives that utilize the silo approach are born of good intentions yet fail to attain the level of cultural congruency needed for effective change.

■ UN SUSTAINABLE DEVELOPMENT GOALS

Following the partial achievement of the MDGs, the UN established the SDGs at the UN summit on September 25, 2015. They implemented the 17 SDGs, known as the *Global Goals*, which are aimed to be achieved by 2030.

- SDG 1: End poverty in all its forms everywhere
- SDG 2: End hunger, achieve food security and improved nutrition, and promote sustainable agriculture

- SDG 3: Ensure healthy lives and promote well-being for all at all ages
- SDG 4: Ensure inclusive and equitable quality education and promote life-long learning opportunities for all
- SDG 5: Achieve gender equality and empower all women and girls
- SDG 6: Ensure availability and sustainable management of water and sanitation for all
- SDG 7: Ensure access to affordable, reliable, sustainable, and modern energy for all
- SDG 8: Promote sustained, inclusive and sustainable economic growth, full and productive employment and decent work for all
- SDG 9: Build resilient infrastructure, promote inclusive and sustainable industrialization and foster innovation
- SDG 10: Reduce inequality within and among countries
- SDG 11: Make cities and human settlements inclusive, safe, resilient, and sustainable
- SDG 12: Ensure sustainable consumption and production patterns
- SDG 13: Take urgent action to combat climate change and its impacts
- SDG 14: Conserve and sustainably use the oceans, seas, and marine resources for sustainable development
- SDG 15: Protect, restore, and promote sustainable use of terrestrial ecosystems, sustainably manage forests, combat desertification, and halt and reverse land degradation and halt biodiversity loss
- SDG 16: Promote peaceful and inclusive societies for sustainable development, provide access to justice for all and build effective, accountable, and inclusive institutions at all levels
- SDG 17: Strengthen the means of implementation and revitalize the global partnership for sustainable development (UN, 2015)

Each of the SDGs are explored for its impact on the health of the world's people and the role of global nursing.

SDG 1 is aimed at *Ending Poverty in All Its Forms Everywhere*. This goal carries forward the overarching goal of the MDGs which were undergirded by an approach aimed at addressing the alleviation of poverty. Although gains were made during the years from 2000 to 2015 within the MDGs, eradication of global poverty remains a critical area for achievement of the goals of the UN. Key areas encompassed are in setting measurable and achievable goals for 2030—the year by which all of the SDGs should be completed.

SDG 2 focuses on *Ending Hunger, Achieving Food Security and Improved Nutrition, and Promotion of Sustainable Agriculture*. This SDG expands upon the MDG goal of ending hunger and also addressing the complex issues of global food security and exploring 21st-century approaches to sustainable agriculture. Access to nutritious foods and developing sustainable agricultural practices will expand global health in resource-limited countries, as well as resource-rich countries.

SDG 3 addresses the importance of *Ensuring Healthy Lives and Promoting Well-Being at All Ages*. The focus on health across the life span is the only goal of the SDGs to specifically address health, although all of the SDGs are aimed at ensuring healthy living and overall well-being.

SDG 4 is *Ensure Inclusive and Equitable Quality Education and Promote Lifelong Learning*. This SDG aims to close the gap on the nearly 57 million children worldwide who lack access to education (UN, 2015). Many of these children live in conflict-prone and impoverished areas. SDG 4 also suggests that there is a need to increase the number of teacher training programs to improve access to education.

SDG 5 aims to *Achieve Gender Equality and Empower All Women and Girls*. Similar to the goal in the MDGs, inequality in gender remains a pressing issue globally. SDG 5 focuses on eradication of all types of inequality and violence including genital mutilation, forced marriage, sexual exploitation, and human trafficking. Adult females should also be more active in global leadership roles and have more economic activities afforded to them. This SDG is key in underscoring the value and importance of women's contributions to the health and welfare of global societies.

SDG 6 addresses *Ensuring Availability and Sustainable Management of Water and Sanitation for All*. This SDG expands more broadly on the MDG 7 aimed at *Ensuring Environmental Stability*. This MDG made great progress by 2015, however, according to the UN, 1.8 billion people obtain drinking water from contaminated sources (UN, 2015). Achievement of SDG 6 will limit the morbidity and mortality of the most vulnerable—infants and children—as well as improve hygiene and increase access to education for women and girls who walk long distances to obtain water.

SDG 7 is *Ensure Access to Affordable, Reliable, Sustainable, and Modern Energy for All*. Twenty percent of the global population lacks access to electricity and the benefits of this access. The goal of having clean, affordable energy and the importance of offering renewable sources of energy is key to advancing our global society. This remains a complex issue since current energy usage worldwide contributes to a large degree of greenhouse gas emissions and influences climate change as discussed in SDG 13.

SDG 8 focuses on *Promoting Sustained, Inclusive and Sustainable Economic Growth, Full and Productive Employment and Decent Work for All*. Lack of access to full and decent employment is one of the major global issues that contributes to poor health of the world. For nurses in global health, the importance of a highly educated healthcare workforce is critical and the need for resilient health systems that support the health of the world's people and employment in the health sector are critical.

SDG 9 aims to *Build Resilient Infrastructure, Promote Inclusive and Sustainable Industrialization and Foster Innovation*. In many resource-limited countries, the need for resilient infrastructure and innovative industrialization are needed for the health and welfare of their societies. While resource-rich countries can foster innovation and industrialization, the importance of this among the marginalized in poorer countries remains key to further development, including in the health sector. Wealthy countries have built technology-driven, innovative health systems, while poorer countries languish in addressing health issues.

SDG 10 focuses on *Reducing Inequality Within and Among Countries*. The inequalities that exist between resource-rich and resource-poor countries are particularly troubling when considered through the lens of health. For example, countries of Africa, in particular, have stark inequalities that are linked with poorer health due to lack of infrastructure, conflict, and political instability. Reducing inequalities is directly linked to improved health of the world's people.

SDG 11 addresses the importance of *Making Cities and Human Settlements Inclusive, Safe, Resilient, and Sustainable*. Similar to SDG 8 focused on employment and economic growth, SDG 11 builds on the need for sustainable urban growth and inclusive human settlement. Urban migration and crowding will greatly impact health systems, and it is critically important to examine the environmental impact of building 21st century innovative communities to achieve global health.

SDGs 12, 13, 14, and 15 are examined collectively since they uniquely overlap related to their application to global health. SDG 12 aims to *Ensure Sustainable Consumption and Production Patterns* and SDG 13 focuses on the need to *Take Urgent Action to Combat Climate Change and Its Impacts*. Both of these SDGs examine the importance of energy production while limiting the carbon footprint that is impacting the health and safety of the world's people. Strategies aimed at mitigation and adaptation related to the health consequences of climate change related to greenhouse gas emissions are critical to the health of the world's people and the roles of nurses in global health. SDG 14 focuses specifically on *Conservation and Sustainable Use of the Oceans, Seas, and Marine Resources for Sustainable Development* since pollution of our water resources, as well as rising sea levels, directly impact global health through lack of access to food sources from oceans and seas, as well as salt water intrusion that impacts people living near oceans and seas. Climate events that impact oceans and seas also have direct negative sequelae for the health of the world's people. SDG 15 aims to *Protect, Restore and Promote Sustainable Use of Terrestrial Ecosystems, Sustainably Manage Forests, Combat Desertification, and Halt and Reverse Land Degradation and Halt Biodiversity Loss.* The importance of addressing deforestation and desertification cannot be underestimated in its link to health. In areas of the world where deforestation has occurred the health of the people has suffered. One example is in Haiti, where desertification and deforestation have limited the ability to sustainably grow crops, which directly affects access to food (U.S. Agency for International Development, 2016).

SDG 16, to *Promote Peaceful and Inclusive Societies for Sustainable Development, Provide Access to Justice for All and Build Effective, Accountable, and Inclusive Institutions at All Levels,* addresses the importance of health communities and directly impacts the health of the world's people. Communities in conflict areas have limited ability to support health, education, and the welfare of its people when violence is pervasive. Displacement of entire populations leads to enormous health challenges in areas around the world. Most notably the war in Syria has led to one of the greatest displacement of people affecting the entire Middle Eastern region and Europe due to mass migration. The health challenges for all, as well as lack of robust educational opportunities for young people, are enormous.

Finally, SDG 17, to *Strengthen the Means of Implementation and Revitalize the Global Partnership for Sustainable Development,* focuses on the importance of global partnerships to achieve all of the SDGs. Reducing global disparities and addressing the health challenges confronted in global locations is key to the success of nurses in global health.

■ HUMAN RIGHTS APPROACH TO HEALTH

Human rights are central to the achievement of the SDGs and perhaps the missing link in many siloed humanitarian efforts. A more comprehensive view of health that includes a reduction in poverty; adequate access to food, water, and education; and economic opportunities has remained elusive in most global health efforts. The cause and effect relationship of poverty and disease and acknowledgment of the impact of structural violence on health mandate a new paradigm for global health delivery. The utilization of a human rights approach to health framework can provide guidance to expand the scope of interventions to address the root causes of poor health.

Applying a human rights approach to health has begun to infiltrate the global health literature and vernacular.

> In a human rights framework, health is a matter of justice—a product of social relations as much as biological or behavioral factors. It is the inequities in these social, and inherently power, relations for which the state (and sometimes other actors) can and should be held accountable from a human rights perspective. (Yamin, 2008, p. 46)

The concept of right to health first gained traction after the atrocities of World War II, and, in 1948, the Universal Declaration of Human Rights was ratified (WHO, 1948). Although simple in concept, there has been no consensus by political or global leaders about the prioritization of health in many nations of the developed or developing worlds. In the United States, health is viewed by policy makers as a privilege not a right, and health as a human right has not been formally recognized. Once the debate of who deserves health is resolved with the acknowledgment of health as a fundamental human right, attention can be directed to addressing the critical issues of access and global health delivery.

■ GLOBAL NURSING

What do we mean by global health nursing practice? Is it nursing that is practiced in other than one's home country? Is it nurses from so-called developed countries travelling for various periods to areas where the density of nurses per population is less than the need? Or is it nurses who would like to spend time in another country for the cultural experience, regardless of the need for nurses' skills or because the compensation and working conditions in the host country exceed those in the donor country? Or is there yet some other definition and description that is apropos for this concept?

Nurses are the foundation of healthcare globally. Thirty-five million nurses are integral to healthcare delivery in every country of the world, but this critical cadre of healthcare professionals is often absent from decision making in global health delivery. Inherent in any discussion of global nursing and midwifery is the acknowledgment of the lack of consistency of education, clinical preparation, and status within the healthcare system and countries as a whole, factors that add to the ambiguity surrounding the impact and importance of the nursing profession (WHO, 2009). Global scope and standards of nursing practice remain elusive and the discussion is further complicated by a lack of consistency in midwifery preparation and its inclusion or exclusion from the realm of nursing. There is little information available on nurse-sensitive indicators in global health delivery, although, interestingly, vaccination coverage is directly linked to the density of nurses and is almost entirely independent of physicians (Global Health Workforce Alliance, 2010). It is essential that we articulate the value of nurses in global health delivery by employing explicit evaluation methods to show improved patient outcomes with quality nursing care.

Nursing is virtually voiceless in higher level global health leadership, and a momentum is growing to demand its representation. In May of 2011, expressing extreme concern at the lack of nursing policy presence within the WHO structures, an emergency resolution was passed by the governing body of the International Council of Nurses (ICN) at its biennial meeting held in Valetta, Malta. The official representatives of ICN member national nurses associations voted unanimously to demand that the WHO director-general empower and finance nursing leadership positions throughout the organization (ICN, 2011). This effort by ICN drew attention within the global nursing community but did not appear to have any impact thus far on changing the current leadership structures. In June of 2017, the new director-general of the World Health Organization, Dr. Tedros Adhanom Ghebreyesus, in a message to the ICN 2017 congress, expressed his gratitude to the nursing profession, recognizing "invaluable contribution and sacrifices at the frontline of health services around the world" (ICN, 2017).

■ DEVELOPMENT OF GLOBAL NURSE LEADERS: ADVANCED PRACTICE ROLES AND A PRACTICE DOCTORATE

Acknowledging the importance of nursing leadership at all levels of international development and the creation of nurse leaders globally is critical. The lack of progress in achieving many of the MDGs is disappointing and in large measure is due to the absence of nursing leadership in influencing health in resource-limited countries. Ketefian (2008) discusses the need for doctoral-prepared nurses as part of this solution and advocates for a movement toward preparation of nurses at the doctoral level. She suggests that "the most important goal of nursing doctoral education is to prepare leaders who can use their expertise to guide and lead country and international efforts to address health, education, and policy needs" (p. 1401). Although relatively new to the global landscape, nurses with clinical/practice doctorates can provide much needed leadership and advance nurses to the forefront in developing new models of care delivery.

Globally, academic nursing continues to evolve. Currently, though the advanced practice/nurse practitioner (NP) role is emerging, it thus far remains limited in many resource-limited settings. "There is a substantive body of international evidence about the positive impact of APN roles for improving patient health outcomes, quality of care and health system efficiency" (Bryant-Lukosius et al., 2017, p. 7). The ICN International Nurse Practitioner/Advanced Practice Nursing Network (INP/APNN) was established in 2000 and supports the roles of NPs and advanced practice registered nurses (APRNs) as they emerge worldwide.

The goals of the network are to become an international resource for nurses practicing in nursing practitioner or advanced nursing practice (ANP) roles and for interested others (e.g. policy makers, educators, regulators, health planners) by

1. Making relevant and timely information about practice, education, role development, research, policy and regulatory developments, and appropriate events widely available
2. Providing a forum for the sharing and exchange of knowledge, expertise, and experience
3. Supporting nurses and countries who are in the process of introducing or developing NP or ANP roles and practice
4. Accessing international resources that are pertinent to this field (http://icn-apnetwork.org)

■ UNIVERSAL HEALTH COVERAGE

Universal health coverage (UHC) is "access to key promotive, preventive, curative and rehabilitative health interventions for all at an affordable cost, thereby achieving equity in access" (WHO, 2005). To achieve UHC, we must address the financial barriers to providing accessible quality healthcare, particularly in countries in the low- to middle-income strata. The WHO has highlighted 10 recommendations for reducing inefficiency in healthcare by nearly 40% (WHO, 2005).

> Our overall conclusion is that there is an alarmingly large degree of inefficiency in the health sector, irrespective of the income level of different regions or countries. At a global level, we put this at between 20%–40% of total health spending, equivalent to a current monetary value that approaches $1.5 trillion per year. (Chisholm & Evans, 2010, p. 28)

To address this significant issue, creative solutions are needed. "At least five of the 10 recommendations could be addressed through the introduction of APRN roles, not just in primary healthcare, but across the health system where needs and inefficiencies exist" (Bryant-Lukosius et al., 2017, p. 5). These five recommendations are related to

1. The overuse of healthcare services
2. Inappropriate and costly staff mix and unmotivated workers

3. Inappropriate hospitalization and length of stay
4. Errors and suboptimal quality of care
5. Inefficient mix or level of health interventions (Bryant-Lukosius et al., 2017, p. 5).

With an overwhelming healthcare worker shortage globally, producing a more efficient, competent, and critical-thinker in nursing is in the best interest of the population as a whole. The role of APNs will continue to evolve and could, if done in conjunction with ministries of health, provide a professional growth opportunity as well as help improve healthcare access.

■ DNPs IN GLOBAL HEALTH

Rolfe and Davies (2009) trace the history of doctoral education in nursing from its beginnings in the 1930s in the United States and in Europe in the 1990s. Although there are PhD-prepared nurses working globally, there are few nurses from the developing world who have had access to doctoral education. Rolfe and Davies join Ellis and Lee (2005) in seeing the value of a clinical doctorate for nurses in global health delivery. "Application to practice is at the philosophical core of the professional doctorates" (Ellis & Lee, 2005, p. 2). The emphasis of the clinical doctorate on systems approaches to practice-oriented problems, quality improvement, and real-time application support the important roles that nurses with clinical doctorates could offer in advancing nursing practice globally.

■ INTERDISCIPLINARY, MULTIDISCIPLINARY, AND TRANSDISCIPLINARY GLOBAL HEALTHCARE DELIVERY

Nowhere is the importance of a team approach to care delivery more applicable than in global health. Commonly used in educational settings, the term "multidisciplinary" may be defined as the teaching of common material to people from different disciplines, while the term "interdisciplinary" curriculum implies learning between students sharing their experiences and unique perspective with those from different disciplines. Less familiar to most in healthcare, "transdisciplinary entails not only a transcendence of disciplinary boundaries, but to some extent the transcendence of the very idea of disciplines" (Rolfe & Davies, 2009, p. 1270). Reluctance to embrace collaborative models of care delivery is an unfortunate reality in the resource-rich and resource-poor worlds. Although there is an increasing rhetoric in healthcare about the need for multiple disciplines to be part of care delivery, rarely does this move beyond mission statements or task forces. Fostering mutual respect and acknowledgment of different but important contributions to health delivery is an ongoing process and emerging models of common content being taught to nursing and medical students as a combined class may be part of the solution. This would require an overhaul of nursing and medical education. "Transprofessional education might be as important as interprofessional education. An examination of the skill mix in selected countries of sub-Saharan African underscores the importance of professionals learning to work with nonprofessionals in health teams" (Frenk et al., 2010, p. 1948). Ability to work with transprofessional teams is of critical importance and is rarely taught or stressed at all in health provider education.

Task-shifting has become a necessary part of global health but is sometimes found to be threatening by different cadres of healthcare workers. Voiced concerns of nurses include the creation of new cadres of healthcare workers, lack of supervision and training of auxiliary workers, and lack of involvement of health professions in decision making about task-shifting (World Health Professionals Alliance [WHPA], 2008). A shift in language to *task-sharing* may better embody the intent of a team approach to healthcare delivery. All members of the team, regardless of position in the healthcare system, should have accountability to the patient with a feedback loop to continually assess patient outcomes. For example, if a task formally done by nurses is shifted to a community health worker (medication delivery), the nurse is still accountable to that patient and health system to uphold the highest quality of patient care possible. Similarly, shifting of the management of antiretroviral medications for patients with HIV from a physician to a nurse does not dissolve the responsibility of the government entities (including a physician in leadership role) to provide adequate staff and training to the nurses now tasked to deliver high-quality HIV treatment and monitoring.

Frenk et al. (2010) discuss their vision for health professionals for a new century: "Individual professions might have distinctive and complementary skills that could be considered the core of their special niche. But there is an imperative for bringing such expertise together into teams for effective patient-centered and population-based health work." Competency-based curriculum and team learning are critical for preparing the next generation of health professionals. This method of education is more easily adapted to a changing global health environment and can include measurement of the impact on the health delivery system. As Frenk continues to urge, the priority for education evaluators must be attainment of specific competencies, and not "turf protection" (p. 1951).

■ DNPs IN GLOBAL HEALTH

The converging realities of the current healthcare worker shortage, lack of global nursing leadership, grim achievements in improvements in the SDGs, and a call for a new model of global healthcare delivery that is based on competencies and transprofessional teams require a shift in the global nursing paradigm. The DNP, the terminal practice degree in nursing, is well-positioned to play a major role in the transformation needed in global health.

The DNP *Essentials*, adopted in 2005, would benefit from updated core elements, particularly those related to DNP education for future global health nursing leaders. As previously discussed, Rolf and Davies's (2009) call for doctoral education in the practice-generated knowledge model of discovery correlates well with the preparation and intent of the DNP degree.

All eight essentials are important and pertain to the global arena, but only essentials II, III, V, VI, and VII are discussed in more detail. The second essential, "organizational and systems leadership for quality improvement and systems thinking," addresses healthcare disparities and a systems approach to care. "These graduates are distinguished by their abilities to conceptualize new care delivery models that are based in contemporary nursing science and that are feasible within current organizational, political, cultural, and economic perspectives" (AACN, 2006). In the context of current and future global health needs, new care delivery models will be critical to the provision of equitable, quality global health.

The convergence of the art and science of nursing is evident in the third essential, "clinical scholarship and analytical methods for evidence-based practice nursing." As new knowledge is being generated in practice settings, it will be critical that the DNP nursing leader be well-versed in evidence-based practice and the application of theory to their practice setting.

Essential V, "health care policy for advocacy in health care," is particularly critical due to the call for more global nursing leaders. Integral to effective system improvement is the political will of national and international government leaders. It is only through persistent and strategic engagement on multiple levels that there can be sustainable and far-reaching policy change. DNPs can play a lead role in advocacy on the individual, family, community, national, and global levels. Utilizing health as a human rights framework can provide guidance to establish priorities for high-quality, equitable, and accessible healthcare.

Regardless of the label used to indicate global cross-discipline and creative healthcare teams, Essential VI, "interprofessional collaboration for improving patient and population health outcomes," will require strong leadership, a role that DNPs are qualified to fill. Maintaining a strong professional nursing identity, DNPs are well positioned to provide the key linkage between different cadres of healthcare workers. Advocating for patient-centered care with multiple layers of accountability will ensure that task-sharing leads to greater access and improved patient outcomes.

Rooted in a holistic approach to patient care, nursing's foundation of care has always been comprehensive. Essential VII, "clinical prevention and population health for improving the nation's health," although specific to national health, can be easily be broadened to incorporate what is more traditionally thought of as global health. Bidirectional learning acknowledges the critical knowledge exchange between healthcare providers in the developing and developed world. Applying successful models of global health delivery from a resource-limited setting to a resource-rich setting is a less accepted practice, but one that may contribute in very meaningful ways. Learning to provide quality care with limited resources will be very important as healthcare costs increase.

■ SUMMARY

The emergence of the DNP in the United States as a practice doctorate has and is preparing nurses to offer significant leadership in the global health arena. Innovative approaches to care delivery, task-sharing, and practice knowledge generation are needed. The call for nursing participation in policy and in global health delivery will require an infusion of nurse leaders best prepared to contribute to the allocation of resources and to the provision of a human rights-based approach to health. By partnering with nurse leaders in developing regions, DNPs can advocate for policy reform to increase nursing's visibility and to prioritize upgrading of the nursing educational system.

A radical transformation in the provision of dignified, equitable, and quality healthcare for the poor is desperately needed. Unfortunately, it is likely that we will continue to be a world of shrinking resources and competing priorities. A fundamental shift in our shared accountability toward each other is critically important as we strive to make global health a priority. There is a Haitian Creole saying, *Tout Moun Se Moun* (we are all human beings). We all must live by this simple, but essential guiding principle.

■ REFERENCES

American Association of Colleges of Nursing. (2006, October). *The essentials of doctoral education for advanced nursing practice.* Retrieved from http://www.aacnnursing.org/Portals/42/Publications/DNPEssentials.pdf

Bryant-Lukosius, D., Valaitis, R., Martin-Misener, R., Donald, F., Moran Pena, L., & Brousseau, L. (2017). Advanced practice nursing: A strategy for achieving Universal Health Coverage and Universal Access to Health. *Rev. Latino-Americana Enfermagem, 25,* e2826. doi:10.1590/1518-8345.1677.2826. Retrieved from http://www.ncbi.nlm.nih.gov.

Central Intelligence Agency. (2017). *The world factbook.* Retrieved from http://www.cia.gov

Chisholm, D., & Evans, D. B. (2010). Improving health system efficiency as a means of moving toward Universal Coverage. *WHO.* Retrieved from http://Cdrwww.Who.Int/Healthsystems/Topics/Financing/Healthreport/28ucefficiency.Pdf

Delobelle, P., Rawlinson, J. L., Ntuli, S., Malatsi, I., Decock, R., & Depoorter, A. M. (2011). Job satisfaction and turnover intent of primary healthcare nurses in rural South Africa: A questionnaire survey. *Journal of Advanced Nursing, 67,* 371–383. doi:10.1111/j.1365-2648.2010.05496.x

Dovlo, D. (2004). Using mid-level cadres as substitutes for internationally mobile health professionals in Africa. A desk review. *Human Resources for Health, 2,* 7. doi:10.1186/1478-4491-2-7

Ellis, L., & Lee, N. (2005). The changing landscape of doctoral education: Introducing the professional doctorate for nurses. *Nurse Education Today, 25*(3), 222–229. doi:10.1016/j.nedt.2005.01.009

Frenk, J., Chen, L., Bhutta, Z. A., Cohen, J., Crisp, N., Evans, T., & Garcia, P. (2010). Health professionals for a new century: Transforming education to strengthen health systems in an interdependent world. *Lancet, 376*(9756), 1923–1958. doi:10.1016/S0140-6736(10)61854-5

Global. (2016). In *The American Heritage dictionary of the English language* (5th ed.). Boston, MA: Houghton Mifflin Harcourt

The Global Fund. (2016). New Strategy for 2017–2022 reflects The Global Fund's evolving approach to health systems strengthening. Retrieved from http://www.aidspan.org/gfo_article/new-strategy-2017-2022-reflects-global-fund%E2%80%99s-evolving-approach-health-systems-0

ICN Nurse Practitioner/Advanced Practice Nursing Network. (2017). Retrieved from http://icn-apnetwork.org/

International Council of Nurses. (2011). Open letter to Dr Margaret Chan, director general of the world health organization from the international council of nurses. [Press release]. Retrieved from http://www.icn.ch/images/stories/documents/news/press_releases/2011_PR_07_Open_Letter__NursingVoiceExcluded_WHO.pdf

Ketefian, S. (2008, October). Doctoral education in the context of international development strategies. *International Journal of Nursing Studies, 45*(10), 1401–1402.

MacDorman, M. F., Martin, J. A., Mathews, T. J., Hoyert, D. L., & Ventura, S. J. (2005). Explaining the 2001–02 infant mortality increase: Data from the linked birth/infant death data set. *National Vital Statistics Reports, 53*(12), 1–22.

Rolfe, G., & Davies, R. (2009). Second generation professional doctorates in nursing. *International of Nursing Studies, 46,* 1265–1273.

Sousa, A., Scheffler, R. M., Nyoni, J., & Boerma, T. (2013). A comprehensive health labour market framework for universal health coverage. *Bulletin of World Health Organization, 91,* 892–894. doi:10.2471/BLT.13.118927

United Nations. (2011). Millennium development goals report 2011. Retrieved from http://www.un.org/millenniumgoals

United Nations. (2015). Sustainable development goals. Retrieved from http://www.un.org/sustainabledevelopment/sustainable-development-goals

U.S. Agency for International Development. (2016). *Environment & climate change fact sheet.* Retrieved from https://www.usaid.gov/sites/default/files/documents/1862/Environment%20Fact%20Sheet%20FINAL%20Jan%202016-2%20page.pdf

Wilson, N. W., Couper, I. D., de Vries, E., Reid, S., Fish, T., & Marais, B. J. (2009). A critical review of interventions to redress the inequitable distribution of healthcare professionals to rural and remote areas. *Rural and Remote Health, 9,* 1060. Retrieved from https://www.rrh.org.au/journal/article/1060

World Health Organization. (1948). *Preamble-Constitution of the world health organization,* 2–3. Retrieved from http://whqlibdoc.who.int/hist/official_records/constitution.pdf

World Health Organization. (2005). World Health Assembly Resolution 58.33: Sustainable health financing, universal coverage and social health insurance. Geneva, Switzerland: Author. Retrieved from http://apps.who.int/medicinedocs/documents/s21475en/s21475en.pdf.

World Health Organization. (2006). *Engaging in health: Eleventh general programme of work 2006–2015: A global health agenda.* Retrieved from http://whqlibdoc.who.int/publications/2006/GPW_eng.pdf

World Health Organization. (2009). *Global standards for the initial education of professional nurses and midwives.* Retrieved from http://apps.who.int/iris/bitstream/10665/44100/1/WHO_HRH_HPN_08.6_eng.pdf

World Health Organization. (2016a). *Global strategic directions for strengthening nursing and midwifery.* Retrieved from http://www.who.int/hrh/nursing_midwifery/global-strategic-midwifery2016-2020.pdf

World Health Organization. (2016b). *Global strategy on human resources for health: Workforce 2030.* Retrieved from http://www.who.int/hrh/resources/global_strategy_workforce2030_14_print.pdf

World Health Organization. (2016c). Nursing and midwifery—WHO global strategic directions for strengthening nursing and midwifery 2016–2020. Retrieved from http://www.who.int/hrh/nursing_midwifery/nursing-midwifery/en

World Health Organization. (2017). *World Health Statistics 2017: Monitoring health for the SDGs.* Retrieved from http://www.who.int/gho/publications/world_health_statistics/2017/en

World Health Professionals Alliance. (2008, March 11). Health professions demand strong principles for task shifting [Press Release]. Retrieved from http://www.whpa.org/pr03_08.htm

Yamin, A. (2008). Will we take suffering seriously? Reflections on what applying a human rights framework to health means and why we should care. *Health And Human Rights: An International Journal, 10*(1). Retrieved from https://cdn2.sph.harvard.edu/wp-content/uploads/sites/125/2013/07/7-Yamin.pdf

Index

Printed in the United States
By Bookmasters

Printed in the United States
By Bookmasters